Institute of Medicine (U.S.), Roundtable on Value & Science-Driven Health Care.

THE LEARNING HEALTHCARE SYSTEM SERIES

ROUNDTABLE ON VALUE & SCIENCE-DRIVEN HEALTH CARE

REDESIGNING THE CLINICAL EFFECTIVENESS RESEARCH PARADIGM

Innovation and Practice-Based Approaches

Workshop Summary

LeighAnne Olsen and J. Michael McGinnis, *Editors*

INSTITUTE OF MEDICINE
OF THE NATIONAL ACADEMIES

THE NATIONAL ACADEMIES PRESS
Washington, D.C.
www.nap.edu

THE NATIONAL ACADEMIES PRESS   500 Fifth Street, N.W.   Washington, DC 20001

NOTICE: The project that is the subject of this report was approved by the Governing Board of the National Research Council, whose members are drawn from the councils of the National Academy of Sciences, the National Academy of Engineering, and the Institute of Medicine.

This project was supported by the Agency for Healthcare Research and Quality, America's Health Insurance Plans, AstraZeneca, Blue Shield of California Foundation, Burroughs Wellcome Fund, California Health Care Foundation, Centers for Medicare & Medicaid Services, Charina Endowment Fund, Department of Veterans Affairs, Food and Drug Administration, Gordon and Betty Moore Foundation, Johnson & Johnson, sanofi-aventis, and Stryker. Any opinions, findings, conclusions, or recommendations expressed in this publication are those of the authors and do not necessarily reflect the view of the organizations or agencies that provided support for this project.

International Standard Book Number 13: 978-0-309-11988-7
International Standard Book Number 10: 0-309-11988-X

Additional copies of this report are available from the National Academies Press, 500 Fifth Street, N.W., Lockbox 285, Washington, DC 20055; (800) 624-6242 or (202) 334-3313 (in the Washington metropolitan area); Internet, http://www.nap.edu.

For more information about the Institute of Medicine, visit the IOM home page at: **www. iom.edu.**

Copyright 2010 by the National Academy of Sciences. All rights reserved.

Printed in the United States of America

The serpent has been a symbol of long life, healing, and knowledge among almost all cultures and religions since the beginning of recorded history. The serpent adopted as a logotype by the Institute of Medicine is a relief carving from ancient Greece, now held by the Staatliche Museen in Berlin.

Suggested citation: IOM (Institute of Medicine). 2010. *Redesigning the Clinical Effectiveness Research Paradigm: Innovation and Practice-Based Approaches: Workshop Summary.* Washington, DC: The National Academies Press.

"Knowing is not enough; we must apply.
Willing is not enough; we must do."
—Goethe

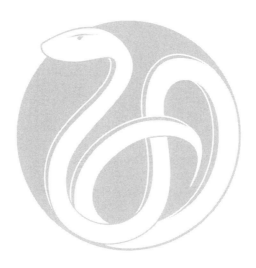

INSTITUTE OF MEDICINE
OF THE NATIONAL ACADEMIES

Advising the Nation. Improving Health.

THE NATIONAL ACADEMIES
Advisers to the Nation on Science, Engineering, and Medicine

The **National Academy of Sciences** is a private, nonprofit, self-perpetuating society of distinguished scholars engaged in scientific and engineering research, dedicated to the furtherance of science and technology and to their use for the general welfare. Upon the authority of the charter granted to it by the Congress in 1863, the Academy has a mandate that requires it to advise the federal government on scientific and technical matters. Dr. Ralph J. Cicerone is president of the National Academy of Sciences.

The **National Academy of Engineering** was established in 1964, under the charter of the National Academy of Sciences, as a parallel organization of outstanding engineers. It is autonomous in its administration and in the selection of its members, sharing with the National Academy of Sciences the responsibility for advising the federal government. The National Academy of Engineering also sponsors engineering programs aimed at meeting national needs, encourages education and research, and recognizes the superior achievements of engineers. Dr. Charles M. Vest is president of the National Academy of Engineering.

The **Institute of Medicine** was established in 1970 by the National Academy of Sciences to secure the services of eminent members of appropriate professions in the examination of policy matters pertaining to the health of the public. The Institute acts under the responsibility given to the National Academy of Sciences by its congressional charter to be an adviser to the federal government and, upon its own initiative, to identify issues of medical care, research, and education. Dr. Harvey V. Fineberg is president of the Institute of Medicine.

The **National Research Council** was organized by the National Academy of Sciences in 1916 to associate the broad community of science and technology with the Academy's purposes of furthering knowledge and advising the federal government. Functioning in accordance with general policies determined by the Academy, the Council has become the principal operating agency of both the National Academy of Sciences and the National Academy of Engineering in providing services to the government, the public, and the scientific and engineering communities. The Council is administered jointly by both Academies and the Institute of Medicine. Dr. Ralph J. Cicerone and Dr. Charles M. Vest are chair and vice chair, respectively, of the National Research Council.

www.national-academies.org

ROUNDTABLE ON VALUE & SCIENCE-DRIVEN HEALTH CARE[1]

---

[1] Formerly the Roundtable on Evidence-Based Medicine. IOM forums and roundtables do not issue, review, or approve individual documents. The responsibility for the published workshop summary rests with the workshop rapporteur and the institution.

Reviewers

This report has been reviewed in draft form by individuals chosen for their diverse perspectives and technical expertise, in accordance with procedures approved by the National Research Council's Report Review Committee. The purpose of this independent review is to provide candid and critical comments that will assist the institution in making its published report as sound as possible and to ensure that the report meets institutional standards for objectivity, evidence, and responsiveness to the study charge. The review comments and draft manuscript remain confidential to protect the integrity of the process. We wish to thank the following individuals for their review of this report:

David Atkins, Department of Veterans Affairs Health Services
Michael S. Lauer, National Institutes of Health
Frank W. Rockhold, GlaxoSmithKline
Brian L. Strom, University of Pennsylvania School of Medicine

Although the reviewers listed above have provided many constructive comments and suggestions, they were not asked to endorse the final draft of the report before its release. The review of this report was overseen by **Richard E. Marshall,** Harvard Vanguard Medical Associates. Appointed by the Institute of Medicine, he was responsible for making certain that an independent examination of this report was carried out in accordance with institutional procedures and that all review comments were carefully considered. Responsibility for the final content of this report rests entirely with the authoring committee and the institution.

Institute of Medicine
Roundtable on Value & Science-Driven Health Care
Charter And Vision Statement

The Institute of Medicine's Roundtable on Value & Science-Driven Health Care has been convened to help transform the way evidence on clinical effectiveness is generated and used to improve health and health care. Participants have set a goal that, by the year 2020, 90 percent of clinical decisions will be supported by accurate, timely, and up-to-date clinical information, and will reflect the best available evidence. Roundtable members work with their colleagues to identify the issues not being adequately addressed, the nature of the barriers and possible solutions, and the priorities for action, and marshal the resources of the sectors represented on the Roundtable to work for sustained public-private cooperation for change.

* *

The Institute of Medicine's Roundtable on Value & Science-Driven Health Care has been convened to help transform the way evidence on clinical effectiveness is generated and used to improve health and health care. We seek the development of a *learning healthcare system* that is designed to generate and apply the best evidence for the collaborative healthcare choices of each patient and provider; to drive the process of discovery as a natural outgrowth of patient care, and to ensure innovation, quality, safety, and value in health care.

Vision: Our vision is for a healthcare system that draws on the best evidence to provide the care most appropriate to each patient, emphasizes prevention and health promotion, delivers the most value, adds to learning throughout the delivery of care, and leads to improvements in the nation's health.

Goal: By the year 2020, 90 percent of clinical decisions will be supported by accurate, timely, and up-to-date clinical information, and will reflect the best available evidence. We feel that this presents a tangible focus for progress toward our vision, that Americans ought to expect at least this level of performance, that it should be feasible with existing resources and emerging tools, and that measures can be developed to track and stimulate progress.

Context: As unprecedented developments in the diagnosis, treatment, and long-term management of disease bring Americans closer than ever to the promise of personalized health care, we are faced with similarly unprecedented challenges to identify and deliver the care most appropriate for individual needs and conditions. Care that is important is often not delivered. Care that is delivered is often not important. In part, this is due to our failure to apply the evidence we have about the medical care that is most effective—a failure related to shortfalls in provider knowledge and accountability, inadequate care coordination and support, lack of insurance, poorly aligned payment incentives, and misplaced patient expectations. Increasingly, it is also a result of our limited capacity for timely generation of evidence on the relative effectiveness, efficiency, and safety of available and emerging interventions. Improving the value of the return on our healthcare investment is a vital imperative that will require much greater capacity to evaluate high priority clinical interventions, stronger links between clinical research and practice, and reorientation of the incentives to apply new insights. We must quicken our efforts to position evidence development and application as natural outgrowths of clinical care—to foster health care that learns.

Approach: The Institute of Medicine's Roundtable on Value & Science-Driven Health Care serves as a forum to facilitate the collaborative assessment and action around issues central to achieving the vision and goal stated. The challenges are myriad and include issues that must be addressed to improve evidence development, evidence application, and the capacity to advance progress on both dimensions. To address these challenges, as leaders in their fields, Roundtable members work with their colleagues to identify the issues not being adequately addressed, the nature of the barriers and possible solutions, and the priorities for action, and marshal the resources of the sectors represented on the Roundtable to work for sustained public–private cooperation for change.

Activities include collaborative exploration of new and expedited approaches to assessing the effectiveness of diagnostic and treatment interventions, better use of the patient care experience to generate evidence on effectiveness and efficacy of care, identification of assessment priorities, and communication strategies to enhance provider and patient understanding and support for interventions proven to work best and deliver value in health care.

Core concepts and principles: For the purpose of the Roundtable activities, we define value and science-driven health care broadly to mean that *to the greatest extent possible, the decisions that shape the health and health care of Americans—by patients, providers, payers, and policy makers alike—will be grounded on a reliable evidence base, will account appropriately for individual variation in patient needs, and will support the generation of new insights on clinical effectiveness.* Evidence is generally considered to be information from clinical experience that has met some established test of validity, and the appropriate standard is determined according to the requirements of the intervention and clinical circumstance. Processes that involve the development and use of evidence should be accessible and transparent to all stakeholders.

A common commitment to certain principles and priorities guides the activities of the Roundtable and its members, including the commitment to the right health care for each person; putting the best evidence into practice; establishing the effectiveness, efficiency, and safety of medical care delivered; building constant measurement into our healthcare investments; the establishment of healthcare data as a public good; shared responsibility distributed equitably across stakeholders, both public and private; collaborative stakeholder involvement in priority setting; transparency in the execution of activities and reporting of results; and subjugation of individual political or stakeholder perspectives in favor of the common good.

Foreword

Recent scientific and technological advances have accelerated our understanding of the causes of disease development and progression, and resulted in innovative treatments and therapies. Ongoing work to elucidate the effects of individual genetic variation on patient outcomes suggests the rapid pace of discovery in the biomedical sciences will only accelerate. However, these advances belie an important and increasing shortfall between the expansion in therapy and treatment options and knowledge about how these interventions might be applied appropriately to individual patients. The impressive gains made in Americans' health over the past decades provide only a preview of what might be possible when data on treatment effects and patient outcomes are systematically captured and used to evaluate their effectiveness. Needed for progress are advances as dramatic as those experienced in biomedicine in our approach to assessing clinical effectiveness.

The establishment in the 1970s of the randomized controlled trial as the Food and Drug Administration's standard in its judgments about efficacy brought greater rigor, through systematic evaluation, to the field of medicine and to the introduction of new interventions. However, in the emerging era of tailored treatments and rapidly evolving practice, ensuring the translation of scientific discovery into improved health outcomes requires a new approach to clinical evaluation. A paradigm that supports a continual learning process about what works best for individual patients will not only take advantage of the rigor of trials, but also incorporate other methods that might bring insights relevant to clinical care and endeavor to match the right method to the question at hand.

The Institute of Medicine Roundtable on Value & Science-Driven Health Care's vision for a learning healthcare system, in which evidence is applied and generated as a natural course of care, is premised on the development of a research capacity that is structured to provide timely and accurate evidence relevant to the clinical decisions faced by patients and providers. Convened in 2006, the Roundtable has considered key opportunities to transform how evidence is generated and applied to improve health and health care. Therefore, on December 12–13, 2007, as part of the Roundtable's Learning Healthcare System series of workshops, clinical researchers, academics, and policy makers gathered for the workshop Redesigning the Clinical Effectiveness Research Paradigm: Innovation and Practice-Based Approaches. Participants explored cutting-edge research designs and methods and discussed strategies for development of a research paradigm to better accommodate the diverse array of emerging data resources, study designs, tools, and techniques. Presentations and discussions are summarized in this volume.

I thank the members of the Roundtable and other workshop participants for their leadership and dedication in addressing the challenging issues needed to advance progress toward a healthcare system that seeks to promote innovation, safety, efficiency, and value. I also thank members of the Roundtable staff for their efforts to coordinate and facilitate Roundtable activities, as well as the sponsors, who make this work possible: the Agency for Healthcare Research and Quality, America's Health Insurance Plans, AstraZeneca, Blue Shield of California Foundation, Burroughs Wellcome Fund, California Health Care Foundation, Centers for Medicare & Medicaid Services, Charina Endowment Fund, Department of Veterans Affairs, Food and Drug Administration, Gordon and Betty Moore Foundation, Johnson & Johnson, sanofi-aventis, and Stryker.

Harvey V. Fineberg, M.D., Ph.D.
President, Institute of Medicine

Preface

As we move toward a healthcare system in which interventions and treatment strategies are increasingly tailored to individual genetic variation, preferences, and circumstances, a similar shift is needed in the way care is delivered and evidence is developed. Endeavoring to provide the treatment most appropriate to each individual requires a commitment to developing the systems of care, capturing the data, and advancing the methods of analysis needed to generate evidence on clinical effectiveness. These efforts will enable researchers to build on the safety and efficacy determinations developed in the approval process and to better assess intervention effects in real- world patients and practice environments.

The Institute of Medicine's (IOM's) Roundtable on Value & Science-Driven Health Care envisions the development of such a system that "draws on best evidence to provide the care most appropriate to each patient, emphasizes prevention and health promotion, delivers the most value, adds to learning throughout the delivery of care, and leads to improvements in the nation's health." To better understand how key healthcare stakeholders—patients, providers, insurers, regulators, and researchers— might help to initiate the work needed to realize this vision, the Roundtable has developed the Learning Healthcare System series of meetings and workshops. The Roundtable's inaugural publication, *The Learning Healthcare System*, provides an overview of the key barriers and opportunities for advancing progress toward the Roundtable's goal that by 2020, 90 percent of clinical decisions will be supported by accurate, timely, and up-to-date clinical information and will reflect the best available evidence.

Chief among the needs identified is the development of a new clinical research paradigm—oriented toward the creation of a more practical and reliable means to gather and assess evidence of clinical effectiveness. Many have suggested that current approaches to developing clinical evidence are inadequate for the need and, given the rapid pace of discovery and technological innovation, may soon become irrelevant. To explore the opportunities presented by new and emerging research methods that can support the development of insights relevant to clinical practice, by taking better advantage of vastly larger databases and other sources of electronically captured data such as electronic health records, the Roundtable convened a workshop titled Redesigning the Clinical Effectiveness Research Paradigm: Innovation and Practice-Based Approaches. This publication, the fifth in the Learning Healthcare System series, summarizes the presentations and discussions of that workshop, which explored the methods, data resources, tools, and techniques that might be deployed collectively as a new generation of studies and serve as foundational elements of a learning healthcare system.

Numerous themes emerged from the workshop discussion on how research tools and methods can be engaged to better address many of the current challenges in clinical effectiveness research related to time and cost constraints, the trade-offs between internal and external validity of study designs, and the need to accommodate for genetic variation among research subjects. An overarching focus over the 2 days of presentations was on the strategies and implications of moving from a paradigm centered on a hierarchy of evidence toward a model of continuous learning and more appropriately matching study designs with circumstances and needs. Also identified by workshop participants were a number of cross-sector follow-up actions proposed for possible Roundtable attention, including greater support for researchers at the cutting edge of methods development; opportunities to bring greater clarity to the field on what constitutes state-of-the-art research methods and how these studies are reported and applied; and help to spur action around the technical, economic, and cultural issues needed to better support the collection of health data at the point of care and apply these data to clinical effectiveness research.

We would like to acknowledge those individuals and organizations who gave valuable time toward the development of this workshop summary. In particular, we acknowledge the contributors to this volume for their presence at the workshop and/or their efforts to further develop their presentations into the manuscripts in this summary. We also would like to acknowledge those who provided counsel by serving on the planning committee for this workshop, including Robert Califf (Duke University), Lynn Etheredge (George Washington University), Kim Gilchrist (Astra-Zeneca LP), Bryan Luce (United BioSource Corporation), Jonathan Perlin

(HCA, Inc.), and Richard Platt (Harvard University).[1] A number of IOM staff were instrumental in coordinating the 2-day workshop in December 2007, including Sarah Bronko and Kristina Shulkin. Roundtable staff, including Katherine Bothner, Alex Goolsby, LeighAnne Olsen, and Daniel O'Neill, helped to translate the workshop proceedings and discussion into this summary. Stephen Pelletier and Laura Penny also contributed substantially to publication development. We would also like to thank Lara Andersen, Michele de la Menardiere, Bronwyn Schrecker, Vilija Teel, and Jackie Turner for helping to coordinate the various aspects of review, production, and publication.

Workshop discussions captured in this publication provide important perspectives for the development of our research enterprise as electronic health data, statistical tools, and innovative study designs expand our abilities. Full application of this capacity will amount to nothing less than a dynamic new clinical research paradigm. The pace of that progress will depend on our success in achieving stronger incentives for stakeholders to embrace the use of practice-based evidence and in fostering a research community galvanized and organized for change.

Denis A. Cortese
Chair, Roundtable on Value & Science-Driven Health Care

J. Michael McGinnis
Executive Director, Roundtable on Value & Science-Driven Health Care

---

[1] IOM planning committees are solely responsible for organizing the workshop, identifying topics, and choosing speakers. The responsibility for the published workshop summary rests with the workshop rapporteur and the institution.

Contents

xix

Summary

INTRODUCTION AND OVERVIEW[1]

Clinical effectiveness research (CER) serves as the bridge between the development of innovative treatments and therapies and their productive application to improve human health. Building on efficacy and safety determinations necessary for regulatory approval, the results of these investigations guide the delivery of appropriate care to individual patients. As the complexity, number, and diversity of treatment options grow, the provision of clinical effectiveness information is increasingly essential for a safe and efficient healthcare system. Currently, the rapid expansion in scientific knowledge is inefficiently translated from scientific lab to clinical practice (Balas and Boren, 2000; McGlynn, 2003). Limited resources play a part in this problem. Of our nation's more than $2 trillion investment in health care, an estimated less than 0.1 percent is devoted to evaluating the relative effectiveness of the various diagnostics, procedures, devices, pharmaceuticals, and other interventions in clinical practice (AcademyHealth, 2005; Moses et al., 2005).

The problem is not merely a question of resources but also of the way they are used. With the information and practice demands at hand, and new tools in the works, a more practical and reliable clinical effectiveness research paradigm is needed. Information relevant to guiding decision making in clinical practice requires the assessment of a broad range of research

---

[1] The planning committee's role was limited to planning the workshop, and the workshop summary has been prepared by Roundtable staff as a factual summary of the issues and presentations discussed at the workshop.

questions (e.g., how, when, for whom, and in what settings are treatments best used?), yet the current research paradigm, based on a hierarchical arrangement of study designs, assigns greater weight or strength to evidence produced from methods higher in the hierarchy, without necessarily considering the appropriateness of the design for the particular question under investigation. For example, the advantages of strong internal validity, a key characteristic of the randomized controlled trial (RCT)—long considered the gold standard in clinical research—are often muted by constraints in time, cost, and limited external validity or applicability of results. And, although the scientific value of well-designed clinical trials has been demonstrated, for certain research questions, this approach is not feasible, ethical, or practical and may not yield the answer needed. Similarly, issues of bias and confounding inherent to observational, simulation, and quasi-experimental approaches may limit their use and enhancement, even for situations and circumstances requiring a greater emphasis on external validity.

Especially given the growing capacity of information technology to capture, store, and use vastly larger amounts of clinically rich data and the importance of improved understanding of an intervention's effect in real-world practice, the advantages of identifying and advancing methods and strategies that draw research closer to practice become even clearer.

Against the backdrop of the growing scope and scale of evidence needs, limits of current approaches, and potential of emerging data resources, the Institute of Medicine (IOM) Roundtable on Evidence-Based Medicine, now the Roundtable on Value & Science-Driven Health Care convened the *Redesigning the Clinical Effectiveness Research Paradigm: Innovation and Practice-Based Approaches* workshop. The issues motivating the meeting's discussions are noted in Box S-1, the first of which is the need for a deeper and broader evidence base for improved clinical decision making. But also important are the needs to improve the efficiency and applicability of the process. Underscoring the timeliness of the discussion is recognition of the challenges presented by the expense, time, and limited generalizability of current approaches, as well as of the opportunities presented by innovative research approaches and broader use of electronic health records that make clinical data more accessible. The overall goal of the meeting was to explore these issues, identify potential approaches, and discuss possible strategies for their engagement.

Participants examined ways to expedite the development of clinical effectiveness information, highlighting the opportunities presented by innovative study designs and new methods of analysis and modeling; the size and expansion of potentially interoperable administrative and clinical datasets; and emerging research networks and data resources. The presentations and discussion emphasized approaches to research and learning that had the potential to supplement, complement, or supersede RCT findings and

> **BOX S-1**
> **Issues Motivating the Discussion**
>
> - Need for substantially improved understanding of the comparative clinical effectiveness of healthcare interventions.
> - Strengths of the randomized controlled trial muted by constraints in time, cost, and limited applicability.
> - Opportunities presented by the size and expansion of potentially interoperable administrative and clinical datasets.
> - Opportunities presented by innovative study designs and statistical tools.
> - Need for innovative approaches leading to a more practical and reliable clinical research paradigm.
> - Need to build a system in which clinical effectiveness research is a more natural by-product of the care process.

suggested opportunities to engage these tools and methods as a new generation of studies that better address current challenges in clinical effectiveness research. Consideration also was given to the policies and infrastructure needed to take greater advantage of existing research capacity.

Current Research Context

Starting points for the workshop's discussion reside in the presentation of what has come to be viewed as the traditional clinical research model, depicted as a pyramid in Figure S-1. In this model, the strongest level of evidence is displayed at the peak of the pyramid: the randomized controlled double blind study. This is often referred to as the "gold standard" of clinical research, and is followed, in a descending sequence of strength or quality, by randomized controlled studies, cohort studies, case control studies, case series, and case reports. The base of the pyramid, the weakest evidence, is reserved for undocumented experience, ideas, and opinions. A brief overview of the range of clinical effectiveness research methods is presented in Table S-1. Approaches are categorized into two groups: experimental and nonexperimental. Experimental studies are those in which the choice and assignment of the intervention is under control of the investigator; the results of a test intervention are compared to the results of an alternative approach by actively monitoring the respective experiences of either individuals or groups receiving or not receiving the intervention. Nonexperimental studies are those in which manipulation or randomiza-

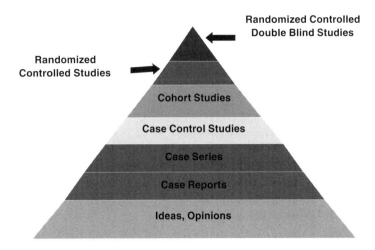

FIGURE S-1 The classic evidence hierarchy.
SOURCE: DeVoto, E., and B. S. Kramer. 2005. Evidence-Based Approach to Oncol-
ogy. In *Oncology an Evidence-Based Approach*. Edited by A. Chang. New York:
Springer. Modified and reprinted with permission of Springer SBM.

tion is generally absent, the choice of an intervention is made in the course
of clinical care, and existing data collected in the course of the care process
are used to draw conclusions about the relative impact of different circumstances or interventions that vary between and among identified groups,
or to construct mathematical models that seek to predict the likelihood of
events in the future based on variables identified in previous studies.

Noted at the workshop was the fact that, as currently practiced, the
randomized controlled and blinded trial is not the gold standard for every
circumstance. While not an exhaustive catalog of methods, Table S-1 provides a sense of the range of clinical research approaches that can be used
to improve understanding of clinical effectiveness. Each method has the
potential to advance understanding of the various aspects of the spectrum
of questions that emerge throughout a product's or intervention's lifecycle
in clinical practice. The issue is therefore not whether internal or external
validity should be the overarching priority for research, but rather which
approach is most appropriate to the particular need. In each case, careful
attention to design and execution studies are vital.

Recent methods development, along with the identification of problems
in generalizing research results to broader populations than those enrolled
in tightly controlled trials, as well as the impressive advances in the potential availability of data through expanded use of electronic health records,
have all prompted re-consideration of research strategies and opportuni-

TABLE S-1 Selected Examples of Clinical Research Study Designs for Clinical Effectiveness Research

Approach	Description	Data types	Randomization
Randomized Controlled Trial (RCT)	Experimental design in which patients are randomly allocated to intervention groups (randomized) and analysis estimates the size of difference in predefined outcomes, under ideal treatment conditions, between intervention groups. RCTs are characterized by a focus on efficacy, internal validity, maximal compliance with the assigned regimen, and, typically, complete follow-up. When feasible and appropriate, trials are "double blind"—i.e., patients and trialists are unaware of treatment assignment throughout the study.	Primary, may include secondary	Required
Pragmatic Clinical Trial (PCT)	Experimental design that is a subset of RCTs because certain criteria are relaxed with the goal of improving the applicability of results for clinical or coverage decision making by accounting for broader patient populations or conditions of real-world clinical practice. For example, PCTs often have fewer patient inclusion/exclusion criteria, and longer term, patient-centered outcome measures.	Primary, may include secondary	Required
Delayed (or Single-Crossover) Design Trial	Experimental design in which a subset of study participants is randomized to receive the intervention at the start of the study and the remaining participants are randomized to receive the intervention after a pre-specified amount of time. By the conclusion of the trial, all participants receive the intervention. This design can be applied to conventional RCTs, cluster randomized and pragmatic designs.	Primary, may include secondary	Required

continued

TABLE S-1 Continued

Approach	Description	Data types	Randomization
Adaptive Design	Experimental design in which the treatment allocation ratio of an RCT is altered based on collected data. Bayesian or Frequentist analyses are based on the accumulated treatment responses of prior participants and used to inform adaptive designs by assessing the probability or frequency, respectively, with which an event of interest occurs (e.g., positive response to a particular treatment).	Primary, some secondary	Required
Cluster Randomized Controlled Trial	Experimental design in which groups (e.g., individuals or patients from entire clinics, schools, or communities), instead of individuals, are randomized to a particular treatment or study arm. This design is useful for a wide array of effectiveness topics but may be required in situations in which individual randomization is not feasible.	Often secondary	Required
N of 1 trial	Experimental design in which an individual is repeatedly switched between two regimens. The sequence of treatment periods is typically determined randomly and there is formal assessment of treatment response. These are often done under double blind conditions and are used to determine if a particular regimen is superior for that individual. N of 1 trials of different individuals can be combined to estimate broader effectiveness of the intervention.	Primary	Required
Interrupted Time Series	Study design used to determine how a specific event affects outcomes of interest in a study population. This design can be experimental or non-experimental depending on whether the event was planned or not. Outcomes occurring during multiple periods before the event are compared to those occurring during multiple periods following the event.	Primary or secondary	Approach dependent

TABLE S-1 Continued

Approach	Description	Data types	Randomization
Cohort Registry Study	Non-experimental approach in which data are prospectively collected on individuals and analyzed to identify trends within a population of interest. This approach is useful when randomization is infeasible. For example, if the disease is rare, or when researchers would like to observe the natural history of a disease or real world practice patterns.	Primary	No
Ecological Study	Non-experimental design in which the unit of observation is the population or community and that looks for associations between disease occurrence and exposure to known or suspected causes. Disease rates and exposures are measured in each of a series of populations and their relation is examined.	Primary or secondary	No
Natural Experiment	Non-experimental design that examines a naturally occurring difference between two or more populations of interest—i.e., instances in which the research design does not affect how patients are treated. Analyses may be retrospective (retrospective data analysis) or conducted on prospectively collected data. This approach is useful when RCTs are infeasible due to ethical concerns, costs, or the length of a trial will lead to results that are not informative.	Primary or Secondary	No
Simulation and Modeling	Non-experimental approach that uses existing data to predict the likelihood of outcome events in a specific group of individuals or over a longer time horizon than was observed in prior studies.	Secondary	No

continued

TABLE S-1 Continued

Approach	Description	Data types	Randomization
Meta Analysis	The combination of data collected in multiple, independent research studies (that meet certain criteria) to determine the overall intervention effect. Meta analyses are useful to provide a quantitative estimate of overall effect size, and to assess the consistency of effect across the separate studies. Because this method relies on previous research, it is only useful if a broad set of studies are available.	Secondary	No

SOURCE: Adapted, with the assistance of Danielle Whicher of the Center for Medical Technology Policy and Richard Platt from Harvard Pilgrim Healthcare, from a white paper developed by Tunis, S. R., *Strategies to Improve Comparative Effectiveness Research Methods and Data Infrastructure*, for June 2009 Brookings workshop, *Implementing Comparative Effectiveness Research: Priorities, Methods, and Impact*.

ties (Kravitz, 2004; Liang, 2005; Rush, 2008; Schneeweiss, 2004; Agency for Healthcare Research and Quality [AHRQ] CER methods and registry issues).

This emerging understanding about limitations in the current approach, with respect to both current and future needs and opportunities, sets the stage for the workshop's discussions.

Clinical Effectiveness Research and the IOM Roundtable

Formed in 2006 as the Roundtable on Value & Science-Driven Health Care brings together key stakeholders from multiple sectors—patients, health providers, payers, employers, health product developers, policy makers, and researchers—for cooperative consideration of the ways that evidence can be better developed and applied to drive improvements in the effectiveness and efficiency of U.S. medical care. Roundtable participants have set the goal that "by the year 2020, 90 percent of clinical decisions will be supported by accurate, timely, and up-to-date clinical information, and will reflect the best available evidence." To achieve this goal, Roundtable members and their colleagues identify issues and priorities for cooperative stakeholder engagements. Central to these efforts is the Learning Healthcare System series of workshops and publications. The series collectively characterizes the key elements of a healthcare system that is designed to generate and apply the best evidence for healthcare choices of patients and providers. A related purpose of these meetings is the identification and engagement of barriers to the development of the learning healthcare system and the key opportunities for progress. Each meeting is summarized in a publication available through The National Academies Press. Workshops in this series include

- The Learning Healthcare System (July 20–21, 2006)
- Judging the Evidence: Standards for Determining Clinical Effectiveness (February 5, 2007)
- Leadership Commitments to Improve Value in Healthcare: Toward Common Ground (July 23–24, 2007)
- Redesigning the Clinical Effectiveness Research Paradigm: Innovation and Practice-Based Approaches (December 12–13, 2007)
- Clinical Data as the Basic Staple of Health Learning: Creating and Protecting a Public Good (February 28–29, 2008)
- Engineering a Learning Healthcare System: A Look to the Future (April 28–29, 2008)
- Learning What Works: Infrastructure Required for Learning Which Care Is Best (July 30–31, 2008)
- Value in Health Care: Accounting for Cost, Quality, Safety, Outcomes and Innovation (November 17–18, 2008)

This publication summarizes the proceedings of the fourth workshop in the Learning Healthcare System series, focused on improving approaches to clinical effectiveness research.

The Roundtable's work is predicated on the principle that "to the greatest extent possible, the decisions that shape the health and health care of Americans—by patients, providers, payers, and policy makers alike—will be grounded on a reliable evidence base, will account appropriately for individual variation in patient needs, and will support the generation of new insights on clinical effectiveness." Well-conducted clinical trials have and will continue to contribute to this evidence base. However, the need for research insights is pressing, and as data are increasingly captured at the point of care and larger stores of data are made available for research, exploration is urgently needed on how to best use these data to ensure care is tailored to circumstance and individual variation.

The workshop's intent was to provide an overview of some of the most promising innovations and approaches to clinical effectiveness research. Opportunities to streamline clinical trials, improve their practical application, and reduce costs were reviewed; however, particular emphasis was placed on reviewing methods that improve our capacity to draw upon data collected at the point of care. Rather than providing a comprehensive review of methods, the discussion in the chapters that follow uses examples to highlight emerging opportunities for improving our capacity to determine what works best for whom.

A synopsis of key points from each session is included in this chapter; more detailed information on session presentations and discussions can be found in the chapters that follow. Day one of the workshop identified key lessons learned from experience (Chapter 2) and important opportunities presented by new tools and techniques (Chapter 3) and emerging data resources (Chapter 4). Discussion and presentations during day two focused on strategies to better plan, develop, and sequence the studies needed (Chapter 5) and concluded with presentations on opportunities to better align policy with research opportunities and a panel discussion on organizing the research community for change (Chapter 6). Keynote presentations provided overviews of the evolution and opportunities for clinical effectiveness research and provided important context for workshop discussions. These presentations and a synopsis of the workshop discussion are included in Chapter 1. The workshop agenda, biographical sketches of the speakers, and a list of workshop participants can be found in Appendixes A, B, and C, respectively.

COMMON THEMES

The Redesigning the Clinical Effectiveness Research Paradigm workshop featured speakers from a wide range of perspectives and sectors in health care. Although many points of view were represented, certain themes emerged from the 2 days of discussion, as summarized below and in Box S-2[2]:

- *Address current limitations in applicability of research results.* Because clinical conditions and their interventions have complex and varying circumstances, there are different implications for the evidence needed, study designs, and the ways lessons are applied: the internal and external validity challenge. In particular given our aging population, often people have multiple conditions—co-morbidities—yet study designs generally focus on people with just one condition, limiting their applicability. In addition, although our assessment of candidate interventions is primarily through pre-market studies, the opportunity for discovery extends throughout the lifecycle of an intervention—development, approval, coverage, and the full period of implementation.

---

[2] The material presented expresses the general views and discussion themes of the participants of the workshop, as summarized by staff, and should not be construed as reflective of conclusions or recommendations of the Roundtable or the Institute of Medicine.

BOX S-2
Redesigning the Clinical Effectiveness Research Paradigm

- Address current limitations in applicability of research results
- Counter inefficiencies in timeliness, costs, and volume
- Define a more strategic use to the clinical experimental model
- Provide stimulus to new research designs, tools, and analytics
- Encourage innovation in clinical effectiveness research conduct
- Promote the notion of effectiveness research as a routine part of practice
- Improve access and use of clinical data as a knowledge resource
- Foster the transformational research potential of information technology
- Engage patients as full partners in the learning culture
- Build toward continuous learning in all aspects of care

- *Counter inefficiencies in timeliness, costs, and volume.* Much of current clinical effectiveness research has inherent limits and inefficiencies related to time, cost, and volume. Small studies may have insufficient reliability or follow-up. Large experimental studies may be expensive and lengthy but have limited applicability to practice circumstances. Studies sponsored by product manufacturers have to overcome perceived conflicts and may not be fully used. Each incremental unit of research time and money may bring greater confidence but also carries greater opportunity costs. There is a strong need for more systematic approaches to better defying how, when, for whom, and in what setting an intervention is best used.

- *Define a more strategic use to the clinical experimental model.* Just as there are limits and challenges to observational data, there are limits to the use of experimental data. Challenges related to the scope of possible inferences, to discrepancies in the ability to detect near-term versus long-term events, to the timeliness of our insights and our ability to keep pace with changes in technology and procedures, all must be managed. Part of the strategy challenge is choosing the right tool at the right time. For the future of clinical effectiveness research, the important issues relate not to whether randomized experimental studies are better than observational studies, or vice versa, but to what's right for the circumstances (clinical and economic) and how the capacity can be systematically improved.

- *Provide stimulus to new research designs, tools, and analytics.* An exciting part of the advancement process has been the development of new tools and resources that may quicken the pace of our learning and add real value by helping to better target, tailor, and refine approaches. Use of innovative research designs, statistical techniques, probability, and other models may accelerate the timeliness and level of research insights. Some interesting approaches using modeling for virtual intervention studies may hold prospects for revolutionary change in certain clinical outcomes research.
- *Encourage innovation in clinical effectiveness research conduct.* The kinds of "safe harbor" opportunities that exist in various fields for developing and testing innovative methodologies for addressing complex problems are rarely found in clinical research. Initiative is needed for the research community to challenge and assess its approaches—a sort of meta-experimental strategy—including those related to analyzing large datasets, in order to learn about the purposes best served by different approaches. Innovation is also needed to counter the inefficiencies related to the volume of studies conducted. How might existing research be more systematically summarized or different research methods be organized, phased, or coordinated to add incremental value to existing evidence?
- *Promote the notion of effectiveness research as a routine part of practice.* Taking full advantage of each clinical experience is the theoretical goal of a learning healthcare system. But for the theory to move closer to the practice, tools and incentives are needed for caregiver engagement. A starting point is with the anchoring of the focus of clinical effectiveness research planning and priority setting on the point of service—the patient–provider interface—as the source of attention, guidance, and involvement on the key questions to engage. The work with patient registries by many specialty groups is an indication of the promise in this respect, but additional emphasis is necessary in anticipation of the access and use of the technology that opens new possibilities.
- *Improve access and use of clinical data as a knowledge resource.* With the development of bigger and more numerous clinical data sets, the potential exists for larger scale data mining for new insights on the effectiveness of interventions. Taking advantage of the prospects will require improvements in data sharing arrangements and platform compatibilities, addressing issues related to real and perceived barriers from interpretation of privacy and patient protection rules, enhanced access for secondary analysis to federally sponsored clinical data (e.g., Medicare part D, pharmaceutical,

clinical trials), the necessary expertise, and stronger capacity to use clinical data for postmarket surveillance.

• *Foster the transformational research potential of information technology.* Broad application and linkage of electronic health records hold the potential to foster movement toward real-time clinical effectiveness research that can generate vastly enhanced insights into the performance of interventions, caregivers, institutions, and systems—and how they vary by patient needs and circumstances. Capturing that potential requires working to better understand and foster the progress possible, through full application of electronic health records, developing and applying standards that facilitate interoperability, agreeing on and adhering to research data collection standards by researchers, developing new search strategies for data mining, and investing patients and caregivers as key supporters in learning.

• *Engage patients as full partners in the learning culture.* With the impact of the information age growing daily, access to up-to-date information by both caregiver and patient changes the state of play in several ways. The patient sometimes has greater time and motivation to access relevant information than the caregiver, and a sharing partnership is to the advantage of both. Taking full advantage of clinical records, even with blinded information, requires a strong level of understanding and support for the work and its importance to improving the quality of health care. This support may be the most important element in the development of the learning enterprise. In addition, the more patients understand and communicate with their caregivers about the evolving nature of evidence, the less disruptive will be the frequency and amplitude of public response to research results that find themselves prematurely, or without appropriate interpretative guidance, in the headlines and the short-term consciousness of Americans.

• *Build toward continuous learning in all aspects of care.* This foundational principle of a learning healthcare system will depend on system and culture change in each element of the care process with the potential to promote interest, activity, and involvement in the knowledge and evidence development process, from health professions education to care delivery and payment.

INCREASING KNOWLEDGE FROM PRACTICE-BASED RESEARCH

Of particular prominence throughout the workshop discussion was the notion of closing the gap between research and practice. Participants emphasized the challenges of ensuring that research is structured to provide information relevant to real-world decisions faced by patients, providers, and policy makers; ensuring the rigor of the research design and execution; and monitoring the safety and effectiveness of new products, with more attention to point-of-care data.

The multifaceted, practice-oriented approach to clinical effectiveness research discussed at the workshop complements and blends with traditional trial-oriented clinical research and may be represented as a continuum in which evidence is continuously produced by a blend of experimental studies with patient assignment (clinical trials); modeling, statistical, and observational studies without patient assignment; and monitored clinical experience (Figure S-2). The ratio of the different approaches varies with the nature of the intervention, as does the weight given to available studies. This enhanced flexibility and range of research resources is facilitated by the development of innovative design and analytic tools, and by the growing potential of electronic health records to allow much broader and structured access to the results of the clinical experience. The ability to draw on real-time clinical insights will naturally improve over time.

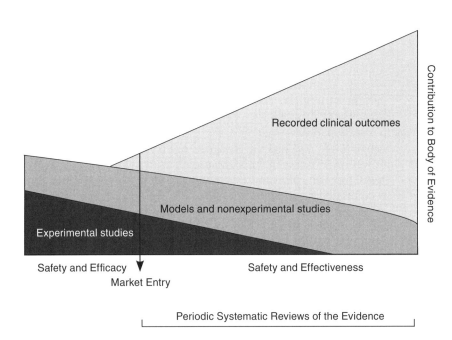

FIGURE S-2 Evidence development in the learning healthcare system.

PRESENTATION AND DISCUSSION SUMMARIES

The workshop presentations and discussions by experts from many areas of health care detailed the current state of clinical effectiveness research, provided examples of promising approaches, and proposed some key challenges and opportunities for improvement. Keynote addresses opened the 2 days of the workshop, previewing and underscoring the conceptual background, issues, and themes. IOM President Harvey V. Fineberg reviewed the evolution of clinical effectiveness research, and Carolyn M. Clancy offered meeting participants a vision for research that is better matched to evidence needs. Workshop discussions and presentations are briefly summarized; expanded discussions are included in the chapters that follow.

Clinical Effectiveness Research: Past, Present, and Future

In his keynote presentation, Fineberg briefly traced the evolution of clinical effectiveness research. From early efforts such as James Lynd's evaluation of treatments for scurvy to 20th-century developments in statistics that strengthen scientific studies to the establishment of RCTs as the standard of Food and Drug Administration (FDA) in making judgments about efficacy in the early 1970s, clinical effectiveness research has developed rapidly and has helped to transform medical care. However, Fineberg suggested that the resulting research paradigm, with randomized controlled double blind trials at the pinnacle, has often left important evidence needs unmet when combined with the costs, complexity, and lack of generalizability of RCTs. These gaps in evidence, he noted, prompt a reevaluation of the current application and require movement toward a strategy that takes better advantage of the range of methodologies to develop evidence that meets the particular need.

Important to the redesign of the research paradigm is the consideration of a set of prior questions that could better shape research design and conduct. For example, understanding the purpose of and vantage point from which these clinical questions are being asked helps to put into perspective the roles and contributions of the study designs that might be employed. Thinking critically about what is being evaluated and mapping what is appropriate, effective, and efficient for the various types of questions is an ongoing and important challenge in clinical effectiveness research. These efforts will also combat the central paradox in health care today: Despite the overwhelming abundance of information available, there is an acute shortage of information that is relevant, timely, appropriate, and useful to clinical decision making.

The critically central question for clinical effectiveness research is what works best in clinical care for the individual patient at the time care is needed. Answering this type of question will require the transformation of current approaches to a system that combines point-of-care focus with an electronic health record (EHR) data system coupled to systems for assembling evidence in a variety of ways. Such a system would combine several components: *evaluation* of learning what works and what does not work in a patient, weighing benefits and costs; *decision support* for the patient that would compensate for the overwhelming amount of evidence and make relevant determinations from the information available while increasing the pool of potentially useful information; *meaningful continuing education* for health professionals—real time, in time, practical, and applied—moving beyond the traditional lecture to learning in place, in real time, in the course of clinical care; and *quality improvement systems* that synthesize information from the three components above—evaluation, decision support, and meaningful continuing education.

Fineberg proposed a meta-experimental strategy, in which researchers not only focus on how well a certain method evaluates a particular kind of problem, in a specific class of patient, from a particular point of view, but also on determining the array of experimental methods that collectively perform in a manner that enables us to make better decisions for the individual and for society. With this approach, future learning opportunities can be structured to provide insights on what works for a particular kind of patient as well as how that strategy of evaluation can be employed to achieve a health system driven by evidence and based on value.

The Path to Research That Meets Evidence Needs

In the second day's keynote address, Carolyn M. Clancy, director of the Agency for Healthcare Research and Quality (AHRQ), shared perspectives in two broad areas: emerging methods that might be applied to meet current challenges in clinical effectiveness research and approaches to turning evidence into action. Stressing the importance of not producing better evidence for its own sake, Clancy challenged researchers to focus on the goal of achieving an information-rich, patient-focused system. Building toward a healthcare system in which actionable information is made available to clinicians and patients and in which evidence is continually refined as a by-product of healthcare delivery will require a broadening of the investigative approaches and methodologies that constitute the research arsenal.

Clancy noted that the traditional evidence hierarchy is being increasingly challenged, in part because it is inadequate to meet the current decision-making needs in health care, prompting calls for a rigorous reassessment of the appropriate roles for randomized and nonrandomized evidence. Recognizing that an intervention can work is a necessary, but not sufficient, requirement for making a treatment decision for an individual patient or for promoting it for a broad population. Even the most rigorously designed randomized trials have limitations, and research methods are needed to explore critical questions related to important trade-offs between risks and benefits of treatments for individual patients.

Although some circumstances may always require randomized trials, nonrandomized studies can complement and extend insights from RCTs in various ways—for example, tracking longer term outcomes, monitoring replicability in broader populations and community settings, and expanding information on potential benefits and harms of a given intervention. From a practical perspective, these approaches can help to evidence match the pace of rapid change and innovation found, for example, in surgical procedures and medical device development. Promising advances include (1) practical clinical trials, in which trial design is based on information needed to make a clinical decision and conduct is embedded into healthcare delivery systems; and (2) the use of cohort study registries to explore heterogeneity of treatment effects due to setting, practitioner, and patient variation, and consequently to turn evidence into action.

Observational studies offer an alternative when trials are impractical or infeasible and also help to accelerate translation of evidence into practice and aid risk management and minimization efforts. The promotion of more transparent, consistent approaches to the assessment of evidence and increased emphasis on the quality of study design and conduct over the type of method used are trends toward research that fit evidence needs, as is the focus on new and improved research methods. Finally, Clancy emphasized that to ensure research impacts practice, attention also is needed to improve approaches to turning evidence into action, and recent efforts by AHRQ and others underscore the research community's commitment to the creation of a system focused on the patient and improving health outcomes.

Cases in Point: Learning from Experience

The second chapter summarizes workshop discussions of case examples of high-profile issues—some linked to application of effective treatments or to premature adoption of unwarranted treatments—from which important lessons might be drawn about the design and interpretation of clinical effectiveness studies. The experiences recounted show that, from randomized trials to observational studies, each investigative approach has limitations. These limitations argue against using a particular approach and suggest that the research community needs more experience with the array of methodologies used to generate insights into clinical effectiveness and structured decision rules to guide the study design choice for particular research circumstances. Improvements can be made across the process, including careful consideration of the methods most appropriate to the question being asked; careful development and conduct of trials or studies to ensure they reflect the "state of the art"; clear communication of results; and exploration of new approaches, such as using a hybrid mix of research approaches.

Hormone Replacement Therapy

The first case was presented by JoAnn E. Manson from Harvard Medical School on the impact of hormone replacement therapy (HRT) on health. Both observational studies and clinical trials have contributed critically important information to elucidate the health effects of HRT with estrogen and progestin and to inform decision making, and they constitute a model suggesting that research findings should be considered in the context of the totality of available evidence and that studies should be designed to complement and extend existing data. Manson noted that observational studies and randomized clinical trials of menopausal HRT and coronary heart disease (CHD) have produced widely divergent results. Observational studies had suggested a 40–50 percent reduction in the risk of CHD among women taking HRT, whereas randomized trials suggested a neutral or even elevated risk of coronary events. Well-recognized limitations of observational studies, including the potential for confounding by lifestyle practices, socioeconomic status, education, and access to medical care, as well as selection factors related to "indications for use," can explain only some of the discrepancies. Other methodologic factors that may help to explain the differences include the limitations of observational studies in assessing short-term or acute risks, which led to incomplete capture of early clinical events after therapy began, and the predominance of follow-up time among compliant long-term users of HRT. In contrast to the greater weighting of long-term use in observational studies, clinical trial results tend to reflect shorter term use. Given that CHD risks related to HRT are highest soon after initiation of therapy, these differences may contribute substantially to the discrepancies observed.

Methodologic differences between observational studies and clinical trials, however, may not fully elucidate the basis for the discrepancies observed. The findings of observational studies and clinical trials are remarkably concordant for other health outcomes, including stroke, venous thromboembolism (blood clot), breast cancer, colorectal cancer, and fracture—outcomes that also should be affected by confounding and selection biases. Indeed, an emerging body of research suggests that the age of menopause or time since menopause critically influences the relationship between HRT and CHD outcomes.

Importantly, observational studies should be designed to capture both short- and long-term risks and should have frequent updating of exposure variables of interest (electronic health and pharmacy records may be useful). Clinical trials must be powered adequately to assess clinically relevant subgroups and to address the possibility of a modulating effect of key clinical variables. Consideration of absolute risks in research presentation and interpretation is critically important. Finally, it may be helpful to incorporate intermediate and surrogate markers into study designs, although such markers can never fully replace clinical event ascertainment.

Drug-Eluting Coronary Stents

Research to date strongly suggests that further understanding of and solutions to the safety issues concerning drug-eluting stents (DES) will likely come from a mix of randomized trials and observational registries conducted in both the premarket and postmarket arenas and a collaborative effort among regulators, industry, and academia. As Ashley B. Boam from the FDA recounted, coronary drug-eluting stents have dramatically changed interventional cardiology practice since their introduction in the United States in 2003. These products—a combination of a metal stent and an antiproliferative drug—have significantly reduced the need for reintervention compared to the previous standard of care, bare metal stents. This substantial improvement has led to widespread adoption of these products and use in patients outside those enrolled in the initial pivotal clinical studies. The desire to bring additional DES technology to the market quickly drove research into the identification of potential surrogate markers for effectiveness. While at least two measures obtained from angiography (i.e., late loss and percentage diameter stenosis of vessel) have been identified as biomarkers with a strong correlation to clinical effectiveness—specifically, the need for a reintervention—no such marker has been identified as a possible surrogate for safety outcomes, such as death or myocardial infarction.

In the last half of 2006 and through 2007, however, the emergence of stent thrombosis—the occurrence of a clot within the stent that often leads to myocardial infarction or death—shifted the focus of DES research significantly from effectiveness to safety. Recent meta-analyses and research from centers in Europe and the United States have indicated that late stent thrombosis may be an ongoing risk to DES patients. Low event rates, less than 1 percent, and late-term occurrence (beyond 1 year postimplantation) have complicated efforts to understand the true incidence and etiology of this noteworthy complication. Confounding the picture is the lack of appropriate studies to optimize prescription of mandatory adjunctive dual antiplatelet therapy, early interruption of which is one known risk factor for stent thrombosis. The issue is challenging in part because what is under consideration is a low frequency event with a late-term appearance, which generally mandates very large and long studies. Randomization, long-term follow-up, concurrent device iterations and new platforms, on-label versus broad clinical use considerations, and the role of resistance to acetylsalicylic acid and/or clopidogrel are among the other challenges.

Bariatric Surgery

Population-based registries—appropriately funded and constructed with clinician engagement—offer a compromise of strengths and limitations and may be the most effective tool for evaluating emerging healthcare technology, argued David R. Flum of the University of Washington. The dichotomy between "effectiveness" and "efficacy" is particularly relevant in evaluating surgical interventions where characteristics of the surgeon (experience, training, and specialty), variations in technical performance, patient selection, practice environments, and publication bias all influence the understanding of healthcare interventions. Case series, often authored by experts in the field, dominate the surgical literature. Despite their limitations, they are strong influences on clinical and policy decisions.

Bariatric interventions include a group of operations that have become increasingly popular with the advent of less-invasive surgical approaches and epidemic obesity. Understanding the safety and efficacy of bariatric interventions has come almost exclusively through single-center case series. A research group based at the University of Washington has worked to expand knowledge in this field through the use of retrospective population-level cohorts using administrative data, clinical registries, and longitudinal prospective cohorts that work to assess effectiveness. These safety data have been helpful in coverage decisions by payers in assessing quality improvement opportunities and in providing more realistic assessments of these interventions. Inherent limitations in effectiveness research include trade-offs among numbers of patients and details on patients, the granularity and accuracy of the data, and limits to the types of outcomes that can be evaluated (i.e., no quality-of-life or functional data).

Antipsychotic Therapeutics

As shown in recent research to ensure that antipsychotic medication use is clinically effective, advances in study designs, databases, and analytic methods provide a toolbox of complementary techniques from which researchers can draw, suggested Phillip S. Wang of the National Institute of Mental Health (NIMH). Antipsychotic medications are now widely used by patients and account for a large proportion of pharmaceutical spending, particularly in public healthcare programs. However, there is a paucity of evidence to help guide clinical, purchasing, and policy decisions regarding antipsychotic medications. The recently completed, NIMH-sponsored comparative effectiveness trials of antipsychotic medications in patients with schizophrenia (the CATIE trial), for example, blends features of efficacy studies and large, simple trials to create a pragmatic trial to provide extensive information about antipsychotic drug effectiveness over a drug course of at least 18 months. Recent advances in databases, designs, and methods can also be brought to bear to improve antipsychotic effectiveness. New study populations and databases have been developed, including practice-based networks that look at psychiatric care. Large administrative datasets are also available, such as Medicaid and useful health maintenance organization (HMO) databases, which are ideal for studying primary care in the setting where most mental health care is actually received.

Other approaches can be employed when trial data are not available. Researchers can use clinical epidemiologic data and methods, which are often a useful addition to the literature. When trials and quasi-experimental and even epidemiologic studies are not possible, researchers can use simulation methods. In addition, researchers have developed new means to deal with threats to validity—both threats to external validity, as in the development of effectiveness research, and threats to internal validity. These include new analytic methods, propensity score adjustments, and instrumental variable techniques.

Cancer Screening

Developing comparative effectiveness information about screening tests is a complex undertaking, as demonstrated by Peter B. Bach of Memorial Sloan-Kettering Cancer Center. The general rationale for screening in the context of clinical medicine or typical practice is that clinical disease usually "presents"—patients arrive with symptoms or signs that define a population that can be screened. Such circumstances actually make a strong argument for looking for preclinical conditions. That is what screening is intended to do—essentially scan an unaffected population to look for people who are at risk for developing some condition. The underlying principle of such an investigation is that theoretically we can decrease morbidity and mortality and other negative outcomes by looking for patients with preclinical conditions. Screening is widely encouraged, and one could argue that it is the dominant activity in much of primary care. Most medical journals, for example, regularly publish tables of screening evaluations, which are lists of questions that physicians should ask their patients to determine their risk for given diseases.

How these screenings impact a patient's health need to be understood better. A recent study found that screening for lung cancer with low-dose computed tomography may increase the rate of lung cancer diagnosis and treatment, but may not meaningfully reduce the risk of advanced lung cancer or death. Until more conclusive data are available, asymptomatic individuals should not be screened outside of clinical research studies that have a reasonable likelihood of further clarifying the potential benefits and risks. There are similar examples—in prostate cancer, in breast cancer with mammography, in renal cell cancer, and in melanoma. A paradoxical reality of the surrogate end-points often used to evaluate effectiveness in these cases is that they are readily available, but can be misleading. Simply stated, screening can often pick up pseudodisease, conditions that are not significant, yet trigger interventions or conditions that cannot be cured that are too often quickly characterized as "early" or "curable." Refuting the principle of "catch it early" is difficult, but there are many approaches to this goal, each with its own advantages and disadvantages.

Taking Advantage of New Tools and Techniques

Clinical effectiveness research can be improved and expedited through better use of existing methods and attention to emerging tools and techniques that enhance study design, conduct, and analysis. Chapter 3 presents discussion of some key opportunities for advancement in effectiveness research, including improved efficiency and result applicability of trials and studies; innovative statistical approaches to analyses of large databases; capture and use of the wealth of data generated in genomic research; and the promise of simulation and predictive modeling.

As each paper notes, the full benefits of these tools and techniques have yet to be fully realized. To enhance clinical effectiveness research, attention is needed in part to developing a shared understanding of these various approaches and clarity on the insights each offer the research enterprise, both alone and in synergy with other approaches. Essential to this discussion will be careful consideration of circumstances and questions for which a particular approach is best suited.

Innovative Approaches to Trials

Clinical trials play an important role in assessing the effects of medical interventions, in particular where observational studies are often inadequate, such as the detection of modest treatment effects or when the risk of an invalid answer is substantial. Robert Califf from Duke University emphasizes the importance of focusing discussion about medical evidence on a serious examination of ways to improve the operational methods of both approaches and of building human systems that take advantage of the power of modern informatics on improving both RCTs and observational studies. In particular, the design and conduct of RCTs needs to evolve to take further advantage of modern informatics and to provide a more flexible and practical tool for clinical effectiveness research. Improvements in the structure, strategy, conduct, analysis, and reporting of RCTs can help to address their perceived limitations related to cost, timeliness, and reduced generalizability.

Innovative approaches discussed including the conduct of trials within "constant registries" and targeting the standard set of rules for the conduct of trials to make them more adaptable and customized to meet research needs. A relevant model is the clinical practice database found at The Society of Thoracic Surgeons. This database has been used for quality reporting and increasingly to evaluate operative issues and technique. An extension of this model would be to develop constant disease registries capable of drawing on multiple EHR systems. The conduct of RCTs within the database would allow researchers to revolutionize the timeframe and costs of clinical trials. Trials also could take better advantage of "natural units of care" with cluster randomization, or provide information more relevant to practice by focusing on research questions based on gaps in clinical practice guidelines or being conducted in real-world practice (e.g., pragmatic clinical trials). Research networks offer the opportunity to enable the needed sharing of protocols, data structures, and other information.

A promising initiative for improvements in the quality and efficiency of clinical trials is the FDA Critical Path public–private partnership: Clinical Trials Transformation Initiative (CTTI). A collaboration of the FDA, industry, academia, patient advocates, and nonacademic clinical researchers, CTTI is designed to enhance regulations that improve the quality of clinical trials, eliminate guidances and practices that increase costs but provide no value, and conduct empirical studies of the value of guidances and practices. Primary barriers to innovation include the lack of appropriately structured financial incentives and the caution toward change that comes with a highly regulated market. To contend with this substantial barrier to ensuring that innovative approaches are implemented in practice, the research community should adopt a model from business of establishing "envelopes of creativity," or environments in which researchers could innovate with a certain creative freedom, and where they would have appropriate financial incentives.

Califf concludes that smarter trials that provide timely information on outcomes that matter most to patients and clinicians at an acceptable cost will become an integral part of practice in learning health systems as trials increasing become embedded into the information systems that form the basis for clinical practice. These systems also will provide the foundation for integrating modern genomics and molecular medicine into the framework of care.

Innovative Analytic Tools for Large Clinical and Administrative Databases

Because healthcare databases record drug use and some health outcomes for increasingly large populations, they will be a useful data resource for timely, comparative analyses that reflect routine care. Confounding is one of the biggest issues facing effectiveness research in the analyses of these large-claims databases. While recognizing that instrumental variable analyses have the drawback of producing certain levels of untestable assumptions, Sebastian Schneeweiss from Harvard Medical School proposes that their use can lead to substantial research improvements, particularly in situations with strong confounding and where it is likely that important confounders remain unmeasured in a data source. Several developments may bring the field closer to acceptable validity, including approaches that exploit the concepts of proxy variables using high-dimensional propensity scores and exploiting provider variation in prescribing preference using instrumental variable analysis.

Epidemiologists have a number of techniques that can control for confounding by measured factors, but instrumental variables are a promising approach to address unmeasured confounders because they are an unconfounded substitute for the actual treatment. In this approach, instead of modeling treatment and outcome, researchers model the instrument—which is unconfounded on the outcome—and then correct the estimate for the correlation between the instrumental variable and the actual treatment. In this respect valid results require the identification of a quasi-random treatment assignment in the real world, such as interruption in medical practice. Recent work has also demonstrated the potential of provider treatment preference as a random component in the treatment choice process, providing an additional instrument worth consideration for comparative drug effectiveness studies.

Instrumental variable analysis is an underused, but very promising, approach compared to effectiveness research using nonrandomized data, and researchers should routinely explore whether an instrument variable analysis is possible in a particular setting. Additional work is underway to develop better methods to assess its validity and to develop systematic screens for instrument candidates.

Adaptive and Bayesian Approaches to Study Design

Adaptive and, particularly, Bayesian approaches to study design offer opportunities to improve on randomization and to facilitate new ways of learning in health care. Donald A. Berry from the University of Texas M.D. Anderson Cancer Center contends that these approaches can be used to make RCTs more flexible by using data developed during a study to guide its conduct and to incorporate different sources of information to strengthen findings related to comparative effectiveness. The historical, frequentist approach, in which a design must be completely designed in advance and the study must be complete before inferences can be made, impedes the ability to continually assess and alter a course of study based on accrued learning. In contrast, the Bayesian approach's ability to calculate probabilities of future observations based on previous observations enables an "online learning" ideal for developing adaptive study designs. Prospective building of adaptive study designs is critical and, except in the simplest situations, requires simulation.

Adaptive designs increase the flexibility of RCTs by enabling modifications—based on interim or other study results—including stopping the study early, changing eligibility criteria, expanding or extending accrual, dropping or adding study arms or doses, switching between clinical phases, or shifting focus to subsets of patient populations. These adaptations not only enable rapid learning about relative therapeutic benefits but also improve the overall efficiency of research. Flexibility with respect to patient accrual, for example, may enable a needed increase in study sample size, potentially minimizing the need for additional follow-on studies.

Inherently a synthetic approach, Bayesian analysis can also enhance our capacity to appropriately aggregate information from multifarious sources. For instance, in addition to use in meta-analyses, this approach has been used recently to help answer complex questions, such as the proportional attribution of mammographic screening and adjuvant treatment with tamoxifen and chemotherapy in a drop in breast cancer mortality in the United States. The results of the Bayesian models used to explore this question were consistent with non-Bayesian models as well as those derived in clinical trials.

In conclusion, Berry notes that although the rigor and inflexibility of the current research paradigm has been important to establishing medicine as a science, new approaches such as Bayesian thinking and methodologies can help to move the field even further by making research more nimble and applicable to patient care, while maintaining scientific rigor.

Simulation and Predictive Modeling

Certain research questions or evidence gaps will be difficult or impractical to answer using clinical trial methods. Although physiology-based or mechanistic models have been used only recently in medicine, as noted by Mark S. Roberts from the University of Pittsburgh and representing Archimedes, Inc., physiology-based models, such at the Archimedes model, have the potential to address these gaps by extending results beyond the narrow spectrum of disease or practice found in most trials. These trials can also reduce the cost and time required to complete RCTs.

Physiology-based models aim to replicate disease processes at a biological level—from individual variables to system-level, whole-organ relationships. The behavior of these elements and effect on health outcomes are modeled using equations derived from and calibrated with data from empirical sources. When properly constructed and independently validated, these models not only can serve as useful tools to identify, set priorities in, or facilitate the design of new trials, but also can be engaged to conduct virtual comparative effectiveness trials. When time, cost, or other factors make doing a trial impossible, an independently validated, physiology-based model provides a useful alternative.

Emerging Genetic Information

At the forefront of discovery research, genomewide association studies permit examination of inherited genetic variability at an unprecedented level of resolution. As described by Teri Manolio of the National Human Genome Research Institute, given 500,000 or even a million SNPs (single-nucleotide polymorphism or differences among individuals within species) scattered across the genome, researchers can capture as many as 95 percent of variations in the population. This capacity enables "agnostic" genome-wide evaluations, whereby a researcher does not need to preformulate hypotheses or to limit examination to specific candidate genes, but rather can scan the entire genome. Following the availability of high-density genotyping platforms, the pace of genomic discovery has accelerated dramatically for an increasingly broad array of traits and diseases. However, examples of genomewide association studies do have drawbacks. Given the large number of comparisons per study, there is an unprecedented potential for false-positive results. Validation of findings through replication of results generally requires expanding studies from a small initial set of individuals to as many as 50,000 participants.

Two prototypes for applying genomic information from genomewide association studies to clinical effectiveness research are genetic variants related to two traits—Type 2 diabetes risk and warfarin dosing. Though both have sufficient scientific foundations and clinical availability, they remain many steps away from clinical application. Gaining more from these types of insights from genomic research will require additional epidemiologic and genomic information and evidence of impact on outcomes of importance. This evidence can be derived by linking genotypic data to phenotypic characteristics in clinical or research databases, an approach being explored by a number of biorepositories. The National Human Genome Research Institute's eMERGE network is applying genotyping to subsets of participants in a number of biorepositories with electronic health records. If the phenotypic measures derived from the EHRs are standardized to increase reliability, these types of linked databases hold significant promise for clinical effectiveness research.

Capacity for research, including the testing and interpretation of results, will require significant laboratory infrastructure, including a valid, readily available, FDA-certified, affordable test, conducted under the auspices of a CLIA (Clinical Laboratory Improvement Amendments)-certified laboratory. Robust electronic health records will also be critical to receive data and provide real-time performance feedback so that patients who receive abnormal results can be given suggestions for how to process that information and proceed from that point. In addition, tools for identifying emerging genomic information with potential clinical applications are needed. In this respect, a useful model is the database of Genotype and Phenotype (dbGaP), an accessible but secure large-scale database that receives, archives, and distributes results of studies of genotype–phenotype associations.

Also of vital importance is infrastructure related to policy and educational needs. For example, there is a pressing need to ensure confidentiality and privacy protection, specifically because the potential for discrimination by employers and insurers might occur if they have access to genomic information. To that end, the recently approved Genetic Information Non-Discrimination Act will be helpful. The research community also needs consensus on what should be reported to patients when abnormalities appear—what to tell them, when to tell them, and how to tell them—and adequate consent policies and procedures as well as consistent Institutional Review Board approaches. A flexible approach to genetic counseling is also needed, including the ability for patients to obtain adequate counseling from someone other than a certified genetic counselor. Also needed is a better educational infrastructure to ensure that these issues are discussed both by physicians and by patients, even during the course of ongoing genomic research; this would include better reporting guidelines for both patients and physicians. Education is needed in medical schools and nursing schools, at professional conferences, and in ongoing professional development and training to ensure that caregivers are "genomically literate." At the same time, we have a responsibility to also educate the general population, so that patients can develop a deeper understanding of genomics. By learning how genomics affects their lives and their health care, patients will know what questions to ask.

Organizing and Improving Data Utility

Vastly larger, electronically accessible health records and administrative and clinical databases currently under development offer previously unimagined resources for researchers and have significant and yet untapped potential to inform clinical effectiveness research. Mining data to expand the base of relevant knowledge and to determine what works for individual patients will use some of the techniques identified in Chapter 3 but will also require tools for organizing and improving these data collections. Chapter 4 provides an overview of the potential for data sources to improve effectiveness research, and identifies opportunities to better define rules of engagement and ensure these emerging data sources are appropriately harnessed. EHR and point-of-care data, enhanced administrative datasets, clinical registries, and distributed data networks are discussed. Collectively these papers illustrate how these approaches can be applied to improve the efficiency and quality of clinical practice; provide meaningful complementary data to existing research findings; accelerate the capture and dissemination of learnings from innovation in practice; and offer a means to process complex information—derived from multiple sources and formats—and develop information that supports clinical practice and informs the research enterprise.

The Electronic Health Record and Care Reengineering: Performance Improvement Redefined

Ronald A. Paulus reported on Geisinger's use of EHRs to transform care delivery to support his contention that there is more potential than currently exploited at the nexus of point-of-care systems and research. When systematically captured, the data produced by these systems can be used to inform and improve clinical practice. Demonstrating the potential of EHRs for impact beyond practice standardization and decision support mechanisms, Geisinger has used these resources in the production of "delivery-based evidence." EHRs capture data directly relevant to real work practice and can therefore provide extensive, longitudinal data. When coupled with an integrated data warehouse, the creation of a unique data resource can be mined for both clinical and economic insights. These data can also facilitate observational studies that address issues of clinical relevance to complement and fill gaps in RCT data. In developing such models, it is expected that more thought needs to be given to aggregating, transforming, and normalizing data in order to conduct productive analysis that will bridge the knowledge creation gap.

To illustrate the power inherent in linking data to clinical care, Paulus reviewed Geisinger's work to enhance performance improvement (PI) initiatives. EHRs and associated data aggregation and analysis to complement PI initiatives are increasingly being adopted in the healthcare setting. At Geisinger, PI has evolved into a continuous process involving data generation, performance measurement, and analysis to transform clinical practice.

Underlying this transformation is an EHR platform fully used across the system. Geisinger's integrated database, including EHR, financial, operational, claims, and patient satisfaction data, serves as the foundation of a Clinical Decision Intelligence System (CDIS) and is used to inform and document the results of PI efforts. PI Architecture draws upon CDIS and other inputs (e.g., evidence-based guidelines, third-party benchmarks) and leverages this information via decision support applications to help the organization answer important questions that could not be addressed before.

Key goals supported by PI Architecture include (1) assessment of PI initiatives' returns on investment (ROIs); (2) simultaneous focus on quality and efficiency; (3) development and refinement of reusable components and modules to support future PI efforts; and (4) elimination of any unnecessary steps in care, automating processes when safe and effective to do so, delegating care to the least cost, competent caregiver, and activating the patient as a participant in her own self-care. The PI Architecture enhances and refines the traditional Plan-Do-Study-Act (PDSA) cycle and yields advantages of reduced cycle time, increased relevance, increased sustainability, increased focus on ROI, and enhanced research capabilities. Key features include (1) use of local data to document the current state of practice and to direct focus on areas of greatest potential improvement; (2) use of electronic record review and simulation to confirm hypotheses and to project the benefits of varying avenues and degrees of change; (3) testing on a small scale, using an iterative approach that builds toward a strategy of rapid escalation; and (4) leveraging of reusable parts from past initiatives to build core infrastructure and accelerate future work.

Administrative Databases in Clinical Effectiveness Research

As described by Alexander M. Walker of Worldwide Health Information Science Consultants and the Harvard School of Public Health, data from health insurance claims form the backbone of many health analytic programs. Although administrative databases are being used more effectively for research, their development and especially their application for generating insights into clinical effectiveness require careful consideration and attention to potential methodologic pitfalls and hazards. Nonetheless, there is extraordinary promise in these resources.

Insurance claims data, derived from government payers or independent health insurers, are comprehensive, population based, and well structured for longitudinal analysis. All services and therapeutics for which there is a payment enter the data system, with easy linkage across providers. The regional or employment-based nature of the populations covered includes medicine as actually provided, not just the care that reflects best practice. The need for multiple providers to interact with multiple insurers or with a government mandate has led to highly standardized data structures supported by regular audit. Finally, these data are available for large numbers of individuals; the largest database with complete information is estimated to include data on 20 million patients.

Although claims data are excellent resources for answering many questions in health services research, they are not always sufficient for clinical research. For example, although labs ordered are recorded, the outcomes or results are not. To address this limitation, research groups have begun to augment their core files—adding laboratory and consumer data, creating the infrastructure for medical record review, implementing methods for automated and quasi-automated examination of masses of data, developing "rapid-cycle" analyses to circumvent the delays of claims processing and adjudication, and opening initiatives to collaborations that respect patients' and institutions' legitimate needs for privacy and confidentiality. These enhanced databases provide the information that allows researchers to trace back to specific patients or providers for additional information.

Enhanced claims databases that have been used to support surveillance programs along with automated and quasi-automated database review provide potential decision support tools for clinical safety and efficacy. Basic issues of confounding remain, however, and much attention is needed on these emerging tools to capture the full potential of these databases.

Clinical Effectiveness Research: The Promise of Registries

The dynamic and highly innovative character of healthcare technologies has been important to improvements in health; however, because intervention capacities often evolve due to iterative improvements or expanded use in practice, assessing their effectiveness presents a substantial challenge to researchers and policy makers. Because clinical registries capture information important to understanding the use of diagnostic and therapeutic interventions throughout their lifecycle, they are particularly valuable resources for assessing real-world health and economic outcomes. Alan J. Moskowitz and Annetine Gelijns from Columbia University suggest that in addition to providing information important to guiding decision making for patient care and setting policy, registries are valuable for assessing the performance of physicians and institutions, such as through the use of risk-adjusted volume–outcome relationship studies, and for increasing the efficiency of RCTs.

Several examples of findings derived from registry data on left ventricular assist devices (LVADs) were presented by Moskowitz to illustrate the potential of registries to improve effectiveness research. He pointed out that in contrast to efficacy trials or administrative databases, registries are able to keep pace with the dynamic process of medical innovation. The premarket setting has limits on what can be learned because of the nature of efficacy trials, which are usually short and conducted in narrow populations and under ideal conditions. Once interventions are introduced into general practice, they are used in broader patient populations and under different practice circumstances. For example, only 4 percent of patients treated with coronary artery bypass grafts in practice meet the eligibility criteria of the initial trials (the elderly, females, and those with co-morbidities were excluded). Expanded use of interventions in clinical practice creates a locus for learning and innovation, with the frequent discovery of new and unexpected indications for use, as well as the accrual of knowledge on the appropriate integration of technology into the care of particular patients. Characterized as an "organized system using observational study methods to collect uniform data to evaluate specified outcomes for a population defined by a particular disease, condition, or exposure, and that serves a predetermined scientific, clinical, or policy purpose," clinical registries collect data information important to learning and innovation. Examples include long-term outcomes and rare adverse events and outcomes achieved when technology is used by a broadened set of providers or patients. Clinical registries also provide comparative effectiveness information.

Registries offer a powerful means to capture innovation and downstream learning that take place in practice and to develop information complementary and supplementary to that produced by randomized trials. Enhancing the value of registries for clinical research requires improving the quality of data obtained, while decreasing costs and other barriers to data access. Special attention needs to be paid to the definition and standardization of target populations and outcomes (e.g., adverse events); efforts to address bias; measures to ensure representative capture of the population; and sound analytical approaches. Incorporating data collected in the usual course of patient care may help to reduce the burden and cost of registries.

Opportunities to address the traditional weaknesses of registries are presented by advances in informatics, analytical techniques, and new models of financing. The potential of registries to improve the efficiency of randomized trials also must be addressed. The development of investment incentives for stakeholders is important to improving the viability of clinical registries. Although registries have been created by public, not-for-profit, or private organizations, public–private partnerships offer a new model for registry support.

Distributed Data Networks

The variety of information created by healthcare delivery has the potential to provide insights to improve care and support clinical research.

Increasingly, these data are held by many organizations in different forms. Although the aggregation of disparate databases into a super dataset may seem desirable for the improved study power and strength of findings provided by larger numbers, such efforts also face significant challenges due to privacy concerns and the proprietary nature of some data. Richard Platt, from Harvard University illustrated how distributed research models circumvent these issues and minimize security risks by allowing the data repositories of multiple parties to remain separately owned and controlled. These models also provide an interface to these stores of highly useful data that allows them to function as a large combined dataset. This approach also takes advantage of local expertise needed to interpret content.

Work at the HMO Research Network has demonstrated the feasibility of this approach for biosurveillance and vaccine safety networks, and several additional models are currently in development. The FDA is calling for the development of a sentinel network to support postmarketing safety research, AHRQ has written a contract to develop a prototype distributed network that will be targeted at comparative effectiveness and safety research, the Robert Wood Johnson Foundation has funded the development of a distributed network that will evaluate quality measures, and the National Institutes of Health (NIH) clinical translational science centers are trying to develop ways for the centers to collaborate with one another in a wide range of clinical research activities. Opportunities to build and use these types of resources also extend to the private sector.

Effective governance models are most pressing for the development and use of these networks. Attention must be given to policies, funding, and further research that supports their development, and to make such work more efficient. Consideration should also be given to developing common standards for distributed research networks so that a single infrastructure might serve multiple functions, even as networks accommodate different kinds of interfaces and governance systems. Overall, governance of such networks, as well as funding for them, will be nontrivial concerns.

Moving to the Next Generation of Studies

In the face of expanding options for diagnostic and treatment options, focus is needed on the development of information that can help guide clinical decision making. Not only are the number of research questions increasing, but current approaches to developing comparative effectiveness information are impractical—making the need to take better advantage of new sources of data and other opportunities to produce evidence relevant to clinical practice more urgent. Many participants noted that in research today, knowledge is expanding much faster than we can effectively translate and process it in ways that can impact patient care. Thus there is a sense that to address gaps in evidence and newly emerging research challenges, the research community needs to support and nurture efforts to develop new approaches to study design and strategies.

In a session focused on moving to the next generation of studies, participants considered a set of interrelated questions: What are the key opportunities and needed advancements to improve our approach to clinical effectiveness research? How might we take better advantage of emerging resources to plan, develop, and sequence studies that are more timely, relevant, efficient, and generalizable? How can we account for lifecycle variation of the conditions and interventions at play? A variety of innovations were presented, including new mathematical models, new ideas for observational studies and hybrid studies, tools for assessing the roots of genetic variation, cooperative research networks, and even innovation in incentives.

Large Data Streams and the Power of Numbers

Data are increasingly generated and captured throughout the research, development, and delivery of healthcare products and services. Sharon-Lise Normand of Harvard Medical School contends that the availability of large data streams holds potential to enhance our capacity to produce clinically useful information, but under the current evidence paradigm, these types of information are often wasted. By treating these data sources as silos of information, opportunities are lost for insights on issues such as treatment heterogeneity, or multiple outcomes and patient subgroups. New analytic strategies are needed to more effectively deploy these resources and improve the efficiency with which the research community produces information.

Taking better advantage of large data streams is important in moving to the next generation of studies. The development and implementation of pooling algorithms are needed, as are inferential tools to detect relationships among diverse data sources and to appropriately combine them. Possible applications include comparative effectiveness research through the enhancement of trial results or inferences derived from single data sources. Moreover, although the research community has some experience in pooling observational data with trial data, study designs that exploit features of the emerging diverse data sources—such as hybrid designs, preference-based designs, and quasi-experimental designs—have not yet been exploited to the full potential.

The number of data sources will only continue to expand, and infrastructure is needed to enable their optimal use, including support for the development of new, innovative analytic strategies and mechanisms for data sharing, documentation, and quality control. Approaches are needed to assess data-pooling strategies, minimize false discoveries, and validate findings. More opportunities are needed to explore approaches to pooling different data sources and employing various study designs. Finally, we need to educate policy makers and researchers in the interpretation of results from the new designs.

Observational Studies

Observational studies add value to the research paradigm through their ability to address the dilemma presented by the costs, slow pace, and other logistical difficulties of conducting RCTs. Additionally, suggested Wayne A. Ray of Vanderbilt University, this approach is essential for answering important clinical questions in which RCTs are not appropriate. Although findings of observational studies are intrinsically more prone to uncertainty than those from randomized trials, abiding by some fundamental epidemiologic principles will allow clinicians to better exploit the wealth of available observational data. Common errors include elementary design mistakes; failure to identify a clinically meaningful t_0, or start to follow-up; exposure and disease misclassification; use of overly broad endpoints for safety studies; confounding by the "healthy drug-user effect"; and marginal sample size. These sources of bias and error can easily lead to the design of a "false-negative" safety study or a "false-positive" efficacy study; upon examination, many controversial or misleading results of observational studies result from such suboptimal methodology.

Although the design of observational studies is a complex subject, opportunities exist to improve their capacity to contribute to clinical effectiveness research. The notion that study design and analysis are quick and inexpensive is misleading. Resources and expertise are needed to support state-of-the-art observational studies—in which consideration is given at the outset of the question at hand and how the various biases might apply. For analyses examining safety, limitations that lead to false results are fairly easy to identify and counteract, and a greater challenge is to address conflicts of interest concerns related to their conduct. For efficacy, a first step is to ensure that the expected benefits of therapy exist for the population as a whole, if not for the individual. Underpinning all of these needed advancements is improved education and training of researchers. Epidemiologists need to become more familiar with the clinical and pharmacological principles that affect the use of observational data and to ensure that these guide the design and conduct of proposed and published studies.

Enhancing the Evidence to Improve Practice: Experimental and Hybrid Studies

Basic scientific research continues to generate advances in treatment options, but bringing a product to market is not enough to ensure its optimal, appropriate, and safe use in clinical practice. In terms of improving health outcomes and use of resources, research to determine how, for whom, when, and in what context a treatment is best used deserves higher emphasis in funding and prioritization. As illustrated by John Rush of the University of Texas Southwestern Medical Center, a variety of methods are available for answering such complex and clinically important questions—such as using observational data obtained when systemic practices are employed (registry/cohort studies), effectiveness trials (practical clinical trials), and hybrid designs. Also of note are new study designs (e.g., equipoise stratified randomized designs; adaptive treatment studies) and posthoc data analyses (e.g., moderator analyses).

The results of a multisite NIMH trial, Sequenced Treatment Alternatives to Relieve Depression (STAR*D), illustrate how a hybrid trial can be employed to provide valuable insights on the optimal use of interventions in clinical practice as well as to improve future research analyses. This investigation helped to answer a host of clinically critical questions, such as the time needed to see a response in treatment; effects of sequence when a course of multiple treatment steps are involved; and effectiveness in a treatment population expanded beyond those in the efficacy trials to include patients with concurrent general medical conditions.

Expanding the evidence base to answer a broader set of questions important to delivering appropriate care—such as those examined in STAR*D—will require the design and use of cost-efficient, rapidly executed studies and the prioritization of research questions. Some key considerations include research that will change practice, enhance outcomes or understanding of the disorder, improve cost efficiency, and/or make treatments safer. Defining and answering these key questions will require the input of relevant stakeholders and care systems reengineered to support research. Finally, once the questions are defined, designs must be identified or developed to obtain the answers. NIH leadership will be essential, as will input and support from clinicians, patients, investigators, and payers. Without these commitments, how, when, for whom, and in what setting a treatment is best will remain the "art of medicine," rather than the science.

Accommodating Genetic Variation as a Standard Feature of Clinical Research

Genomics is poised to have a significant impact on clinical care, and likewise, the medical system could, if adequately harnessed, dramatically transform our understanding of the role of genetic variation on disease development and progression. A significant threat to genomic medicine lies in its potential to generate a large number of spurious findings. To contend with this issue, the research community seeks approaches that garner a large number of patients needed to obtain reproducible linkages between disease characteristics and rare events or weak effects measured for common genetic variants. Given the potential offered by large-scale genomic studies, developing efficient and inexpensive approaches to obtain data of needed quality and quantity is of utmost importance. Issac S. Kohane of Harvard Medical School suggests three prongs of instrumentation of the health system in particular that will help to efficiently produce the large N needed: high-throughput genotyping, phenotyping, and sample acquisition.

Although the costs of high-throughput genotyping are rapidly dropping, the cost of assembling, phenotyping, and studying large populations is an estimated $3 billion for 500,000 individuals. Fortunately, the informational by-products of routine clinical care can be used to bring phenotyping and sample acquisition to the same high-throughput, commodity price point as is currently true of genotyping costs. Kohane discussed recent efforts to contend with challenges related to identifying relevant patient populations and obtaining biosamples from any phenotyped population. First, advances in automated natural language processing has allowed the evaluation of online health record text to quickly, reproducibly, and accurately stratify 96,000 out of 2.5 million patients for disease severity, pharmacoresponsiveness, and exposures. If expanded across many delivery systems, high-throughput phenotyping will be achievable at the national level. Second, a system currently being pilot-tested takes advantage of the many biosamples collected by laboratories in the course of care that are usually discarded. These samples present the opportunity to develop a potentially rich set of clinically relevant information (e.g., genomic composition, identification of biomarkers, effects of new treatments) that can be linked to previously phenotyped populations. A focus on instrumenting the health enterprise will not only contribute to advances in genomic studies but also provide an opportunity to learn from care delivery, if the appropriate security procedures are assured. The detection of cardiovascular risk in patients taking Vioxx was enabled by the development of large-scale databases and datamarts and is one example of how the healthcare system can be used for both discovery research and surveillance.

The most important step toward this goal is to create a safe harbor for methodological testing that challenges researchers to experiment with large datasets analysis. Open and transparent discussion is needed about the strengths and weaknesses of various methodological approaches; data should be made more broadly available so that researchers can test the data and methodologies and replicate findings. Progress will require increased investment in information technology—particularly to increase the quality of secondary uses of electronically captured data; addressing, through policy and education, various aspects of the Health Insurance Portability and Accountability Act (HIPAA) that prevent broader implementation of these systems and approaches; and the development of an informatics-savvy healthcare research workforce that understands relationships among health information, genomics, and biology.

Phased Introduction and Payment for Interventions Under Protocol

Clinical effectiveness research draws on experience gained in the post-market setting. Because this research is distinct from that required for FDA approval and market entry, innovative policies that encourage and facilitate these types of investigations will be needed. Wade Aubry from the Center for Medical Technology Policy described coverage with evidence development (CED) as an example of how policy can be used to contend with an essential problem in medical care—that for many clinical situations, evidence is insufficient to inform decision making. A brief history of how concepts evolved since CED's initial use in the 1990s, as well as some lessons learned, is discussed.

An important early example of CED is of the support of commercial payers such as Blue Cross Blue Shield plans for patient care costs of high-priority, National Cancer Institute (NCI)-sponsored randomized clinical trials evaluating high-dose chemotherapy with autologous bone marrow transplantation. Other examples in Medicare include the FDA/Centers for Medicare & Medicaid Services (CMS) interagency agreement allowing for coverage of Category B investigational devices, coverage of lung volume reduction surgery for bullous emphysema under an NIH protocol, and the Medicare clinical trials policy, under which qualifying clinical trials receive Medicare coverage for patient care costs under an approved protocol. Over the past 4 years, Medicare CED has been formalized by CMS with guidance documents for CED policies on (1) implantable cardioverter defibrillators for prevention of sudden cardiac death, and (2) positron emission tomography for diagnosis of Alzheimer's disease.

The application of CED to commercial health plans has grown in interest over the past year as part of the debate over whether a national comparative effectiveness institute should be established. Despite this progress, significant barriers to further development of this concept in the private sector remain. These include health plan Evidence of Coverage (EOC) language defining medical necessity, ethical issues, the difficulty in achieving multistakeholder consensus, lack of a clear definition of "adequate" evidence compared to "ideal" evidence, timing of CED in regard to existing coverage without restrictions, and limitations of the number of studies that can be implemented under CED.

Research Networks

Successful initiatives such as the Cooperative Oncology Groups, HMO Research Network, Center for Education and Research in Therapeutics, the Framingham Heart Study, and others provide useful models for how the clinical effectiveness paradigm might be redesigned to be more timely, relevant, efficient, and generalizable. As noted by Eric B. Larson from the Group Health Cooperative, similar emerging research networks embedded in the healthcare system provide an important anchoring element for a new generation of effectiveness studies. Certain characteristics of research networks make them particularly suited to produce good research on which to base clinical decisions.

Research conducted in a functioning delivery system is generally population based, with greater generalizability and relevance than research in convenience samples or highly selected, specialized populations. This research infrastructure also allows for better accounting for ecological factors in a real, live organization that can affect applicability of research. A well-constructed healthcare system not only enables more efficient conduct of trials and studies but also continuously pioneers technological and structural advancements to improve care. Such advancements are not the focus of traditional research but often significantly improve the quality of care.

Working in a functioning delivery system promotes another key characteristic: the "bidirectionality" of research. Research ideas often emerge from advances in more rarefied research settings when they may be ready for application to practice. Research ideas often surface because of real-world problems that need solutions or because innovative ideas emerge from the practice environment that need refinement and testing. Rather than thinking of only bench to bedside, the best research networks will perform bidirectional research and follow-up, so that there is, in essence, both an afferent and efferent limb to the research. Research networks are ideal for pragmatic and efficient clinical trials and, if population based, assessment of generalizability is ideal. That said, research networks placed in well-constructed healthcare systems will need to (and can) develop other, robust methods such as cluster randomized trials, disease registries, inception cohort studies and time series, and quasi-experimental use of observational data that can be helpful to a learning healthcare organization. Such research will also inform the field in general, especially if population based, allowing one to infer its generalizabilty. Research networks in well-characterized populations that are enrolled in an organized delivery system are ideal to reduce the time from research to translation, particularly in emerging research areas such as genomic/personalized medicine and use of electronic health records to efficiently determine phenotypes.

We are beginning to realize the potential of bringing together research networks in integrated healthcare systems with university-based scientists. One outcome of the NIH Roadmap has been development of NIH-funded programs under the Clinical and Translational Science Awards (CTSAs). The CTSA program aims to "develop a national system of interconnected clinical research networks capable of more quickly and efficiently mounting large-scale studies." One consequence of this effort is a nascent culture change and, in places, work by institutions choosing to "reengineer" their clinical and translational research programs. A redesign of the clinical effectiveness research paradigm ideally would address challenges the NIH will face as it aims to reengineer the massive U.S. biomedical research enterprise. To achieve this culture change, both human and technical factors must be addressed: For CTSAs to work together, we will need a baseline level of interoperability to facilitate data exchange. It is also important to consider how CTSAs might seamlessly partner with other networks. Additionally, the research community needs to articulate and conscientiously attend to the challenges of building and sustaining strong collaborative teams.

Aligning Policy with Research Opportunities

Reform in clinical effectiveness research will require action beyond the development of new and improved methodologies. The healthcare sectors contain substantial talent and leadership, and many opportunities to better harness and direct these resources to improvement in clinical care might emerge with broader engagement and stakeholder commitment to these efforts. Opportunities for cross-sectoral collaboration are necessary to create a focus and set priorities for these efforts, to clarify the questions that must be addressed, and to marshal the resources that reform requires. Chapter 6 identifies some policy changes that can drive innovative research and explores how government, industry, and consumers can contribute to and build support for clinical effectiveness work.

Course-of-Care Data

Clinical systems increasingly capture data on the experience of each patient and clinician in a structured and quantifiable manner. These data resources present a major opportunity for "rapid learning" about the effectiveness of various treatments in the clinical practice setting. Greg Pawlson from the National Committee for Quality Assurance notes that although these data offer the opportunity to bridge the chasm between clinical practice and clinical or health services investigations, much work is needed to make these data available and useful for research. Key barriers to progress include insufficient funding for the development of the health information technology (HIT) infrastructure needed for rapid learning; the influence of HIPAA protections and the proprietary nature of these data on the research questions and approaches pursued; and the structure of the EHR.

Important to enabling the full potential of EHR and other course-of-care data resources will require greater focus on designing and developing EHR systems for research—beginning with the development of data standards and increased funding for the development of HIT infrastructure to facilitate access and use of data. Suggested policy interventions include:

- Better coordinating how the private and public sectors fund research, clinical learning, and HIT development;
- Increasing the proportion of funding dedicated to improving the quality and quantity of secondary database analyses;
- Creating incentives for collecting and structuring data useful for research;
- Providing more open and affordable access to data held by health plans and others;
- Engaging both the private and public sectors in an effort to set standards for how and what data are entered and retrieved from EHRs;
- Modifying HIPAA regulations to remove the major barriers imposed on research while balancing privacy concerns; and
- Improving medical education to better prepare health professionals to use individual and aggregated data for the care of patients.

Pharmaceutical Industry Data

As the healthcare system becomes more complex, the pharmaceutical industry is increasingly challenged to meet regulatory, payer, and patient demands for demonstration of the value of their products. Such assessments of risk–benefit, long-term safety, and comparative effectiveness often require postmarket clinical trial and database commitments. Peter Honig of Merck reflected on the difficult balance between the data transparency and data access needed to support the necessary epidemiologic, pharmacovigilance, and outcomes research with the increasingly commoditized and proprietary nature of data sources. Additional barriers to efficient use of these data include the decentralized nature of most utilization and claims outcome data and needed improvements in study and trial methods.

These issues are of particular interest to the industry in light of the high risk and high costs of the drug development process. Honig discusses several important initiatives underway to address these challenges. The FDA's Critical Path initiative is advocating for public–private partnerships in the precompetitive space to address challenges in drug discovery and development, comparators other than placebo are being increasingly incorporated into clinical postapproval (Phase IV) trials, and structured methods are being developed to provide risk–benefit information that aids clinicians, payers, and regulators in making important decisions about safety, indicated use, and effectiveness. Industry acceptance of an ongoing, learning paradigm for evidence development has increased. Increasing rigor in pharmacoepidemiologic and risk–benefit standards is an asset to the field and the patient. The use of registries, both sentinel and population based, may provide a better method for pharmacovigilance. Increasing use of Bayesian statistical approaches, use of spontaneous and population-based data mining for postmarketing surveillance, and development of sophisticated data analysis tools to improve database output are all advances toward a smarter data collection system. To ensure these data add value to how care is delivered, educational efforts are also needed to improve the translation of generated knowledge into behavior.

Regulatory Requirements and Data Generation

Data developed and collected to satisfy regulatory requirements offer a rich resource and a driving force for improvements in our capacity for clinical effectiveness research. Mark B. McClellan of the Brookings Institution reports on two examples of how we might begin to take better advantage of these resources to enhance the healthcare system's capacity to routinely generate and use data to learn what works in practice. The recently passed Food and Drug Administration Amendment Act of 2007 envisions the development of a postmarket surveillance system that actively monitors for suspected safety problems with medical products. However, it also has the potential to lead to the development of infrastructure built into the healthcare system that can be used to address questions of effectiveness and use of products in different types of patients and populations. To take advantage of the opportunity presented, attention is needed to developing standards and consistent methods for defining adverse events and pooling relevant summary data from large-scale analyses, as well as contending with issues that impeded data sharing.

Medicare's CED policy has also helped to develop the data needed to better inform coverage and clinical decisions by supporting the conduct of trials or the development of registries that collect and house sophisticated sets of clinical data about the use and impact of several medical technologies on patient outcomes. McClellan pointed out that clarification by Congress of CMS's authority to use these methods is needed to support efforts currently underway and to encourage similar efforts taking place in the private sector.

These efforts seek to build the capacity to develop better evidence into the healthcare system, an approach that will become increasingly important to contend with the vast scope and scale of current and future knowledge gaps. The majority of these gaps are in areas for which it has been particularly challenging to develop evidence—such as assessing the effects of the many subtle and built-in differences in medical practice for patients with chronic disease. Because such information is critically important to improving outcomes, and will not be derived from traditional RCTs, priority efforts are needed to enhance the healthcare system's capacity to generate data as a routine part of care and to use these data to learn what works in practice. Additional support is needed for the infrastructure, data aggregation, and analysis, and for improving the relevant statistical methods.

Ensuring Optimal Use of Data Generated by Public Investment

Though large amounts of data exist and have the potential to inform clinical and comparative effectiveness assessment, substantial barriers prevent optimal use of these data. Many innovative opportunities are possible from these publicly supported and generated data, such as the ability to inform clinical practice and policy. However, the restrictive interpretation of HIPAA and related privacy concerns, the growth of Medicare HMOs, and the fragmentation and commercialization of private-sector clinical databases all limit effectiveness research and threaten effectiveness findings. J. Sanford Schwartz referred to this as the paradox of available but inaccessible data and called for more attention to reducing the barriers to data use until they do not impede research effectiveness.

Enhanced coordination in the development of publicly generated data both within and across agencies can mitigate overlap and redundancy; the government should expand the RCT registry to include all comparative effectiveness research to further the range of issues addressed and information available. Access to data generated by public investment, including those by publicly funded investigators, should be expanded through the development of effective technical and support mechanisms. To move past the barriers presented by HIPAA, Medicare HMOs, and private-sector databases, Schwartz urged establishing practical, less burdensome policies for secondary data that protect patient confidentiality, expand Medicare claims files to incorporate new types and sources of data, and develop more cost-effective access to private-sector, secondary clinical data for publicly funded studies.

Building the Research Infrastructure

Given that evidence-based medicine requires integration of clinical expertise and research and depends on an infrastructure that includes human capital and organizational platforms, the NIH's Alan M. Krensky said the NIH is committed to supporting a stable, sustainable scientific workforce. Continuity in the pipeline and the increasing age at which new investigators obtain independent funding are the major threats to a stable workforce. To address these concerns, the NIH is developing new programs that target first-time R01-equivalent awardees with programs such as the Pathway to Independence and NIH Director's New Innovator Awards, with more than 1,600 new R01 investigators funded in 2007. NIH-based organizational platforms are intra- and interinstitutional. CTSAs fund academic health centers to create homes for clinical and translational science, from informatics to trial design, regulatory support, education, and community involvement. The NIH is in the midst of building a national consortium of CTSAs that will serve as a platform for transforming how clinical and translational research is conducted. The Immune Tolerance Network (ITN), funded by the National Institute of Allergy and Infectious Diseases, the National Institute of Diabetes and Digestive and Kidney Diseases, and the Juvenile Diabetes Research Foundation, is an international collaboration focused on critical path research from translation to clinical development. The ITN conducts scientific review, clinical trials planning and implementation, tolerance assays, data analysis, and identification of biomarkers, while also providing scientific support in informatics, trial management, and communications. Centralization, standardization, and the development of industry partnerships allow extensive data mining and specimen collection. Most recently, the Immune Tolerance Institute, a nonprofit, was created at the intersection of academia and industry to quickly transform scientific discoveries into marketable therapeutics. Policies aimed at building a sustainable research infrastructure are central to support evidence-based medicine.

Engaging Consumers

Conducting meaningful clinical effectiveness research requires collecting, sharing, and analyzing large quantities of health information from many individuals, potentially for long periods of time. To be successful, this research will need the support and active participation of patients. The relationship between researcher and research participant, as defined by current practice, is ill suited to successfully leverage such active participation. As reported by Kathy Hudson of Johns Hopkins University, however, public engagement efforts in biomedical research, while still in their infancy, suggest some key challenges and opportunities for cultivating active public participation in clinical effectiveness research.

The biomedical community—and the science and technology community more generally—traditionally have viewed the linear progression from public education to public understanding to public support as an accurate model through which to cultivate a public enthusiastically supportive of and involved in research. As the flaws in this philosophy have become more apparent, research-performing institutions increasingly are turning to public engagement and public consultation approaches to enlist public support. Unlike unidirectional and hierarchal communications that characterize past efforts, public engagement involves symmetric flow of information using transparent processes and often results in demonstrable shifts in attitudes among participants (though not always in the direction one might expect or prefer). The outcome is different, as well: Rather than aspiring for or insisting on the public's deeper understanding of science, a primary goal of public engagement is the scientists' deeper understanding of the public's preferences and values.

ORGANIZING THE RESEARCH COMMUNITY FOR CHANGE

Most issues here require the attention of the research community in order to drive change, with some of the most pressing concerns in areas such as methods improvement, data quality and accessibility, incentive alignment, and infrastructure. Much work is already underway to enhance and accelerate clinical effectiveness research, but efforts are needed to ensure stronger coordination, efficiencies, and economies of scale within the research community. Participants in the final panel, composed of sector thought leaders, were asked to consider how the research community might be best organized to develop and promote the needed change and to offer suggestions on immediate opportunities for progress not contingent on expanded funding or legislative action.

Panelists characterized the current research paradigm, infrastructure, funding approaches, and policies—some more than 50 years old—as in need of overhauling and emendation. Discussion highlighted the need for principles to guide reform, including a clarification of the mission of research as centered on patient outcomes, identification of priority areas for collective focus, a research paradigm that emphasizes best practices in methodologies, and a greater emphasis on supporting innovation. Apart from a need for stronger coordination, collaboration, and the setting of priorities for questions to address and the studies to be undertaken, there is a need to develop systems that inherently integrate the needs and interests of patients and healthcare providers. The lifecycle approach to evidence development in which trials and studies are staged or sequenced to better monitor the effectiveness of an intervention as it moves into the postmarket environment was also suggested as an approach that could support the development of up-to-date best evidence. Finally, participants suggested immediate opportunities to build on existing infrastructure that could support the continual assessment approach to evidence development, including broader support of clinical registries and networked resources such as CTSAs, as well as the FDA's efforts to develop a sustainable system for safety surveillance.

ISSUES FOR POSSIBLE ROUNDTABLE FOLLOW-UP

Among the range of issues engaged in the workshop's discussion were a number that could serve as candidates for the sort of multistakeholder consideration and engagement represented by the Roundtable on Value & Science-Driven Health Care, its members, and their colleagues.

Clinical Effectiveness Research

- *Methodologies.* How do various research approaches best align to different study circumstances—e.g., nature of the condition, the type of intervention, the existing body of evidence? Should Roundtable participants develop a taxonomy to help to identify the priority research advances needed to strengthen and streamline current methodologies, and to consider approaches for their advancement and adoption?
- *Priorities.* What are the most compelling priorities for comparative effectiveness studies and how might providers and patients be engaged in helping to identify them and to set the stage for research strategies and funding partnerships?
- *Coordination.* Given the oft-stated need for stronger coordination in the identification, priority setting, design, and implementation of clinical effectiveness research, what might Roundtable members do to facilitate evolution of the capacity?
- *Clustering.* The NCI is exploring the clustering of clinical studies to make the process of study consideration and launching quicker and more efficient. Should this be explored as a model for others?
- *Registry collaboration.* Since registries offer the most immediate prospects for broader "real-time" learning, can Roundtable participants work with interested organizations on periodic convening

of those involved in maintaining clinical registries, exploring additional opportunities for combined efforts and shared learning?

- *Phased intervention with evaluation.* How can progress be accelerated in the adoption by public and private payers of approaches to allow phased implementation and reimbursement for promising interventions for which effectiveness and relative advantage has not been firmly established? What sort of neutral venue would work best for a multistakeholder effort through existing research networks (e.g., CTSAs, HMO Research Network [HMORNs])?

- *Patient preferences and perspectives.* What approaches might help to refine practical instruments to determine patient preferences— such as NIH's PROMIS (Patient-Reported Outcomes Measurement Information System)—and apply them as central elements of outcome measurement?

- *Public–private collaboration.* What administrative vehicles might enhance opportunities for academic medicine, industry, and government to engage cooperatively in clinical effectiveness research? Would development of common contract language be helpful in facilitating public–private partnerships?

- *Clinician engagement.* Should a venue be established for periodic convening of primary care and specialty physician groups to explore clinical effectiveness research priorities, progress in practice-based research, opportunities to engage in registry-related research, and improved approaches to clinical guideline development and application?

- *Academic health center engagement.* With academic institutions setting the pattern for the predominant approach to clinical research, drawing prevailing patterns closer to broader practice bases will require increasing the engagement with community-based facilities and private practices for practice-based research. How might Roundtable stakeholders partner with the Association of American Medical Colleges and Association of Academic Health Centers to foster the necessary changes?

- *Incentives for practice-based research.* Might an employer–payer working group from the Roundtable be useful in exploring economic incentives to accelerate progress in using clinical data for new insights by rewarding providers and related groups that are working to improve knowledge generation and application throughout the care process?

- *Condition-specific high-priority effectiveness research targets.* Might the Roundtable develop a working group to characterize the gap between current results and what should be expected, based on

current treatment knowledge, strategies for closing the gap, and collaborative approaches (e.g., registries) for the following conditions:
— Adult oncology
— Orthopedic procedures
— Management of co-occurring chronic diseases

Clinical Data

- *Secondary use of clinical data.* Successful use of clinical data as a reliable resource for clinical effectiveness evidence development requires the development of standards and approaches that assure the quality of the work. How might Roundtable members encourage or foster work of this sort?
- *Privacy and security.* What can be done within the existing structures and institutions to clarify definitions and to reduce the tendencies for unnecessarily restrictive interpretations on clinical data access, in particular related to secondary use of data?
- *Collaborative data mining.* Are there ways that Roundtable member initiatives might facilitate the progress of EHR data-mining networks working on strategies, statistical expertise, and training needs to improve and accelerate post-market surveillance and clinical research?
- *Research-related EHR standards.* How might EHR standard-setting groups be best engaged to ensure that standards developed are research-friendly, developed with the research utility in mind, and have the flexibility to adapt as research tools expand?
- *Transparency and access.* What vehicles, approaches, and stewardship structures might best improve the receptivity of the clinical data marketplace to enhanced data sharing, including making federally sponsored clinical data more widely available for secondary analysis (data from federally supported research, as well as Medicare-related data)?

Communication

- *Research results.* Since part of the challenge in public misunderstanding of research results is a product of "hyping" by the research community, how might the Roundtable productively explore the options for "self-regulatory guidelines" on announcing and working with media on research results?
- *Patient involvement in the evidence process.* If progress in patient outcomes depends on deeper citizen understanding and engagement as full participants in the learning healthcare system—both

as partners with caregivers in their own care, and as supporters of the use of protected clinical data to enhance learning—what steps can accelerate and enhance patient involvement?

As interested parties consider these issues, it is important to remember that the focus of the research discussed at the workshop is, ultimately, for and about the patient. The goals of the work are fundamentally oriented to bringing the right care to the right person at the right time at the right price. The fundamental questions to answer for any healthcare intervention are straightforward: Can it work? Will it work—for *this* patient, in *this* setting? Is it worth it? Do the benefits outweigh any harms? Do the benefits justify the costs? Do the possible changes offer important advantages over existing alternatives?

Finally, despite the custom of referring to "our healthcare system," the research community in practice functions as a diverse set of elements that often seem to connect productively only by happenstance. Because shortfalls in coordination and communication impinge on the funding, effectiveness, and efficiency of the clinical research process—not to mention its progress as a key element of the learning healthcare system—the notion of working productively together is vital for both patients and the healthcare community. Better coordination, collaboration, public–private partnerships, and priority setting are compelling priorities, and the attention and awareness generated in the course of this meeting are important to the Roundtable's focus on redesigning the clinical effectiveness research paradigm.

REFERENCES

AcademyHealth. 2005. Placement, coordination, and funding of health services research within the federal government. In *Academyhealth Report*. Washington, DC.
———. 2008. *Health Services Research (HSR) Methods*. [cited June 18, 2008]. http://www. hsrmethods.org/ (accessed June 21, 2010).
DeVoto, E., and B. S. Kramer. 2006. Evidence-based approach to oncology. In *Oncology: An Evidence-Based Approach*, edited by A. E. Chang, P. A. Ganz, D. F. Hayes, T. Kinsella, H. I. Pass, J. H. Schiller, R. M. Stone, and V. Strecher. New York: Springer.
Hartung, D. M., and D. Touchette. Overview of clinical research design. *American Journal of Health-System Pharmacy* 66:398-408.
Kravitz, R. L., N. Duan, and J. Braslow. 2004. Evidence-based medicine, heterogeneity of treatment effects, and the trouble with averages. *Milbank Quarterly* 82(4):661-687.
Liang, L. 2007 (March/April). The gap between evidence and practice. *Health Affairs* 26(2): w119-w121.
Lohr, K. N. 2007. Emerging methods in comparative effectiveness and safety: Symposium overview and summary. *Medical Care* 45(10):55-58.
Moses, H., 3rd, E. R. Dorsey, D. H. Matheson, and S. O. Thier. 2005. Financial anatomy of biomedical research. *Journal of the American Medical Association* 294(11):1333-1342.
Rush, A. J. 2008. Developing the evidence for evidence-based practice. *Canadian Medical Association Journal* 178:1313-1315.

Sackett, D. L., R. Brian Haynes, G. H. Guyatt, and P. Tugwell. 2006. Dealing with the media. *Journal of Clinical Epidemiology* 59(9):907-913.

Schneeweiss, S. 2007. Developments in post-marketing comparative effectiveness research. *Clinical Pharmacology and Therapeutics* 82(2):143-156.

1

Evidence Development for Healthcare Decisions: Improving Timeliness, Reliability, and Efficiency

INTRODUCTION

The rapid growth of medical research and technology development has vastly improved the health of Americans. Nonetheless, a significant knowledge gap affects their care, and it continues to expand: the gap in knowledge about what approaches work best, under what circumstances, and for whom. The dynamic nature of product innovation and the increased emphasis on treatments tailored to the individual—whether tailored for genetics, circumstances, or patient preferences—present significant challenges to our capability to develop clinical effectiveness information that helps health professionals provide the right care at the right time for each individual patient.

Developments in health information technology, study methods, and statistical analysis, and the development of research infrastructure offer opportunities to meet these challenges. Information systems are capturing much larger quantities of data at the point of care; new techniques are being tested and used to analyze these rich datasets and to develop insights on what works for whom; and research networks are being used to streamline clinical trials and conduct studies previously not feasible. An examination of how these innovations might be used to improve understanding of clinical effectiveness of healthcare interventions is central to the Roundtable on Value & Science-Driven Health Care's aim to help transform how evidence is developed and used to improve health and health care.

EBM AND CLINICAL EFFECTIVENESS RESEARCH

The Roundtable has defined evidence-based medicine (EBM) broadly to mean that, "to the greatest extent possible, the decisions that shape the health and health care of Americans—by patients, providers, payers, and policy makers alike—will be grounded on a reliable evidence base, will account appropriately for individual variation in patient needs, and will support the generation of new insights on clinical effectiveness." This definition embraces and emphasizes the dynamic nature of the evidence base and the research process, noting not only the importance of ensuring that clinical decisions are based on the best evidence for a given patient, but that the care experience be reliably captured to generate new evidence.

The need to find new approaches to accelerate the development of clinical evidence and to improve its applicability drove discussion at the Roundtable's workshop on December 12–13, 2007, Redesigning the Clinical Effectiveness Research Paradigm. The issues motivating the meeting's discussions are noted in Box 1-1, the first of which is the need for a deeper and broader evidence base for improved clinical decision making. But also important are the needs to improve the efficiency and applicability of the process. Underscoring the timeliness of the discussion is recognition of the challenges presented by the expense, time, and limited generalizability of current approaches, as well as of the opportunities presented by innovative research approaches and broader use of electronic health records that make clinical data more accessible. The overall goal of the meeting was to explore these issues, identify potential approaches, and discuss possible strategies

---

BOX 1-1
Issues Motivating the Discussion

- Need for substantially improved understanding of the comparative clinical effectiveness of healthcare interventions.
- Strengths of the randomized controlled trial muted by constraints in time, cost, and limited applicability.
- Opportunities presented by the size and expansion of potentially interoperable administrative and clinical datasets.
- Opportunities presented by innovative study designs and statistical tools.
- Need for innovative approaches leading to a more practical and reliable clinical research paradigm.
- Need to build a system in which clinical effectiveness research is a more natural by-product of the care process.

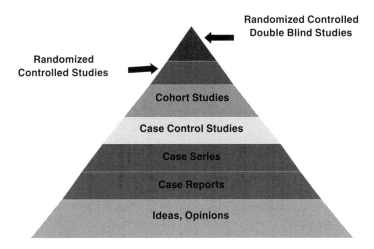

FIGURE 1-1 The classic evidence hierarchy.
SOURCE: DeVoto, E., and B. S. Kramer. 2005. Evidence-Based Approach to Oncology. In *Oncology an Evidence-Based Approach*. Edited by A. Chang. New York: Springer. Modified and reprinted with permission of Springer SBM.

for their engagement. Key contextual issues covered in the presentations and open workshop discussions are reviewed in this chapter.

Background: Current Research Context

Starting points for the workshop's discussion reside in the presentation of what has come to be viewed as the traditional clinical research model, depicted as a pyramid in Figure 1-1. In this model, the strongest level of evidence is displayed at the peak of the pyramid: the randomized controlled double blind study. This is often referred to as the "gold standard" of clinical research, and is followed, in a descending sequence of strength or quality, by randomized controlled studies, cohort studies, case control studies, case series, and case reports. The base of the pyramid, the weakest evidence, is reserved for undocumented experience, ideas and opinions. Noted at the workshop was the fact that, as currently practiced the randomized controlled and blinded trial is not the gold standard for every circumstance.

The development in recent years of a broad range of clinical research approaches, along with the identification of problems in generalizing research results to populations broader than those enrolled in tightly controlled trials, as well as the impressive advances in the potential availability of data through expanded use of electronic health records, have all prompted re-consideration of research strategies and opportunities (Kravitz, 2004; Schneeweiss, 2004; Liang, 2005; Lohr, 2007; Rush, 2008).

Table 1-1 provides brief descriptions of the many approaches to clinical effectiveness research discussed during the workshop—and these methods can be generally characterized as either experimental or non-experimental. Experimental studies are those in which the choice and assignment of the intervention is under control of the investigator; and the results of a test intervention are compared to the results of an alternative approach by actively monitoring the respective experience of either individuals or groups receiving the intervention or not. Non-experimental studies are those in which either manipulation or randomization is absent, the choice of an intervention is made in the course of clinical care, and existing data, that was collected in the course of the care process, is used to draw conclusions about the relative impact of different circumstances or interventions that vary between and among identified groups, or to construct mathematical models that seek to predict the likelihood of events in the future based on variables identified in previous studies. The data used to reach study conclusions, can be characterized as primary (generated during the conduct of the study); or secondary (originally generated for other purposes, e.g., administrative or claims data).

While not an exhaustive catalog of methods, Table 1-1 provides a sense of the range of clinical research approaches that can be used to improve understanding of clinical effectiveness. Noted at the workshop was the fact that each method has the potential to advance understanding on different aspects of the many questions that emerge throughout a product or intervention's lifecycle in clinical practice. The issue is therefore not one of whether internal or external validity should be the overarching priority for research, but rather which approach is most appropriate to the particular need. In each case, careful attention to design and execution studies are vital.

Bridging the Research–Practice Divide

A key theme of the meeting was that it is important to draw clinical research closer to practice. Without this capacity, the need to personalize clinical care will be limited. For example, information on possible heterogeneity of treatment effects in patient populations—due to individual genetics, circumstance, or co-morbidities—is rarely available in a form that is timely, readily accessible, and applicable. To address this issue, the assessment of a healthcare intervention must go beyond determinations of efficacy (whether an intervention can work under ideal circumstances) to an understanding of effectiveness (how an intervention works in practice), which compels grounding of the assessment effort in practice records. To understand effec-

TABLE 1-1 Selected Examples of Clinical Research Study Designs for Clinical Effectiveness Research

Approach	Description	Data types	Randomization
Randomized Controlled Trial (RCT)	Experimental design in which patients are randomly allocated to intervention groups (randomized) and analysis estimates the size of difference in predefined outcomes, under ideal treatment conditions, between intervention groups. RCTs are characterized by a focus on efficacy, internal validity, maximal compliance with the assigned regimen, and, typically, complete follow-up. When feasible and appropriate, trials are "double blind"—i.e., patients and trialists are unaware of treatment assignment throughout the study.	Primary, may include secondary	Required
Pragmatic Clinical Trial (PCT)	Experimental design that is a subset of RCTs because certain criteria are relaxed with the goal of improving the applicability of results for clinical or coverage decision making by accounting for broader patient populations or conditions of real-world clinical practice. For example, PCTs often have fewer patient inclusion/exclusion criteria, and longer term, patient-centered outcome measures.	Primary, may include secondary	Required
Delayed (or Single-Crossover) Design Trial	Experimental design in which a subset of study participants is randomized to receive the intervention at the start of the study and the remaining participants are randomized to receive the intervention after a pre-specified amount of time. By the conclusion of the trial, all participants receive the intervention. This design can be applied to conventional RCTs, cluster randomized and pragmatic designs.	Primary, may include secondary	Required

continued

TABLE 1-1 Continued

Approach	Description	Data types	Randomization
Adaptive Design	Experimental design in which the treatment allocation ratio of an RCT is altered based on collected data. Bayesian or Frequentist analyses are based on the accumulated treatment responses of prior participants and used to inform adaptive designs by assessing the probability or frequency, respectively, with which an event of interest occurs (e.g., positive response to a particular treatment).	Primary, some secondary	Required
Cluster Randomized Controlled Trial	Experimental design in which groups (e.g., individuals or patients from entire clinics, schools, or communities), instead of individuals, are randomized to a particular treatment or study arm. This design is useful for a wide array of effectiveness topics but may be required in situations in which individual randomization is not feasible.	Often secondary	Required
N of 1 trial	Experimental design in which an individual is repeatedly switched between two regimens. The sequence of treatment periods is typically determined randomly and there is formal assessment of treatment response. These are often done under double blind conditions and are used to determine if a particular regimen is superior for that individual. N of 1 trials of different individuals can be combined to estimate broader effectiveness of the intervention.	Primary	Required
Interrupted Time Series	Study design used to determine how a specific event affects outcomes of interest in a study population. This design can be experimental or non-experimental depending on whether the event was planned or not. Outcomes occurring during multiple periods before the event are compared to those occurring during multiple periods following the event.	Primary or secondary	Approach dependent

TABLE 1-1 Continued

Approach	Description	Data types	Randomization
Cohort Registry Study	Non-experimental approach in which data are prospectively collected on individuals and analyzed to identify trends within a population of interest. This approach is useful when randomization is infeasible. For example, if the disease is rare, or when researchers would like to observe the natural history of a disease or real world practice patterns.	Primary	No
Ecological Study	Non-experimental design in which the unit of observation is the population or community and that looks for associations between disease occurrence and exposure to known or suspected causes. Disease rates and exposures are measured in each of a series of populations and their relation is examined.	Primary or secondary	No
Natural Experiment	Non-experimental design that examines a naturally occurring difference between two or more populations of interest—i.e., instances in which the research design does not affect how patients are treated. Analyses may be retrospective (retrospective data analysis) or conducted on prospectively collected data. This approach is useful when RCTs are infeasible due to ethical concerns, costs, or the length of a trial will lead to results that are not informative.	Primary or Secondary	No
Simulation and Modeling	Non-experimental approach that uses existing data to predict the likelihood of outcome events in a specific group of individuals or over a longer time horizon than was observed in prior studies.	Secondary	No

continued

TABLE 1-1 Continued

Approach	Description	Data types	Randomization
Meta Analysis	The combination of data collected in multiple, independent research studies (that meet certain criteria) to determine the overall intervention effect. Meta analyses are useful to provide a quantitative estimate of overall effect size, and to assess the consistency of effect across the separate studies. Because this method relies on previous research, it is only useful if a broad set of studies are available.	Secondary	No

SOURCE: Adapted, with the assistance of Danielle Whicher of the Center for Medical Technology Policy and Richard Platt from Harvard Pilgrim Healthcare, from a white paper developed by Tunis, S. R., *Strategies to Improve Comparative Effectiveness Research Methods and Data Infrastructure*, for June 2009 Brookings workshop, *Implementing Comparative Effectiveness Research: Priorities, Methods, and Impact.*

tiveness, feedback is crucial on how well new products and interventions work in broad patient populations, including who those populations are and under what circumstances they are treated.

Redesigning the Clinical Effectiveness Research Paradigm

Growing opportunities for practice-based clinical research are presented by work to develop information systems and data repositories that enable greater learning from practice. Moreover, there is a need to develop a research approach that can address the questions that arise in the course of practice. As noted in Table 1-1, many research methods can be used to improve understanding of clinical effectiveness, but their use must be carefully tailored to the circumstances. For example, despite the increased external validity offered by observational approaches, the uncertainty inherent in such studies due to bias and confounding often undermine confidence in these approaches. Likewise, the limitations of the randomized controlled trial (RCT) often mute its considerable research value. Those limitations may be a sample size that is too small; a drug dose that is too low to fully assess the drug's safety; follow-up that is too short to show long-term benefits; underrepresentation or exclusion of vulnerable patient groups, including elderly patients with multiple co-morbidities, children, and young women; conduct of the trial in a highly controlled environment; and/or high cost and time investments. The issue is not one of RCTs versus non-experimental studies but one of which is most appropriate to the particular need.

Retrospective population-level cohorts using administrative data, clinical registries, and longitudinal prospective cohorts have, for example, been valuable in assessing effectiveness and useful in helping payers to make coverage decisions, assessing quality improvement opportunities, and providing more realistic assessments of interventions. Population-based registries—appropriately funded and constructed with clinician engagement—offer a compromise to the strengths and limitations of, for example, cohort studies, and can assess "real-world" health and economic outcomes to help guide decision making for patient care and policy setting. Furthermore, they are a valuable tool for assessing and driving improvements in the performance of physicians and institutions.

When trials, quasi-experimental studies, and even epidemiologic studies are not possible, researchers may also be able to use simulation methods, if current prototypes prove broadly applicable. Physiology-based models, for example, have the potential to augment knowledge gained from trials and can be used to fill in "gaps" that are difficult or impractical to answer using clinical trial methods. In particular, they will be increasingly useful to provide estimates of key biomarkers and clinical findings. When properly constructed, they replicate the results of the studies used to build them, not only at an outcome level but also at the level of change in biomarkers and clinical findings. Physiology-based modeling has been used to enhance and extend existing clinical trials, to validate RCT results, and to conduct virtual comparative effectiveness trials.

In part, this is a taxonomy and classification challenge. To strengthen these various methods, participants suggested work to define the "state of the art" for their design, conduct, reporting, and validation; improve the quality of data used; and identify strategies to take better advantage of the complementary nature of results obtained. As participants observed, these methods can enhance understanding of an intervention's value in many dimensions—exploring effects of variation (e.g., practice setting, providers, patients) and extending assessment to long-term outcomes related to benefits, rare events, or safety risks—collectively providing a more comprehensive assessment of the trade-offs between potential risks and benefits for individual patients.

It is also an infrastructure challenge. The efficiency, quality, and reliability of research requires infrastructure improvements that allow greater data linkage and collaboration by researchers. Research networks offer a unique opportunity to begin to build an integrated, learning healthcare system. As the research community hones its capacity to collect, store, and study data, enormous untapped capacity for data analysis is emerging. Thus, the mining of large databases has become the focus of considerable interest and enthusiasm in the research community. Researchers can approach such data using clinical epidemiologic methods—potentially using data collected over many years, on millions of patients, to generate insights on real-world intervention use and health outcomes. It was this potential that set the stage for the discussion.

PERSPECTIVES ON CLINICAL EFFECTIVENESS RESEARCH

Keynote addresses opened discussions during the 2-day workshop. Together the addresses and discussions provide a conceptual framework for many of the meeting's complex themes. IOM President Harvey V. Fineberg provides an insightful briefing on how clinical effectiveness research has evolved over the past 2.5 centuries and offers compelling questions for the workshop to consider. Urging participants to stay focused on better understanding patient needs and to keep the fundamental values of health care in perspective, Fineberg proposes a meta-experimental strategy, advocating for experiments with experiments to better understand their respective utilities, power, and applicability as well as some key elements of a system to support patient care and research. Carolyn M. Clancy, director of the Agency for Healthcare Research and Quality, offers a vision for 21st-century health care in which actionable information is available to clinicians and patients and evidence is continually refined as care is delivered. She provides a thoughtful overview of how emerging methods will expand the research arsenal and can address many key challenges in clinical effectiveness research. Emphasis is also given to the potential gains in quality and effectiveness of care, with greater focus on how to translate research findings into practice.

CLINICAL EFFECTIVENESS RESEARCH: PAST, PRESENT, AND FUTURE

Harvey V. Fineberg, M.D., Ph.D.
President, Institute of Medicine

An increasingly important focus of the clinical effectiveness research paradigm is the efficient development of relevant and reliable information on what works best for individual patients. A brief look at the past, present, and future of clinical effectiveness research establishes some informative touchstones on the development and evolution of the current research paradigm, as well as on how new approaches and directions might dramatically improve our ability to generate insights into what works in a clinical context.

Evolution of Clinical Effectiveness Research

Among the milestones in evidence-based medicine, one of the earliest examples of the use of comparison groups in a clinical experiment is laid out in a summary written in 1747 by James Lind detailing what works and what does not work in the treatment of scurvy. With 12 subjects, Lind tried to make a systematic comparison to discern what agents might be helpful to prevent and treat the disease. Through experimentation, he learned that the intervention that seemed to work best to help sailors recover most quickly from scurvy was the consumption of oranges, limes, and other citrus fruits. Many other interventions, including vinegar and sea water, were also tested, but only the citrus fruits demonstrated benefit. What is interesting about that experiment and relevant for our discussions of evidence-based medicine today is that it took the Royal Navy more than a century to adopt a policy to issue citrus to its sailors. When we talk about the delay between new knowledge and its application in practice in clinical medicine, we therefore have ample precedent, going back to the very beginning of systematic comparisons.

Another milestone comes in the middle of the 19th century, with the first systematic use of statistics in medicine. During the Crimean War (1853–1856), Florence Nightingale collected mortality statistics in hospitals and used those data to help discern where the problems were and what might be done to improve performance and outcomes. Nightingale's tables were the first systematic collection in a clinical setting of extensive data on outcomes in patients that were recorded and then used for the purpose of evaluation.

It was not until the early part of the 20th century that statistics in its modern form began to take hold. The 1920s and 1930s saw the development of statistical methods and accounting for the role of chance in scientific studies. R. A. Fisher (Fisher, 1953) is widely credited as one of the seminal figures in the development of statistical science. His classic work, *The Design of Experiments* (1935), focused on agricultural comparisons but articulated many of the critical principles in the design of controlled trials that are a hallmark of current clinical trials. It would not be until after World War II, that the first clinical trial on a medical intervention would be recorded. A 1948 study by Bradford Hill on the use of streptomycin in the treatment of tuberculosis was the original randomized controlled trial. Interestingly, the contemporary use of penicillin to treat pneumonia was never subjected to similar, rigorous testing—perhaps owing to the therapy's dramatic benefit to patients.

Over the ensuing decades, trials began to appear in the literature with increased frequency. Along the way they also became codified and almost deified as the standard for care. In 1962, after the thalidomide scandals, efficacy was introduced as a requirement for new drug applications in the Kefauver amendments to the Federal Food, Drug, and Cosmetic Act. But it was not until the early 1970s, that a decision of the Sixth Circuit Court certified RCTs as the standard of the Food and Drug Administration (FDA) in its judgments about efficacy. Subsequently, organizations like the Cochrane Collaboration have developed ways of integrating RCT information with data from other types of methods and from multiple sources, codifying and putting these results forward for use in clinical decision making.

The classic evidence hierarchy that starts at the bottom with somebody's opinion—one might call that "eminence-based medicine"—and rises through different methodologies to the pinnacle, randomized controlled double blind trials. If double masked trials were universal, if they were easy, if they were inexpensive, and if their results were applicable to all patient groups, we probably would not have a need for discussion on redesigning the clinical effectiveness paradigm. Unfortunately, despite the huge number of randomized trials being conducted a number of needs are not being met by the current "randomized trial only" strategy.

Effectiveness Research to Inform Clinical Decision Making

Archie Cochrane, the inspiration for the Cochrane Collaboration, posed three deceptively simple yet critical questions for assessing clinical evidence. First, Can it work? Implied in this question is an assumption of ideal conditions. More recently, the Office of Technology Assessment popularized the terms efficacy and effectiveness to distinguish between the effects of an intervention in ideal and real-world conditions, respectively. The question "Can it work?" is a question of an intervention's efficacy. Cochrane's second question, "Will it work?," is one of effectiveness. That is, how and for whom does an intervention work in practice—under usual circumstances, deployed in the field, and utilized under actual clinical care conditions with real patients and providers.

The third of Cochrane's questions asks, "Is it worth it?" This can not only be applied to the balance of safety, benefit, and risk to an individual patient, but also can be applied to the society as a whole, for which the balance of costs and effectiveness also come into play. This final question introduces important considerations with respect to assessing different approaches and strategies in clinical effectiveness—the purpose of and vantage point from which these questions are being asked. Because of the significant range and number of perspectives involved in healthcare decision making, addressing these issues introduces many additional questions to consider upstream of those posed by Cochrane.

When assessing the vast array of strategies and approaches to evaluation, these prior questions are particularly helpful to put into perspective the roles and contributions of each. Many dimensions of health care deserve to be considered in evaluation, particularly if we start with the idea of prevention and the predictive elements prior to an actual clinical experience. The scope of an evaluation might be at the level of the intervention (e.g., diagnostic, therapeutic, rehabilitative, etc.), the clinician (specialty, training, profession, etc.) or organization of service, institutional performance, and the patient's role. Thinking critically about what is being evaluated and mapping what is appropriate, effective, and efficient, for the various types of questions, is an ongoing and important challenge in clinical effectiveness research.

Certain clinical questions drive very different design challenges. Evaluation of a diagnostic intervention, for example, involves the consideration of a panoply of factors: The performance of the diagnostic technology in terms of the usual measures of sensitivity and specificity, and the way in which one can reach judgments, make trade-offs, and deal with both false-positive and false-negative results. One also has to be thinking of the whole cascade of events, through clinical intervention and outcomes that may follow. For example, thought should be given to whether results enhance subsequent decisions for therapy, or whether the focus is on patient reassurance or other measurable outcomes, and how these decisions might affect judgments or influence the ultimate outcome of the patient. Considerations such as these are important for evaluating an intervention but are very different from those aimed at assessing system performance (e.g., clinician and health professionals' performance, organizational approaches to service). These differences apply not only to methodologies and strategies but also to information needs. The same kinds of data used to evaluate a targeted, individual, time-specified intervention are not the same as those needed if the goal is to compare various strategies of organization or different classes of providers.

A related set of considerations revolves around this question: For whom—or for what patient group, are we attempting to make an evaluation? The limitations of randomized controlled trials, in terms of external validity, often reduce the relevance of findings for clinical decisions faced by physicians for their patients. For example, the attributes of real-world patients may differ significantly from that of the trial population (e.g., age, sex, other diagnoses, risk factors), with implications for the appropriateness of a given therapy for patients. Early consideration of "for whom" will help to identify those specific methods that can produce needed determinations, or add value by complementing information from clinical trials.

Finally, we must also consider point of view: For any given purpose, from whose point of view are we attempting to carry out this evaluation? For example, is the purpose motivated by one's interest in a clinical benefit, safety, cost, acceptability, convenience, implementability, or some other factor? Is it representing the patient or the pool of patients, the payers of the services, the clinicians who provide the services, the manufacturers? Does the motivation come from a regulatory need for decisions about permissions or restrictions, and if so, under what circumstances? These perspectives all extend differences to what kind of method will be suitable for what kind of question in what kind of circumstance. The questions of what it is we are evaluating, for whom, and with whose perspective and purpose in mind are decidedly nontrivial, and in fact they can be important guides as we reflect on the strengths and weaknesses of a variety of approaches and formulate better approaches to clinical effectiveness research.

Several key challenges drive the need for better methods and strategies for developing clinical effectiveness information. First, it is evident to anyone who has spent an hour in a clinic or has attempted to keep up-to-date with current medical practices that the amount of information that may be relevant to a particular patient and the number of potential interventions and technologies can be simply overwhelming. In fact, it is estimated that the number of published clinical trials now exceeds 10,000 per year. A conscientious clinician trying to stay current with RCTs could read three scientific papers a day and at the end of a year would be approximately 2 years behind in reading. This constant flow of information is one side of a central paradox in heath care today: Despite the overwhelming abundance of information available, there is an acute shortage of information that is relevant, timely, appropriate, and useful to clinical decision making. This is true for caregivers, payers, regulators, providers, and patients. Reconciling those two seemingly differently vectored phenomena is one of the leading challenges today.

Additional barriers and issues include contending with the dizzying array of new and complex technologies, the high cost of trials as a primary means of information acquisition, as well as a complex matrix of ethical, legal, practical, and economic issues associated with fast-moving developments in genetic information and the rise of personalized medicine. These issues are compounded by the seemingly increased divergence of purpose between manufacturers, regulators, payers, clinicians, and patients. Finally, there is the challenge to improve how knowledge is applied in practice. In part this is related to the culture of medicine, the demands of practice, and information overload, but improvements to the system and incentives will be of critical importance moving forward.

Innovative Strategies and Approaches

Fortunately, researchers are developing many innovative strategies in response to these challenges. Some of these build on, some displace, and some complement the traditional array of strategies in the classic evidence hierarchy. Across the research community, for example, investigators are developing improved data sources—larger and potentially interoperable clinical and administrative databases, clinical registries, and electronic health records and other systems that capture relevant data at the point of care (sometimes called "the point of service"). We are seeing also the evolution of new statistical tools and techniques, such as adaptive designs, simulation and modeling, large database analyses, and data mining. Some of these are adaptations of tools used in other areas; others are truly novel and driven by the peculiar requirements of the human clinical trial. The papers that follow offer insights on adaptive designs, simulation and modeling approaches, and the various analytic approaches that can take adequate account of very large databases.

In particular, discerning meaningfully relevant information in the health context begs for closer attention, and strategies for innovative approaches to data mining are emerging—strategies analogous, if you will, to the way that Internet search engines apply some order to the vast disarray of undifferentiated information spread across the terabyte-laden database of the World Wide Web.

We are also seeing the development of innovative trial and study methodologies that aim to compensate for some of the weaknesses of clinical trials with respect to external validity. Such methods also hold promise for addressing some of the cost-related and logistical challenges in the classic formulation of trials. New approaches to accommodate physiologic and genetic information speak to the emergence of personalized medicine. At the same time, there are emerging networks of research that can amplify and accelerate, in efficiency and time, the gathering and accumulation of relevant information and a variety of models that mix and match these strategies.

Regardless of the approaches taken and the variety of perspectives considered, we must ultimately return to confront the critically central question of clinical care for the individual patient in need, at a moment in time, and determine what works best for this patient. In this regard, we might ideally move toward a system that would combine a point-of-care focus with an electronic record data system that is coupled with systems for assembling evidence in a variety of ways. Such a system would accomplish a quadrafecta, if you will—a four-part achievement of goals important to improving the system as a whole. Component goals would include enabling the *evaluation and learning* of what works and what does not work for individual patients that includes weighing benefits and costs; providing *decision support* for the specific patient in front of a clinician—identifying relevant pieces of evidence in the available information, while also contributing to the pool of potentially useable information for future patients; providing *meaningful continuing education* for health professionals—moving beyond the traditional lecture approach to one that enables learning in place, occurs in real-time, and is practical and applied in the course of clinical care; and finally, collectively providing a foundation for *quality improvement systems*. If we can achieve this kind of integration—point of service, patient-centered understanding, robust data systems on the clinical side, coupled with relevant analytic elements—we can, potentially, simultaneously, advance on the four critical goals of evaluation, decision support, continuing education, and quality improvement.

As we move in this direction, it is worth considering whether the ultimate goal is to understand what works and what doesn't work in an "N of 1." After all, this reflects the ultimate in individualized care. Granted, for those steeped in thinking about probability, Bayesian analysis, and decision theory, this seems a rather extreme notion. But if we consider for a moment that probability is an expression of uncertainty and ignorance, a key consideration becomes: What parts of uncertainty in health care are reducible?

Consider the classic example of the coin toss—flip a coin, the likelihood of it landing heads or tails is approximately 50/50. In such an experiment, what forces are constant and what forces are variable in determining what happens to that coin? Gravity, obviously, is a fairly reliable constant, and the coin's size, weight, and balance can be standardized. What varies is the exact place where the coin is tossed, the exact height of the toss, the exact force with which the coin is flipped, the exact surface on which it falls, and the force that the impact imparts to the coin. Imagine, therefore, that instead of just taking a coin out of a pocket, flipping it, and letting it fall on the floor, we instead had a vacuum chamber that was precisely a given height, with a perfectly absorptive surface, and that the coin was placed in a special lever in the vacuum chamber with a special device to flip it with exactly the same force in exactly the same location every time it strikes that perfectly balanced coin. Instead of falling 50/50 heads or tails, how the coin falls will be determined almost entirely by how it is placed in the vacuum chamber and tossed by the lever.

If we apply that analogy to individual patients, the expression of uncertainty about what happens to patients and groupings of patients should be resolvable to the individual attribute at the genetic, physiologic, functional, and historical level. If resolution to the level of individual patients is not possible, an appropriate objective might be to understand an intervention's impact in increasingly refined subgroups of patients. In point of fact, we are already seeing signs of such movement, for example, in the form of different predictive ability for patients who have particular genetic endowments.

As we consider the array of methods and develop strategies for their use in clinical effectiveness research, a guiding notion might be "a meta-experimental strategy" that aids the determination of which new methods and approaches to learning what works, and for what specific purposes, enables the assessment of several strategies, separately and in concert, and develops information on how the various methods and strategies can be deployed successfully. In other words, rather than focusing on how well a particular strategy evaluates a particular kind of problem, in a particular class of patient, from this particular point of view, with these particular endpoints in mind, we might ask what is the array of experimental methods that collectively perform in a manner that enables us to make better decisions for the individual and better decisions for society. What is the experiment of experiments? And how could we structure our future learning opportunity so that as we are learning what works for a particular kind of patient, we are also learning the way in which that strategy of evaluation can be employed to achieve a health system that is driven by evidence and based on value.

THE PATH TO RESEARCH THAT MEETS EVIDENCE NEEDS

Carolyn M. Clancy, M.D.
Agency for Healthcare Research and Quality

All of us share a common passion for developing better evidence so we can improve health care, improve the value of health care, and provide clinicians, patients, and other relevant parties with better information to make health decisions. In that context, this paper explores a central question: How can our approach to clinical effectiveness research take better advantage of emerging tools and study designs to address such challenges as generalizability, heterogeneity of treatment effects, multiple co-morbidities, and translating evidence into practice? This paper focuses on emerging methods in effectiveness research and approaches to turning evidence into action and concludes with some thoughts about health care in the 21st century.

Emerging Methods in Effectiveness Research

Early in the development of evidence-based medicine, discussions of methods were rarely linked to translating evidence into everyday clinical practice. Today, however, that principle is front and center, in part because of the urgency that so many of us feel about bringing evidence more squarely into healthcare delivery. Evidence is a tool for making better decisions, and health care is a process of ongoing decision making. The National Business Group on Health recently issued a survey suggesting that a growing number of consumers—primarily people on the healthier end of the spectrum, but also including some 11 percent of individuals with a chronic illness—say that they turn to sources other than their doctors for information. Some, for example, are even going to YouTube—not yet an outlet for our work, but who knows what the future might bring? If there is a lesson there, it is that evidence that we are developing has to be valid, broadly available, and relevant.

Traditional Hierarchies of Evidence: Randomized Controlled Trials

Traditional hierarchies of evidence have by definition placed the randomized controlled trial (RCT) at the top of the pyramid of evidence, regardless of the skill and precision with which an RCT is conducted. Such hierarchies, however, are inadequate for the variety of today's decisions in health care and are increasingly being challenged. RCTs obviously remain a very strong tool in our research armamentarium. Yet, we need a much more rigorous look at their appropriate role—as well as more scrutiny of the role of nonrandomized or quasi-experimental evidence. As we talk about the production of better evidence, we must keep the demand side squarely in our sights. Clearly a path to the future lies ultimately in the production of evidence that can be readily embedded in the delivery of care itself—a "Learning Healthcare Organization"—a Holy Grail that is not yet a reality.

The ultimate questions are fairly straightforward for a particular intervention, product, tool, or test: Can it work? Will it work—for this patient, in this setting? Is it worth it? Do the benefits outweigh any harms? Do the benefits justify the costs? Does it offer important advantages over existing alternatives? The last question in particular can be deceptively tricky. In some respects, the discussion is really a discussion of value. Given the increases in health expenditures over the past few years alone, the issue of value cannot be dismissed.

Clinicians know, of course, that clearly what is right for one person does not necessarily work for the next person. The balance of benefits versus harms is influenced by baseline risk, patient preferences, and a variety of other factors. The reality of medicine today is that for many treatment decisions, two or more options are available. What is not so clear is determining with the patient what the right choice is, in a given case, for that particular person. (As an aside, we probably do not give individual patients as much support as we should when they choose to take a path that differs from what we recommend.)

Even the most rigorously designed randomized trial has limitations, as we are all acutely aware. Knowing that an intervention can work is necessary but not sufficient for making a treatment decision for an individual patient or to promote it for a broad population. Additional types of research can clearly shed light on such critical questions as who is most likely to benefit from a treatment and what the important trade-offs are.

Nonrandomized Studies: An Important Complement to RCTs

Nonrandomized studies will never entirely supplant the need for rigorously conducted trials, but they can be a very important complement to RCTs. They can help us examine whether trial results are replicable in community settings; explore sources of differences in safety or effectiveness arising from variation among patients, clinicians, and settings; and produce a more complete picture of the potential benefits and harms of a clinical decision for individual patients or health systems. In short, nonrandomized studies can enrich our understanding of how patient treatments in practice differ from those in trials. A good case in point are two studies published in the 1980s by the Lipid Research Clinics showing that treatment to lower cholesterol can reduce the risk of coronary heart disease in middle-aged men (The Lipid Research Clinics Coronary Primary Prevention Trial Results. I. Reduction in Incidence of Coronary Heart Disease, 1984; The Lipid Research Clinics Coronary Primary Prevention Trial Results. II. The Relationship of Reduction in Incidence of Coronary Heart Disease to Cholesterol Lowering, 1984).

The researchers gave us an invaluable look at middle-aged, mostly white men who had one risk factor for coronary artery disease and were stunningly compliant with very unpleasant medicines, such as cholestyramine. The field had never had such specific data before, and, although the study was informative, patients rarely reflect the study population, at least in my experience as most come with additional risk factors and infrequently adhere to unpleasant medicines.

My colleague David Atkins recently alluded to an important nuance of RCTs that bears mention here. He observed that "trials often provide the strong strands that create the central structure, but the strength of the completed web relies on a variety of supporting cross strands made up of evidence from a more diverse array of studies"(Atkins, 2007). In other words, if clinical trials are the main strands in a web of evidence, it is important to remember that they are not the entire web.

For example, recent Agency for Healthcare Research and Quality (AHRQ) reports that have relied exclusively on nonrandomized evidence include one on total knee replacement and one on the value of islet cell transplantation. The latter study found that 50–90 percent of those who had the procedure achieved insulin independence, but it raised questions about the *duration* of effect. Another study on bariatric surgery found the surgery resulted in a 20–30 kilogram weight loss, versus a 2–3 kilogram loss via medicine, but raised questions about safety. Available nonrandomized studies are adequate to demonstrate "it can work," but may not be able to answer the question, "Is it worth it?"

Nonrandomized studies complement clinical trials in several ways.

Because most trials are fairly expensive, requiring development and implementation of a fairly elaborate infrastructure, their duration is more likely to be short term rather than long term. One finding from the initial *Evidence Report on Treatment of Depression—New Pharmacotherapies*, which compared older with newer antidepressants, was that at that time the vast majority of studies followed patients for no longer than 3 months (Agency for Healthcare Policy and Research, 2008d). This situation has changed since then thanks to investments made by the National Institute of Mental Health.

Nonrandomized trials also help researchers to pursue the similarities and differences between the trial population and the typical target population, and between trial intervention and typical interventions. Nonrandomized trials enable researchers to examine the heterogeneity of treatment effects in a patient population that in some ways or for some components may not look very much like the trial population. This, in turn, may create a capacity to modify the recommendations as they are implemented. Finally, nonrandomized trials enable researchers to study harm and safety issues in less selective patient populations and subgroups.

One example is the National Emphysema Treatment Trial, the first multicenter clinical trial designed to determine the role, safety, and effectiveness of bilateral lung volume reduction surgery (LVRS) in the treatment of emphysema. An AHRQ technology assessment of LVRS concluded that the data on the risks and benefits of LVRS were too inconclusive to justify unrestricted Medicare reimbursement for the surgery. However, the study also found that some patients benefited from the procedure. This prompted the recommendation that a trial evaluating the effectiveness of the surgery be conducted. The National Emphysema Treatment Trial followed to evaluate the safety and effectiveness of the best available medical treatment alone and in conjunction with LVRS. A number of interesting occurrences transpired within this study. First, people were not randomized to medicine versus surgery—all patients went through a course of maximum medical therapy or state-of-the-art pulmonary rehabilitation, after which they were randomized to continue rehab or to be enrolled in the surgical part of the trial.

With many patients, this was their first experience with very aggressive pulmonary rehab. Because many felt very good after the rehab, at the end of the first course of treatment many patients pulled out of the study. That extended the time it took for study enrollment. Thereafter, some of the study's basic findings were unexpected. Two or 3 years into the study, a paper in the *New England Journal of Medicine* effectively identified a high-risk subgroup whose mortality was higher after surgery. The talk of increased mortality further impeded study enrollment rates, which of course further delayed the results. Today, the number of LVRS procedures is very low. The reason for the decline is an open question—perhaps it is a matter of patients' perspectives or perhaps the trial took so long that one could argue that it was almost anti-innovation. Regardless, the example illustrates both that trials can take a long time and that they may not provide the magic bullet for making specific decisions.

The Challenge of Heterogeneity of Treatment Effects

In terms of the approval of products, clinical trials may not always represent the relevant patient population, setting, intervention, or comparison. Efficacy trials may exaggerate typical benefits, minimize typical harms, or overestimate net benefits. Clearly, external validity becomes a problem or a challenge, and that dilemma has been the subject of many lively debates. As noted by Nicholas Longford, "clinical trials are good experiments but poor surveys." In a paper a few years ago in the *Milbank Quarterly*, Richard Kravitz and colleagues suggested that the distribution of specific aspects and treatment effects in any particular trial for approval could result in a very different sense of the expected treatment effect in broader populations (Kravitz et al., 2004).

Discussing the difficulties of applying global evidence to individual patients or groups that might depart from the population average, the paper argues that clinical trials "can be misleading and fail to reveal the potentially complex mixture of substantial benefits for some, little benefit for many, and harm for a few. Heterogeneity of treatment effects reflects patient diversity in risk of disease, responsiveness to treatment, vulnerability to adverse effects, and utility for different outcomes." By recognizing these factors, the paper suggests, researchers can design studies that better characterize who will benefit from medical treatments, and clinicians and policy makers can make better use of the results.

A relevant area of study that has received a great deal of attention in this regard has been the use of carotid artery surgery and endarterectomy. Figure 1-2 shows 30-day mortality in older patients who had undergone an endarterectomy. The vertical values show what happened for Medicare patients in trial hospitals as well as hospitals with high, low, and medium patient volume. The lower horizontal line shows, by contrast, mortality in the Asymptomatic Carotid Artery Surgery (ACAS) trial; the line above it represents mortality in the North American Symptomatic Carotid Endarterectomy Trial (NASCET). Clearly, generalizing the results observed in the trials to the community would have been mistaken in terms of mortality rates.

The limitations of approval trials for individual decision making are well known, such as the previously mentioned LRC trial. In point of fact, a trial may represent neither the specific setting and intervention nor the individual patient. Issues of applicability and external validity really come

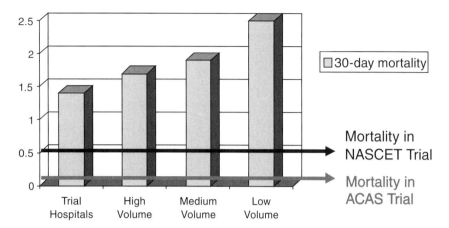

FIGURE 1-2 Thirty-day mortality in older patients undergoing endarterectomy (versus trials and by annual volume).
SOURCE: Derived from McGrath et al., 2000.

into focus, because essentially what we are reporting from trials is the average effect, and for an individual that may or may not be specifically relevant. In addition, of course, the heterogeneity of treatment effects seen in a trial becomes very important. One can come to very different conclusions depending on the distribution of the net treatment benefit and how narrow that distribution is (see Figure 1-3, for example), and yet we don't often know that with the first trial that has been done for approval.

An ongoing challenge and debate is the extent to which we can count on subgroup analysis to gain a more complete picture and information that is more relevant to a heterogeneous treatment population. In terms of such analyses, we need to be cautious in individual trials. Subgroup analyses are not reported regularly enough for individual patient meta-analyses. Moreover, we need to look beyond RCTs to inform judgments about the applicability and heterogeneity of treatment effects. Several years ago, AHRQ was asked to produce a systematic review of what was known about the effectiveness of diagnosis and treatment for women with coronary artery disease. A critical body of evidence existed, because it was a requirement of federal trials that women and minorities be enrolled in all clinical studies. We found, however, that it was extremely difficult to combine results across those studies, which underscores how difficult it is to combine data across trials as a basis for meta-analysis or any other quantitative technique.

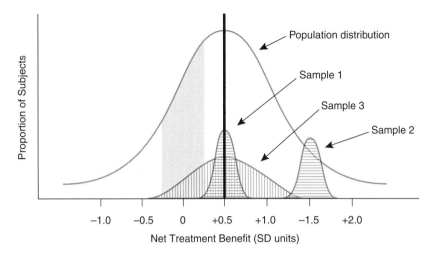

FIGURE 1-3 Treatment benefit distribution of different sample population subgroups for a clinical trial.
NOTE: Reprinted, with permission, from John Wiley & Sons, Inc., 2008.
SOURCE: Kravitz et al., 2004.

Practical Clinical Trials: Embedding Research into Care Delivery

Another interesting set of considerations revolves around the differences between practical (or pragmatic) clinical trials (PCTs) versus explanatory clinical trials and how PCTs might move the field closer to the notion of embedding research into care delivery and contending directly with issues confronting clinicians. In PCTs, hypotheses and study design are formulated based on information needed to make a clinical decision; explanatory trials are designed to better understand how and why an intervention works. Also, while practical trials address risks, benefits, and costs of an intervention as they would occur in routine clinical practice, explanatory trials maximize the chance that the biological effect of a new treatment will be revealed by the study (Tunis et al., 2003).

Another example comes from a systematic review of treatments for allergic rhinitis and sinusitis. For patients with either diagnosis there is a considerable body of information. The real challenge, though, is that in primary care settings most patients are not really interested in the kinds of procedures that one needs to make a definitive diagnosis. Thus, clinicians and patients typically do not have a lot of practical information to work with, even with data from the systematic study reviews. Practical clinical trials would address risks, benefits, and causes of interventions as they occur in routine clinical practice rather than trying to determine whether, for example, a particular mechanism actually provides a definitive diagnosis. Comparisons of practical versus explanatory trials date back to the 1960s, perhaps not surprisingly, in the context of the value of various types of psychotherapy. Since then, however, the literature seems to have gone silent on such issues. It would be a useful activity to revisit these questions and actually develop an inventory of what we know about practical clinical trials and how difficult they can be.

Different study designs contribute different effects. Looking at the variety of study designs, we can move down a continuum from efficacy trials, the least biased estimate of effect under ideal conditions, where we have maximum internal validity; to effectiveness trials, which provide a more representative estimate of the benefits and harms in the real world and presumably have increased external validity; to systematic review of trials that have used the same end-points, outcomes meta-analysis, or other quantitative techniques. The latter types of trials provide the best estimate of overall effect, investigate questions of heterogeneity of treatment effect, and explore uncommon outcomes.

Collaborative Registries

We can also use cohort studies registries, which use risk prediction to target treatment and are effective in reaching underrepresented populations, and case control studies, which can be particularly helpful in detecting relatively rare harms or adverse events that were not known or not expected. There is a substantial, growing interest among a number of physician specialties in creating registries. Registries provide a way to explore longer term outcomes, adverse effects, and practice variations, and they provide an avenue for the investigation of the heterogeneity of a treatment effect. The Society for Thoracic Surgeons is probably the best (and most familiar) model, but other surgical societies also are currently developing registries of their own. It will be a very interesting challenge to determine how, when, and where registries fit into the overall context of study designs, and how information from registries fits within the broader web of evidence-based medicine. AHRQ is using patient registry data as one approach to turning evidence into action, which is discussed in the next section.

Indeed, in the world of evidence-based medicine, two of the key challenges are the translation of evidence into everyday clinical practice, and how to manage situations when existing evidence is insufficient. Virtually every day, AHRQ receives telephone calls that focus on the fact that lack of evidence of effect is not the same thing as saying that a treatment is ineffective. Similarly, what is equivalent for the group is not necessarily equivalent for the individual. Measuring and weighing outcomes such as quality of life and convenience is obviously not a feature of most standardized clinical trials. Moreover, in considerations of such issues, we need to keep in mind the downstream effects of policy applications, such as diffusion of technology, effects on innovation, and unintended consequences. For example, one of the reasons that RCTs are such a poor fit for evaluating devices or any evolving technology is that the devices change all the time. One of the challenges that AHRQ hears regularly is that we invested all of this money and it took years to complete this trial, and we answered a question that is no longer relevant.

Observational Studies

This leads to the question of whether observational studies can reduce the need for randomized trials. Clearly observational studies are a preferred alternative when clinical trials are impractical, not possible, or unethical (we seem to debate that question a lot even though we are not particularly clear about what it means). Last year, a paper defended the value of observational studies. The authors asserted that observational studies can be a very useful tool when one examines something with a stable or predictable background course that is associated with a large, consistent, temporal effect, with rate ratios over 10, and where one can demonstrate dose response, specific effects, and biological plausibility (Glasziou et al., 2007). Observational studies are also of value when the potential for bias is low.

The advantages of observational studies are worth considering. First, most clinical trials are not sufficiently powered to detect adverse drug effects. AHRQ felt the effect of this design weakness when a report it sponsored on the benefits and harms of a variety of antidepressants was published. The report concluded that there was insufficient useful information to say anything definitive about the comparative risk profiles of newer and older antidepressants. The fact that the report had nothing to say about side effects drew a flood of protests from passionate constituents. Among other drawbacks, clinical trials clearly are limited by poor external validity in many situations; they may not be generalized to many subgroups that are of great interest to clinicians. On the other hand, longer term follow-up, not the rule for clinical trials, can be a strong advantage of observational studies. Moreover, observational studies clearly facilitate risk management and risk minimization and may indeed facilitate translation of evidence into practice. There are those who argue that all clinical trials should have an observational component, and in fact the field is starting to see some of that in trials. Comparing surgery to medical treatments for low back pain, for example, the Spine Patient Outcomes Research Trial (SPORT) randomized people if their preferences were neutral. Both patients and clinicians had to be neutral about the value of medicine versus surgery, and those people who were not neutral were followed in a registry.

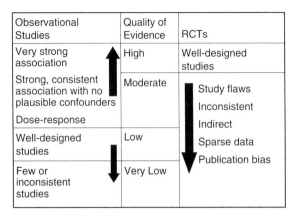

Observational Studies	Quality of Evidence	RCTs
Very strong association	High	Well-designed studies
Strong, consistent association with no plausible confounders	Moderate	Study flaws
Dose-response		Inconsistent
		Indirect
Well-designed studies	Low	Sparse data
		Publication bias
Few or inconsistent studies	Very Low	

FIGURE 1-4 Evidence levels—Grades of Recommendation, Assessment, Development and Evaluation (GRADE).

Grading Evidence and Recommendations

A notable and exciting development is the GRADE (Grades of Recommendation, Assessment, Development and Evaluation) collaborative, whose goal is to promote a more consistent and transparent approach to grading evidence and recommendations.[1] This approach considers that how well a study is done is at least as important as the type of study it is. GRADE evidence levels, as summarized in Figure 1-4, suggest that randomized trials that are flawed in their execution should not be at the top of the pyramid in any hierarchy of evidence. Similarly, observational studies that meet the criteria shown in the figure (and perhaps others as well), and which are done very well, might in some instances be considered better evidence than a randomized trial, if a randomized trial is poorly done. These standards are being adopted by the American Colleges of Physicians, American College of Chest Physicians, National Institute for Clinical Excellence, and World Health Organization, among others.

All of us imagine a near-term future where there is going to be much greater access to high-quality data. However, in order to take full advantage of that, we need to continue to advance work in improving methodological research. Why is this necessary? We need more comprehensive data to guide Medicare coverage decisions and to understand the wider range of outcomes. We need to address the gap when data from results of well-designed RCTs are either not available or incomplete. Finally, there are significant

---

[1] See www.gradeworkinggroup.org.

quality, eligibility, and cost implications of coverage decisions (e.g., consider implantable cardioverter defibrillators).

To help advance the agenda for improving methodology, a series of 23 articles on emerging methods in comparative effectiveness and safety were published in October 2007 in a special supplement to the journal *Medical Care*. These papers are a valuable new resource for scientists who are committed to advancing the comparative effectiveness and safety research, and this is an area in which AHRQ intends to continue to push.[2]

Approaches to Turning Evidence Into Action

The Agency for Healthcare Research and Quality has several programs directed at turning evidence into action. AHRQ's program on comparative effectiveness was authorized by Congress as part of the Medicare Modernization Act and funded through an appropriation starting in 2005. This Effective Health Care Program (EHCP) is essentially trying to produce evidence for a variety of audiences, based on unbiased information, so that people can make head-to-head comparisons as they endeavor to understand which interventions add value, which offer minimal benefit above current choices, which fail to reached their potential, and which work for some patients but not for others. The overarching goal is to develop and disseminate better evidence about benefits and risks of alternative treatments, which is also important for policy discussions. The statute is silent on cost effectiveness, although it does say that the Medicare program may not use the information to deny coverage. Less clear is whether prescription drug plans can use EHCP information in such a way; again, the statute is silent.

The AHRQ EHCP has three core components. One is synthesizing existing evidence through Evidence-Based Practice Centers (EPCs), which AHRQ has supported since 1997. The purpose is to systematically review, synthesize, and compare existing evidence on treatment effectiveness, and to identify relevant knowledge gaps. (Anyone who has ever conducted a systematic or even casual review knows that if you are searching through a pile of studies, inevitably you will have unanswered questions—questions that are related to but not quite the main focus of the particular search that you are doing.)

The second component is to generate evidence—to develop new scientific knowledge to address knowledge gaps—and to accelerate practical studies. To address critical unanswered questions or to close particular

---

[2] All of the articles are available for free download at the website www.effectivehealthcare. ahrq.gov/reports/med-care-report.cfm or can be ordered as Pub. No. OM07-0085 from AHRQ's clearinghouse.

research gaps, AHRQ relies on the DEcIDE (Developing Evidence to Inform Decisions about Effectiveness) network, a group of research partners who work under task-order contracts and who have access to large electronic clinical databases of patient information. The Centers for Education & Research on Therapeutics (CERTs) is a peer-reviewed program that conducts state-of-the-art research to increase awareness of new uses of drugs, biological products, and devices; to improve the effective use of drugs, biological products, and devices; to identify risks of new uses; and to identify risks of combinations of drugs and biological products.

Finally, AHRQ also works to advance the communication of evidence and its translation into care improvements. Many researchers will recall that our colleague John Eisenberg always talked about telling the story of health services research. Named in his honor, the John M. Eisenberg Clinical Decisions and Communications Science Center, based at Oregon Health Sciences University, is devoted to developing tools to help consumers, clinicians, and policy makers make decisions about health care. The Eisenberg Center translates knowledge about effective health care into summaries that use plain, easy-to-understand, and actionable language, which can be used to assess treatments, medications, and technologies. The guides are designed to help people to use scientific information to maximize the benefits of health care, minimize harm, and optimize the use of healthcare resources. Center activities also focus on decision support and other approaches to getting information to the point of care for clinicians, as well as on making information relevant and useful to patients and consumers.

The Eisenberg Center is developing two new translational guides, the *Guide to Comparative Effectiveness Reviews* and *Effectiveness and Off-Label Use of Recombinant Factor VIIa*. In April 2007, AHRQ also published *Registries for Evaluating Patient Outcomes: A User's Guide*, co-funded by AHRQ and the Centers for Medicare & Medicaid Services (CMS), the first government-supported handbook for establishing, managing, and analyzing patient registries. This resource is designed so that patient registry data can be used to evaluate the real-life impact of healthcare treatments and can truly be considered a milestone in growing efforts to better understand what treatments actually work best and for whom (Agency for Healthcare Research and Quality, 2008c).

Clearly, there are a variety of problems that no healthcare system is large enough or has sufficient data to address on its own. Many researchers envision creation of a common research infrastructure, a federated network prototype that would support the secure analyses of electronic information across multiple organizations to study risks, effects, and outcomes of various medical therapies. This would not be a centralized database—data would stay with individual organizations. However, through the use of common research definitions and terms, the collaborative would create a large network that would expand capabilities far beyond the capacity of any one individual system.

The long-term goal is a coordinated partnership of multiple research networks that provide information that can be quickly queried and analyzed for conducting comparative effectiveness research. There are enormous opportunities here, but to come to fruition the effort will take considerable difficult work upfront. In that regard, AHRQ has funded contracts to support two important models of distributed research networks. One model being evaluated leverages partnerships of a practice-based research network to study utilization and outcomes of diabetes treatment in ambulatory care. This project is led by investigators from the University of Colorado DEcIDE center and the American Academy of Family Physicians to develop the Distributed Ambulatory Research in Therapeutics Network (DARTNet), using electronic health record data from 8 organizations representing more than 200 clinicians and over 350,000 patients (Agency for Healthcare Research and Quality, 2008a). The second model is established within a consortium of managed care organizations to study therapies for hypertension. This project is led by the HMO Research Network (HMORN) and the University of Pennsylvania DEcIDE centers (Agency for Healthcare Research and Quality, 2008a). It will develop a "Virtual Data Warehouse" to assess the effectiveness and safety of different anti-hypertensive medications used by 5.5 to 6 million individuals cared for by six health plans.

Both projects will be conducted in four phases over a period of approximately 18 months, with quarterly reports posted on AHRQ's website. These reports will describe the design specifications for each network prototype; the evaluation of the prototype; research findings from the hypertension and diabetes studies; and the major features of each prototype in the format of a prospectus or blueprint so that the model may be replicated and publicly evaluated.

In addition to the AHRQ efforts, others are also supporting activities in this arena. Under the leadership of Mark McClellan, the Quality Alliance Steering Committee at the Engelberg Center for Health Care Reform at the Brookings Institution is engaged in work to effectively aggregate data across multiple health insurance plans for the purposes of reporting on physician performance. Effectively the plans will each be producing information on a particular physician, and its weighted average will be computed and added to the same information derived from using Medicare data. The strategy is that data would stay with individual plans, but would be accessed using a common algorithm. As recent efforts to aggregate data for the purposes of quality measurement across plans have found, this is truly difficult but important work.

Among other efforts, the nonprofit eHealth Initiative Foundation has started a research program designed to improve drug safety for patients. The eHI Connecting Communities for Drug Safety Collaboration is a public- and private-sector effort designed to test new approaches and to develop replicable tools for assessing both the risks and the benefits of new drug treatments through the use of health information technology. Results will be placed in the public domain to accelerate the timeliness and effectiveness of drug safety efforts. Another important ongoing effort is the Food and Drug Administration's work to link private- and public-sector postmarket safety efforts to create a virtual, integrated, electronic "Sentinel Network." Such a network would integrate existing and planned efforts to collect, analyze, and disseminate medical product safety information to healthcare practitioners and patients at the point of care. These efforts underscore the commitment by many in the research community to creating better data and linking those data with better methods to translate them into more effective health care.

Health Care in the 21st Century

We must make sure that we do not lose sight of the importance of translating evidence into practice. For all of our excitement about current and anticipated breakthroughs leading to a world of personalized health care in the next decade, probably larger gain in terms of saving lives and reducing morbidity is likely to come from more effective translation. Researcher Steven Woolf and colleagues published interesting observations on this topic in 2005 (Figure 1-5) (Woolf and Johnson, 2005). They showed that if 100,000 patients are destined to die from a disease, a drug that reduces death rates by 20 percent will save 16,000 lives if delivered to 80 percent of the patients; increase the drug delivery to 100 percent of patients and you save an additional 4,000 lives. To compensate for that in improved efficacy you would have to have something that is 25 percent more efficacious. Thus, in the next decade, translation of the scientific evidence we already have is likely to have a much bigger impact on health outcomes than breakthroughs coming on the horizon.

The clinical research enterprise has talked a lot about phase 1 and 2 translation research (T1 and T2). Yet, we need to think about T3: the "how" of high-quality care. We need to transcend thinking about translation as an example of efficacy and think instead about translation as encompassing measurements and accountability, system redesign, scaling and spread, learning networks, and implementation and research beyond the academic center (Dougherty and Conway, 2008). Figure 1-6 outlines the three translational steps that form the 3T's road map for transforming the healthcare system. Figure 1-7 suggests a progression for the evolution of translational research.

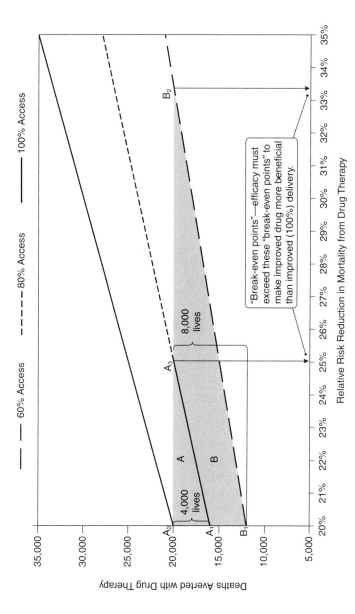

FIGURE 1-5 Potential lives saved through quality improvement—The "break-even point" for a drug that reduces mortality by 20 percent.
SOURCE: Woolf, S. H., and R. E. Johnson. 2005. The break-even point: When medical advances are less important than improving the fidelity with which they are delivered. *Annals of Family Medicine* 3(6):545-552. Reprinted with permission from American Academy of Family Physicians, Copyright © 2005.

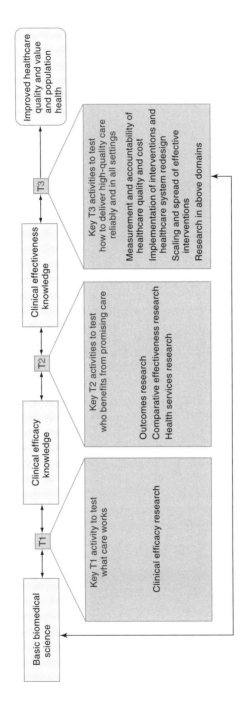

FIGURE 1-6 The 3T's roadmap.

NOTE: T indicates translation. T1, T2, and T3 represent the three major translational steps in the proposed framework to transform the healthcare system. The activities in each translational step test the discoveries of prior research activities in progressively broader settings to advance discoveries originating in basic science research through clinical research and eventually to widespread implementation through transformation of healthcare delivery. Double-headed arrows represent the essential need for feedback loops between and across the parts of the transformation framework.

SOURCE: *Journal of the American Medical Association* 299(19):2319-2321. Copyright © 2008 American Medical Association. All rights reserved.

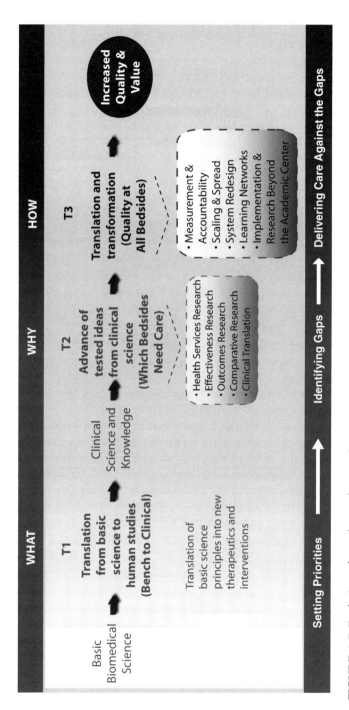

FIGURE 1-7 Evolution of translational research.

Improving quality by promoting a culture of safety through Value-Driven Health Care

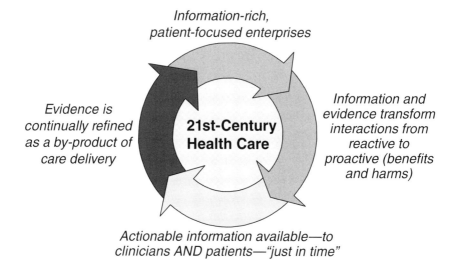

FIGURE 1-8 Model for 21st-century health care.

This area is clearly still under development and in need of more focused attention from researchers

In closing, we can no doubt all agree that the kind of healthcare system we would want to provide our own care would be information rich but patient focused, in which information and evidence transform interactions from the reactive to the proactive (benefits and harms). Figure 1-8 summarizes a vision for 21st-century health care. In this ideal system, actionable information would be available—to clinicians *and* patients—"just in time," and evidence would be continually refined as a by-product of healthcare delivery. The goal is not producing better evidence for its own sake, although the challenges and debates about how to do that are sufficiently invigorating on their own that we can almost forget what the real goals are. Achieving an information-rich, patient-focused system is *the* challenge that is at the core of our work together in the Value & Science-Driven Health Care Roundtable. Where we are ultimately headed, of course, is to establish the notion, discussed widely over the past several years, of a learning healthcare system. This is a system in which evidence is generated as a by-product of providing care and actually fed back to those who are providing care, so that we become more skilled and smarter over time.

REFERENCES

AcademyHealth. 2008. *Health Services Research (HSR) Methods* [cited June 15, 2008]. http:// www.hsrmethods.org/ (accessed June 21, 2010).

Agency for Healthcare Research and Quality. 2008a. *Developing a Distributed Research Network to Conduct Population-based Studies and Safety Surveillance 2009* [cited June 15, 2008]. http://effectivehealthcare.ahrq.gov/index.cfm/search-for-guides-reviews-and-reports/?pageaction=displayproduct&productID=150 (accessed June 21, 2010).

———. 2008b. *Distributed Network for Ambulatory Research in Therapeutics* [cited June 15, 2008]. http://effectivehealthcare.ahrq.gov/index.cfm/search-for-guides-reviews-and-reports/?pageaction=displayproduct&productID=317 (accessed June 21, 2010).

———. 2008c. *Effective Health Care Home* [cited June 15, 2008]. http://effectivehealthcare. ahrq.gov (accessed June 21, 2010).

———. 2008d. *Evidence Report on Treatment of Depression-New Pharmacotherapies: Summary* (Pub. No. 99-E013) [cited June 15, 2008]. http://archive.ahrq.gov/clinic/epcsums/ deprsumm.htm (accessed June 21, 2010).

Atkins, D. 2007. Creating and synthesizing evidence with decision makers in mind: Integrating evidence from clinical trials and other study designs. *Medical Care* 45(10 Supl 2): S16-S22.

DeVoto, E., and B. S. Kramer. 2006. Evidence-based approach to oncology. In *Oncology: An Evidence-Based Approach*, edited by A. E. Chang, P. A. Ganz, D. F. Hayes, T. Kinsella, H. I. Pass, J. H. Schiller, R. M. Stone, and V. Strecher. New York: Springer.

Dougherty, D., and P. H. Conway. 2008. The "3T's" road map to transform US health care: the "how" of high-quality care. *Journal of the American Medical Association* 299(19):2319-2321.

Fisher, R. A. 1953. *The Design of Experiments*. London: Oliver and Boyd.

Glasziou, P., I. Chalmers, M. Rawlins, and P. McCulloch. 2007. When are randomised trials unnecessary? Picking signal from noise. *British Medical Journal* 334(7589):349-351.

Kravitz, R. L., N. Duan, and J. Braslow. 2004. Evidence-based medicine, heterogeneity of treatment effects, and the trouble with averages. *Milbank Quarterly* 82(4):661-687.

Liang, L. 2007 (March/April). The gap between evidence and practice. *Health Affairs* 26(2): w119-w121.

The Lipid Research Clinics Coronary Primary Prevention Trial Results. I. 1984. Reduction in incidence of coronary heart disease. *Journal of the American Medical Association* 251(3):351-364.

The Lipid Research Clinics Coronary Primary Prevention Trial Results. II. 1984. The relationship of reduction in incidence of coronary heart disease to cholesterol lowering. *Journal of the American Medical Association* 251(3):365-374.

Lohr, K. N. 2007. Emerging methods in comparative effectiveness and safety: Symposium overview and summary. *Medical Care* 45(10):55-58.

McGrath, P. D., D. E. Wennberg, J. D. Dickens, Jr., A. E. Siewers, F. L. Lucas, D. J. Malenka, M. A. Kellett, Jr., and T. J. Ryan, Jr. 2000. Relation between operator and hospital volume and outcomes following percutaneous coronary interventions in the era of the coronary stent. *Journal of the American Medical Association* 284(24):3139-3144.

Rush, A. J. 2008. Developing the evidence for evidence-based practice. *Canadian Medical Association Journal* 178:1313-1315.

Sackett, D. L., R. Brian Haynes, G. H. Guyatt, and P. Tugwell. 2006. Dealing with the media. *Journal of Clinical Epidemiology* 59(9):907-913.

Schneeweiss, S. 2007. Developments in post-marketing comparative effectiveness research. *Clinical Pharmacology and Therapeutics* 82(2):143-156.

Tunis, S. R., D. B. Stryer, and C. M. Clancy. 2003. Practical clinical trials: Increasing the value of clinical research for decision making in clinical and health policy. *Journal of the American Medical Association* 290(12):1624-1632.

Woolf, S. H., and R. E. Johnson. 2005. The break-even point: When medical advances are less important than improving the fidelity with which they are delivered. *Annals of Family Medicine* 3(6):545-552.

2

Cases in Point:
Learning from Experience

INTRODUCTION

Media accounts of medical research breakthroughs are full of examples of trial and study results that make headlines because of their potential to improve patient health or even save lives—but those headlines are sometimes misleading or limited in relevance to real-world care. This cycle has caused confusion and distrust among patients and consumers of health care. At the other end of the spectrum, researchers discount the value of some methodologies used to evaluate clinical effectiveness. In part these findings reflect the constantly evolving nature of scientific inquiry; but as illustrated in this chapter, these experiences offer lessons on the improvements needed in the design and interpretation of clinical effectiveness studies.

By reviewing examples of high-profile studies and trials that evaluated the effectiveness of hormone replacement therapy, drug-eluting coronary stents, bariatric surgery, antipsychotic medications, and lung cancer screening, this chapter illustrates the range of issues facing current effectiveness research. Examples of these issues include capturing important health outcomes throughout the lifecycle of an intervention; contending with the biologic complexity of disease and disease progression and rapid evolution of devices or surgical procedures or rapid uptake and application in broader patient populations. This chapter also illustrates the variety of questions that are vital to ensuring effective use of medical interventions and how these issues might require trials with ever-increasing sample sizes that can be completed in a reasonable time period.

The strengths and weaknesses of observational studies and randomized trials are reviewed. Also reviewed are well-recognized limitations of observational studies due to the potential for confounding by a variety of factors as well as their limited capacity to assess short-term or acute risks. Although randomized controlled trials (RCTs) have the advantage of minimizing confounding, RCTs are often constrained by higher costs, shorter duration of follow-up, and limited applicability to populations of greatest clinical relevance. However, mixed experiences with different investigative approaches do not argue for total cessation of any one approach in favor of another. Rather, as the authors in this chapter suggest, the research community needs to be more receptive to the use of alternative methodologies to generate insights into clinical effectiveness, and we need to determine which approach we use for a given question with full recognition of what is right for particular research circumstances. Collectively these experiences suggest the availability of a powerful array of methods, and when results are combined they produce more nuanced information needed to guide treatment decisions. Opportunities to strengthen these methods are discussed and, overall, greater attention is needed to define state-of-the-art methods so the quality of research is readily discernible regardless of study approach. In addition to methods, data and data system improvements are needed. Electronic health records and data registry approaches offer the opportunity to better systematically capture, track, and report outcomes. Moreover, there is the suggestion that a mix of research approaches, using the best advantages of particular designs, offers untapped promise and that researchers should be more open to adopting such approaches. Greater engagement by the healthcare system is imperative in the evaluation of effectiveness.

JoAnn E. Manson from Harvard Medical School reviews the divergent results of observational studies and RCTs, evaluating the effect of menopausal hormone replacement therapy (HRT) on coronary heart disease (CHD). Despite this divergence, both have contributed critically important information on the therapies' effectiveness and implications for healthcare decision making. Building on this experience, Manson discusses factors that might have contributed to the different findings. She suggests that because the short- and long-term effects of a clinical intervention may differ, both observational studies and clinical trial design must have benefits to offer researchers. Perhaps, she says, we should consider research findings in the context of all of the available evidence and design studies to complement and extend existing data. Large-scale studies involving networks of electronic databases could facilitate evidence development. Due to the high cost and generally short duration of clinical trials, information about long-term risk may rely heavily on observational sources.

The Food and Drug Administration's (FDA's) Ashley B. Boam recounts the differences in findings between initial pivotal clinical studies of drug-eluting coronary stents and subsequent studies using other methodology. She observes that further understanding of drug-eluting stents (DES) will likely come from a mix of randomized trials and observational registries, conducted both premarket and postmarket and involving a collaborative effort among regulators, industry, and academia. The next author, David R. Flum, a surgeon from the University of Washington, discusses the dichotomy between "effectiveness" and "efficacy" and the applicability of case series in the context of bariatric surgical interventions. He concludes that population-based registries—appropriately funded and constructed with clinician engagement—offer a compromise of strengths and limitations and may be the most effective tool for evaluating emerging healthcare technology.

Philip S. Wang from the National Institute of Mental Health (NIMH) discusses the recently completed, NIMH-sponsored comparative effectiveness trials of antipsychotic medications in patients with schizophrenia (the CATIE trial) as a model for a hybrid approach to study design that blends advantageous features of efficacy studies and large, simple trials. Wang reviews new data resources that may offer important opportunities to effectiveness research, practical clinical trials, adaptive designs, and cluster randomization when trials are not feasible, affordable, or in some cases, ethical.

In the context of cancer research, Peter B. Bach from Memorial Sloan-Kettering Cancer Center discusses issues in the evaluation of screening tests, particularly the use of surrogate measures of benefit. He reviews the results of a computer simulation model to determine the value of lung cancer screening tests to illustrate some of the key challenges and the need for better approaches to ensure the consistent evaluation of the effectiveness of screening tests prior to widespread adoption. In particular, he suggests the use of coverage and payment as effective means to generate population-based longitudinal data on outcomes among screened groups.

HORMONE REPLACEMENT THERAPY

JoAnn E. Manson, M.D., Dr.P.H.
Harvard Medical School

Observational studies and randomized clinical trials of menopausal hormone therapy (HT) and coronary heart disease have produced widely divergent results. In aggregate, observational studies indicate that women who take estrogen after menopause are 35–50 percent less likely to develop CHD than women who do not take estrogen (Grodstein and Stampfer, 2002), whereas randomized trials suggest a neutral or even elevated risk of coronary events with menopausal HT (Anderson et al., 2004; Hulley et al., 1998; Manson et al., 2003; Rossouw et al., 2002). The cardiovascular findings from the two HT trials (estrogen plus progestin and estrogen-alone) in the Women's Health Initiative (WHI) are presented in Table 2-1. Understanding the basis for the discordant findings may provide important lessons for the design of future studies and may suggest strategies for improving the reliability and quality of clinical research. Detailed analyses from observational studies and randomized clinical trials have elucidated both methodological and biological explanations for the divergent findings, suggesting avenues for additional research to advance evidence development and improve clinical decision making (Grodstein et al., 2000, 2003; Manson and Bassuk, 2007b; Manson et al., 2006; Michels and Manson, 2003; Prentice et al., 2006). It is hoped that lessons learned from the discrepant results, which have provided insights into the strengths and weaknesses of different sources of evidence, will serve as a springboard to the development of more reliable, efficient, and innovative designs for evaluating clinical interventions.

Methodological Factors That Contribute to the Divergent Findings

The potential role of methodologic factors must be considered in understanding the more favorable findings for HT in relation to CHD risk in observational studies than in clinical trials (Table 2-2). Well-recognized limitations of observational studies, including the potential for confounding by lifestyle practices, socioeconomic status, education, and access to medical care, as well as selection factors related to "indications for use," can explain some—but not all—of the discrepancies (Grodstein et al., 2003; Manson et al., 2006; Michels and Manson, 2003; Prentice et al., 2006).

TABLE 2-1 Hazard Ratios and 95 Percent Confidence Intervals for Cardiovascular Outcomes and Total Mortality in the Overall Study Population of Women Aged 50–79 in the Women's Health Initiative (WHI) Trials of Menopausal Hormone Therapy

WHI Hormone Therapy Trials	Estrogen + Progestin (N = 16,608)	Estrogen alone (N = 10,739)
Coronary heart disease	1.24 (1.00–1.54)	0.95 (0.78–1.16)
Stroke	1.31 (1.03–1.68)	1.33 (1.05–1.68)
All-cause mortality	1.00 (0.83–1.19)	1.04 (0.88–1.22)

SOURCES: Derived from Manson, J. E., J. Hsia, K. C. Johnson, et al. 2003. Estrogen plus progestin and the risk of coronary heart disease. *New England Journal of Medicine* 349:523-534; Rossouw, J. E., R. L. Prentice, J. E. Manson, et al. 2007. Postmenopausal hormone therapy and risk of cardiovascular disease by age and years since menopause. *Journal of the American Medical Association* 297:1465-1477.

TABLE 2-2 Postmenopausal Hormone Therapy and CHD: Potential Explanations for Divergent Findings from Clinical Trials and Observational Studies

Potential Explanations for the Divergent Findings

- Methodological Differences
  — Confounding ("healthy user") bias
  — Compliance bias
  — Incomplete capture of early clinical events

- Biological Differences
  — Characteristics of study population (time since menopause, stage of atherosclerosis)
  — Hormone regimen (formulation and dose)

SOURCE: Derived from Grodstein, F., T. B. Clarkson, and J. E. Manson. 2003. Understanding the divergent data on postmenopausal hormone therapy. *New England Journal of Medicine* 348:645-650.

Confounding by healthful lifestyle practices and "healthy user bias" among women taking HT may have led to an overestimation of the CHD benefits, but most studies examining this issue suggest that careful adjustments for these factors (such as smoking, other CHD risk factors, body mass index, physical activity, and diet) attenuate—but do not eliminate— the inverse associations between HT and CHD risk (Grodstein et al., 2000, 2003; Manson et al., 2006). Moreover, the Nurses' Health Study, a large-scale cohort relatively homogeneous for educational attainment, occupation, and access to medical care, showed substantial reductions in CHD risk among HT users, compared to nonusers (Grodstein et al., 2000).

Another methodologic factor that has received less attention is the limitation of most observational studies in assessing short-term or acute risks (due to infrequent updates of exposures), leading to incomplete capture of early clinical events after initiation of therapy and the predominance of follow-up time among compliant long-term users of HT (Grodstein et al., 2003; Manson and Bassuk, 2007b). In contrast to the greater weighting of long-term use in observational studies, clinical trial results tend to reflect shorter term use. Given that CHD risks related to HT are greatest soon after initiation of therapy (Hulley et al., 1998; Manson et al., 2003) and reductions in risk may emerge with longer term use (discussed below) (Michels and Manson, 2003; Prentice et al., 2006; Rossouw et al., 2002), these differences may contribute to the discrepancies observed. Indeed, comparative analyses of HT and CHD in the observational and clinical trial components of the Women's Health Initiative, with stratification by duration of treatment (comparing short-term versus long-term users), indicated greater convergence of study results when examining similar durations of use (Prentice et al., 2006). For example, both the observational and clinical trial cohorts in the WHI suggested an increased risk of CHD during the first several years of HT use but a reduced risk with longer duration (>5 years) of use (Table 2-3).

Moreover, observational studies that have utilized electronic health and pharmacy records, which provide frequent updating of exposure (HT use) information via prescription records and facilitate the capture of both short- and long-term health outcomes, have tended to show less pronounced reductions in CHD risk related to HT use (Heckbert et al., 2001; Lemaitre et al., 2006). In a study utilizing computerized pharmacy records and outcomes databases (Group Health Cooperative), the associations between HT and CHD risk were similar to those observed in the WHI for women of comparable age and health status (Heckbert et al., 2001). However, substantial reductions in mortality among women with long-term use of HT have been observed even in studies using electronic pharmacy and health records (Ettinger et al., 1996).

Thus, methodologic differences between observational studies and clinical trials may not fully elucidate the basis for the discrepancies observed. Although large-scale randomized trials, the gold standard of clinical research, have the advantage of minimizing confounding by lifestyle practices, socioeconomic status, and other factors, they are often constrained by higher costs, shorter duration of follow-up, and, at times, limited applicability to populations of greatest clinical relevance. Furthermore, the findings of observational studies and clinical trials of HT are remarkably concordant

TABLE 2-3 Hazard Ratios (HR) and 95 Percent Confidence Intervals (CIs) in the Women's Health Initative (WHI), According to Duration of HT Use

Comparison of Results from the WHI Clinical Trial (CT) and Observational Study (OS) for HT and CHD, According to Duration of Use

Years since HT Initiation	Estrogen + Progestin HR (95% CI)		Estrogen Alone HR (95% CI)	
	CT	OS	CT	OS
<2	1.68 (1.15–2.45)	1.12 (0.46–2.74)	1.07 (0.68–1.68)	1.20 (0.49–2.94)
2–5	1.25 (0.87–1.79)	1.05 (0.70–1.58)	1.13 (0.70–1.58)	1.09 (0.75–1.60)
>5	0.66 (0.36–1.21)	0.83 (0.67–1.01)	0.80 (0.57–1.12)	0.73 (0.61–0.84)

SOURCE: Derived from Prentice, R., R. D. Langer, M. L. Stefanick, et al. 2006. Combined analysis of Women's Health Initiative observational and clinical trial data on postmenopausal hormone treatment and cardiovascular disease. *American Journal of Epidemiology* 163(7):589-599.

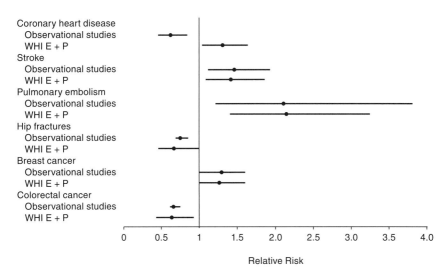

FIGURE 2-1 Relative risks and 95 percent confidence intervals for observational and clinical trial findings on hormone therapy (estrogen + progestin).
SOURCE: Michels, K. B., and J. E. Manson. 2003. Postmenopausal hormone therapy: A reversal of fortune. *Circulation* 107:1830-1833. Reprinted with permission from Michels and Manson, *Circulation*, 2003.

for non-CHD health outcomes, including stroke, venous thromboembolism, breast cancer, colorectal cancer, and fracture (Figure 2-1)—results that should also be affected by confounding and selection biases (Grodstein et al., 2003; Manson et al., 2006; Michels and Manson, 2003).

An emerging body of evidence supports the hypothesis that age or time since menopause critically influences the relationship between HT and CHD outcomes (Estrogen and progestogen use in peri- and postmenopausal women: March 2007 position statement of the North American Menopause Society, 2007; Grodstein et al., 2003; Manson et al., 2006). Women who participate in observational studies tend to be younger and closer to onset of menopause at the time of HT initiation than women in randomized trials (the latter are, on average, more than a decade past menopause onset at randomization). Thus, women in HT clinical trials tend to have later stages of atherosclerosis than their counterparts in observational studies and a possibly greater vulnerability to the adverse vascular effects of HT (Estrogen and progestogen use in peri- and postmenopausal women: March 2007 position statement of the North American Menopause Society, 2007; Manson et al., 2006). In contrast, if estrogen slows early stages of atherosclerosis, as suggested by basic research, animal studies, and imaging findings, recently menopausal women with healthy vascular endothelium may be more likely to have a favorable coronary outcome than women more distant from menopause (Manson et al., 2007; Mendelsohn and Karas, 2005; Mikkola and Clarkson, 2002). Moreover, absolute rates of adverse events and risks attributable to HT are lower in younger than older women, suggesting that the risk:benefit ratio may vary substantially by age and proximity to menopause onset (Estrogen and progestogen use in peri- and postmenopausal women: March 2007 position statement of the North American Menopause Society, 2007; Manson and Bassuk, 2007b). It is important to emphasize that the implication of the "timing hypothesis" is *not* that recently menopausal women be given HT for CHD prevention but rather that clinicians can be reassured about cardiac risks when considering short-term use of HT for vasomotor symptom management in such women. The theory that the influence of estrogen on atherosclerosis and coronary events may vary according to the underlying health of the vasculature and the evidence that a woman's age and time since menopause onset may modulate CHD outcomes with HT, as well as implications for future research, are discussed below.

Biological Factors That May Contribute to the Divergent Findings

As noted above, randomized trials testing the effect of HT on clinical coronary outcomes have not confirmed the cardioprotective effect suggested by most observational studies. In the Heart and Estrogen/progestin Replacement Study (HERS), the 4-year incidence of major coronary events among women with a mean age of 67 years and with preexisting CHD was similar in the HT (oral conjugated equine estrogens [CEE] and medroxy-progesterone acetate [MPA]) and the placebo groups (Hulley et al., 1998). The HT group had a 50 percent increase in risk of CHD events during the first year of the trial, although this elevation was offset by a decreased risk in later years (Grady et al., 2002; Hulley et al., 1998). The Women's Health Initiative examined the effects of oral CEE with or without MPA in healthy postmenopausal women aged 50–79 (mean age 63) (Anderson et al., 2004; Rossouw et al., 2002); participants had either an intact uterus (N = 16,608) or prior hysterectomy (N = 10,739), respectively. Women assigned to CEE + MPA for an average of 5.6 years were more likely to experience a CHD event than those assigned to placebo (relative risk [RR] = 1.24; 95 percent confidence interval [CI]: 1.00, 1.54), with the highest risk during the first year (Manson et al., 2003). Women assigned to CEE alone for an average of 6.8 years also experienced no overall reduction in CHD risk (RR = 0.95; 95 percent CI: 0.78, 1.16) (Prentice et al., 2006). Both WHI trials were stopped early—the CEE + MPA trial because of an increased risk of breast cancer and an unfavorable benefit–risk balance (Rossouw et al., 2002) and the CEE-alone trial because of an increased stroke risk that was not offset by a reduced CHD risk (Anderson et al., 2004). Although most randomized clinical trials have tested the commonly used HT formulations of CEE + MPA or CEE alone, clinical trials using estradiol and other formulations of estrogen and/or progestin have also failed to demonstrate cardioprotection (Grodstein et al., 2003; Manson et al., 2006; Michels and Manson, 2003).

A key difference between participants in observational studies and those in clinical trials of HT is the timing of initiation of treatment in relation to menopause onset, which occurs on average at age 51 in the United States. Hormone users in observational studies typically start therapy in early menopause, whereas trial participants are often randomized to hormones more than a decade after cessation of menses. For example, in the Nurses' Health Study cohort, about 80 percent of women who used HT began treatment within 2–3 years of menopause onset (Grodstein et al., 2003; Manson and Bassuk, 2007b). In contrast, WHI participants, with a mean baseline age of 63, were an average of at least 12 years past menopause at the time of trial enrollment and likely had more extensive atherosclerosis than newly menopausal women. In HERS, the mean age was 67 at baseline, and all participants had been previously diagnosed with CHD. It has been hypothesized that estrogen has diverse and opposing actions, slowing the earlier stages of atherosclerosis through favorable effects on the lipid profile and endothelial function, but triggering acute coronary events through prothrombotic and inflammatory mechanisms and plaque destabilization when advanced lesions are present (Estrogen and progestogen use in peri- and postmenopausal women: March 2007 position statement of the North American Menopause Society, 2007; Grodstein et al., 2003; Manson et al., 2006; Mendelsohn and Karas, 2005) (Figure 2-2).

This hypothesis is supported by several lines of evidence from basic and clinical studies. First, trials in humans show complex effects of exogenous estrogen on cardiovascular biomarkers (Estrogen and progestogen use in peri- and postmenopausal women: March 2007 position statement of the North American Menopause Society, 2007; Manson et al., 2006; Mendelsohn and Karas, 2005). Oral estrogen lowers low-density lipoprotein (LDL) cholesterol, lipoprotein(a), glucose, insulin, and homocysteine levels; inhibits oxidation of LDL cholesterol; increases high-density lipoprotein cholesterol; reverses postmenopausal increases in fibrinogen and plasminogen-activator inhibitor type 1; and improves endothelial function—all effects expected to *lower* coronary risk. However, oral estrogen also increases triglycerides, coagulation factors (factor VII, prothrombin fragments 1 and 2, and fibrinopeptide A), C-reactive protein, and matrix metalloproteinases—effects expected to *raise* coronary risk. Additionally, certain progestogens may offset some of estrogen's benefits.

Data from controlled experiments in nonhuman primates also support the theory that the coronary effects of HT depend on the initial health of the vasculature. Conjugated estrogen (with or without a progestin) did not

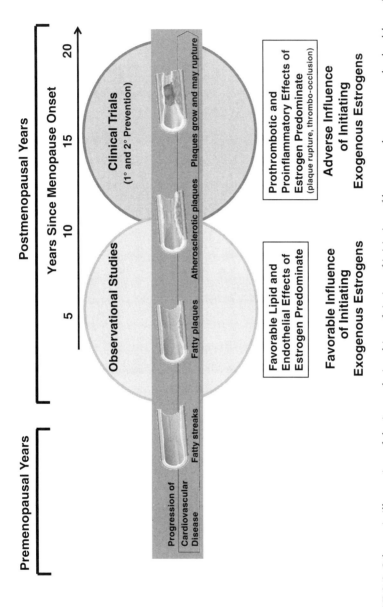

FIGURE 2-2 Schematic illustration of the interrelationships of timing of initiation of hormone therapy, vascular health, and clinical CHD outcomes.
SOURCE: Manson, J. E., S. S. Bassuk, S. M. Harman, et al. 2006. Postmenopausal hormone therapy: New questions and the case for new clinical trials. *Menopause* 13(1):139-147.

affect the extent of coronary artery plaque in cynomolgus monkeys started on this treatment at 2 years (~6 human years) after oophorectomy and well after the establishment of atherosclerosis, but such therapy reduced plaque by 70 percent when initiated immediately after oophorectomy during the early stages of atherosclerosis (Mikkola and Clarkson, 2002) (Figure 2-3).

Similarly, imaging trials in women with significant coronary lesions at baseline have found estrogen to be ineffective in slowing the rate of arterial narrowing (Angerer et al., 2001; Herrington et al., 2000; Hodis et al., 2003; Waters et al., 2002). However, in an imaging trial that did not require participants to have significant vascular disease at entry, estrogen impeded progression of carotid atherosclerosis (Hodis et al., 2001).

When the WHI trials were initiated in the early 1990s, it was not well recognized that age or vascular health might be an important determinant of the effect of HT on coronary or other outcomes; thus, focused subgroup analyses were not emphasized at the outset, nor were the trials powered to detect potential interactions. However, given the striking discrepancies between findings from earlier observational studies and more recent randomized trials (including data from the large trials with hard clinical endpoints, smaller imaging studies, and experimental studies in animals), WHI investigators pursued more detailed analyses of the data to examine whether the timing hypothesis might account for the seemingly contradictory evidence on coronary effects of HT.

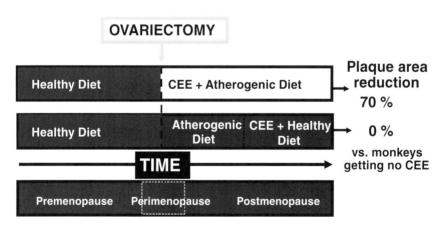

FIGURE 2-3 Role of timing of conjugated equine estrogen (CEE) initiation in relationship to ovariectomy in nonhuman primates.
NOTE: Modified and reprinted with permission from the European Society of Cardiology, Copyright © 2002.
SOURCE: Mikkola, T. S., and T. B. Clarkson. 2002. Estrogen replacement therapy, atherosclerosis, and vascular function. *Cardiovasc Res* 53:605-619.

The results of subgroup analyses of WHI data are consistent with the possibility that age or time since menopause influences the HT-CHD association. Subgroup analyses have been reported for the CEE + MPA (Manson et al., 2003) and CEE-alone (Hsia et al., 2006) trials individually and for a combined analysis of the two trials (Rossouw et al., 2007). The following section focuses primarily on the joint analysis that combined data from both trials, resulting in a large number of confirmed CHD end-points and increased statistical power (Rossouw et al., 2007). However, all of the above reports showed similar patterns.

In the WHI, the HT-associated risk of CHD (defined as myocardial infarction [MI] or coronary death) steadily increased with years since menopause.

In analyses that combined data from both trials, RRs were 0.76, 1.10, and 1.28 for women who were <10, 10–19, and ≥20 years past menopause at study entry, respectively (p, trend = 0.02) (Rossouw et al., 2007). Indeed, a pattern of increasing RRs with greater distance from menopause onset was apparent in both the estrogen-alone (E-alone) and estrogen-progestin (E + P) trials, and a similar gradient of relative risks was seen with increasing age (Rossouw et al., 2007) (Table 2-4). Among women aged 50–59,

TABLE 2-4 Hazard Ratios and 95 Percent Confidence Intervals for Selected Outcomes in the Women's Health Initiative (WHI) Trials of Menopausal Hormone Therapy (joint analysis of the E + P and E-alone trials)

Combined Trials (Joint Analysis of the Two HT Trials in the WHI)			
	Years Since Menopause		
	<10	10–19	≥20	p, trend
Coronary heart disease	0.76 (0.50–1.16)	1.10 (0.84–1.45)	1.28 (1.03–1.58)	0.02
Total mortality	0.76 (0.53–1.09)	0.98 (0.78–1.24)	1.14 (0.96–1.36)	0.51
Global index[a]	1.05 (0.86–1.27)	1.12 (0.98–1.27)	1.09 (0.98–1.22)	0.82
	Age (years)		
	50–59	60–69	70–79	p, trend
Coronary heart disease	0.93 (0.65–1.33)	0.98 (0.79–1.21)	1.26 (1.00–1.59)	0.16
Total mortality	0.70 (0.51–0.96)	1.05 (0.87–1.26)	1.14 (0.94–1.37)	0.06
Global index[a]	0.96 (0.81–1.14)	1.08 (0.97–1.20)	1.14 (1.02–1.29)	0.09

[a]The global index is a composite outcome of coronary heart disease, stroke, pulmonary embolism, breast cancer, colorectal cancer, endometrial cancer, hip fracture, and mortality.
SOURCE: Derived from Rossouw, J. E., R. L. Prentice, J. E. Manson, et al. 2007. Postmenopausal hormone therapy and risk of cardiovascular disease by age and years since menopause. *JAMA* 297:1465-1477.

TABLE 2-5 Hazard Ratios and 95 Percent Confidence Intervals for CHD Outcomes in the Women's Health Initiative (WHI) Estrogen-Alone Trial, According to Age

	WHI Estrogen–Alone Trial: Detailed CHD Results According to Age at Randomization		
Outcome	50–59	60–69	70–79
MI or CHD death	0.63	0.94	1.11
(N = 418)	(0.36–1.08)	(0.71–1.24)	(0.82–1.52)
CABG or PCI	0.55	0.99	1.04
(N = 529)	(0.35–0.86)	(0.78–1.27)	(0.78–1.39)
Composite	0.66	1.02	1.08
MI/CABG/PCI	(0.44–0.97)	(0.83–1.25)	(0.85–1.38)
(N = 728)			

NOTES: CABG = coronary artery bypass grafting; MI = myocardial infarction;. PCI = percutaneous coronary intervention.
SOURCE: Derived from Hsia, J., R. D. Langer, J. E. Manson, et al. 2006. Conjugated equine estrogens and the risk of coronary heart disease: The Women's Health Initiative. *Archives of Internal Medicine* 166:357-365.

assignment to estrogen alone was associated with significant reductions in the secondary end-point of coronary revascularization (RR = 0.55; 95 percent CI: 0.35, 0.86) and a composite end-point of MI, coronary death, or coronary revascularization (RR = 0.66; 95 percent CI: 0.44, 0.97) (Hsia et al., 2006) (Table 2-5). Taken together, the pattern of WHI results suggests a beneficial or neutral effect of HT on CHD risk among women closer to menopause (who are likely to have less atherosclerosis) but an adverse impact in later years. Similar results according to age or time since menopause have been obtained in observational studies and small clinical trials (Brownley et al., 2004; Grodstein et al., 2006; Lobo, 2004).

Salpeter et al. combined data from 22 smaller randomized trials with data from the WHI to provide the most comprehensive assessment to date of the influence of age on the relation between HT and CHD (Salpeter et al., 2006). Their analysis showed that in trials that enrolled predominantly younger participants (women aged <60 or within 10 years of menopause), HT was associated with a 30–40 percent reduction in CHD risk. In contrast, in trials with predominantly older participants, HT had little effect on such risk. A previous meta-analysis had not explicitly examined the effect of age (Hemminki and McPherson, 1997).

In the WHI, age influenced not only the relation between HT and CHD but also appeared to modulate the effect of HT on all-cause mortality and a composite outcome ("global index") (Table 2-4). In an analysis that combined data from the two HT trials in the WHI, HT was associated with a significant reduction in mortality (RR = 0.70; 95 percent CI: 0.51, 0.96) among women in their 50s but not among women aged 60 or older (Rossouw et al., 2007). A 2003 meta-analysis of 30 randomized trials, including the WHI CEE + MPA trial, found that HT was associated with a nearly 40 percent reduction in mortality in trials in which the mean age of participants was <60 but had no effect on mortality in other trials (Salpeter et al., 2004).

In an ancillary study of coronary artery calcium (CAC) measurements in the WHI CEE trial, conducted among women who were aged 50–59 at WHI enrollment, levels of CAC following trial completion were lower among women randomized to estrogen than those randomized to placebo (Manson et al., 2007). Odds ratios for the prevalence of high CAC (scores ≥100) were 0.69 (95 percent CI: 0.48, 0.98) overall and 0.46 (0.29, 0.73) among women with ≥80 percent adherence to study pills. High CAC correlates with a greater atherosclerotic plaque burden and has been shown to predict risk of future coronary events (Hecht et al., 2006). These findings further support the hypothesis that estrogen therapy reduces progression of atherosclerosis and subclinical coronary artery disease in younger women who are closer to the onset of menopause.

Thus, the existing evidence in support of the timing hypothesis is compelling, although the data are not yet conclusive and would *not* justify the use of HT for cardioprotection. However, even if the hypothesis is ultimately disproved and HT-associated RRs for CHD are shown to be similar across groups defined by age or time since menopause, the much lower absolute baseline risks of CHD and other events in younger or recently menopausal women translate to much lower absolute excess risks associated with HT use in these women as compared with women who are older or further past menopause. Estimates of such risks based on WHI data (for CHD, total mortality, and the global index) are provided in Table 2-6.

New trials are in progress to assess the possible differential effects of HT on the progression of atherosclerosis according to age at initiation (Hodis, 2007) and type of therapy (Harman et al., 2005).

Implications of the Timing Hypothesis for Clinical Decision Making

There is a clear consensus among mainstream health organizations and most healthcare providers that the use of HT should be limited to management of moderate-to-severe menopausal symptoms. Most of the current guidelines recommend against the use of HT at any age to prevent CHD and other chronic diseases (Estrogen and progestogen use in peri- and postmenopausal women: March 2007 position statement of the North American Menopause Society, 2007; Executive summary. Hormone therapy, 2004; Hormone therapy for the prevention of chronic conditions in postmenopausal women: Recommendations from the U.S. Preventive Services

TABLE 2-6 Attributable Risks (Cases per 10,000 Women Per Year) for Selected Outcomes in a Combined Analysis of the Women's Health Initiative (WHI) E + P and E-alone Trials

Absolute Excess Risks (cases per 10,000 person years) by Age and Years Since Menopause in the Combined Trials (E + P and E-Alone) of the WHI

Outcome	Age (years)			Years Since Menopause		
	50–59	60–69	70–79	<10	10–19	≥20
CHD	−2	−1	+19[a]	−6	+4	+17[a]
Total mortality	−10	−4	+16[a]	−7	−1	+14
Global index[b]	−4	+15	+43	+5	+20	+23

[a]$P = 0.03$ compared with age 50–59 years or <10 years since menopause.
[b]Global index is a composite outcome of CHD, stroke, pulmonary embolism, breast cancer, colorectal cancer, endometrial cancer, hip fracture, and mortality.
SOURCE: Derived from Rossouw, J. E., R. L. Prentice, J. E. Manson, et al. 2007. Postmenopausal hormone therapy and risk of cardiovascular disease by age and years since menopause. *Journal of the American Medical Association* 297:1465-1477.

Task Force, 2005; Mosca et al., 2007; Wathen et al., 2004), due to other known risks of HT. Although HT should never be prescribed specifically for coronary protection, the timing hypothesis can—and should—inform clinical decision making regarding the use of systemic HT for treatment of hot flashes and night sweats that are severe or frequent enough to disrupt sleep or quality of life—the classic and currently only compelling indications for such therapy (Estrogen and progestogen use in peri- and postmenopausal women: March 2007 position statement of the North American Menopause Society, 2007; Manson and Bassuk, 2007a). The timing hypothesis suggests that women in early menopause and at low baseline risk of CHD are unlikely to experience HT-associated coronary events and would have a more favorable benefit–risk profile on HT than older women.

Lessons Learned from the Hormone Therapy Controversies

The divergent findings on hormone therapy underscore the strengths and limitations of both observational and clinical trial research and suggest important strategies for improving the design of future studies. Understanding the basis for the discrepancies, and the relative convergence of findings after accounting for methodological and biological factors, provides lessons for improving the reliability and quality of research on clinical interventions. The key lessons and their implications for study design are as follows:

- Short- and long-term effects of a clinical intervention may differ and clinical studies must be designed to capture time-varying effects. A strength of clinical trials is the ability to pinpoint the onset of an exposure/intervention and to capture early events, whereas observational studies often miss acute or short-term effects unless exposure information is updated frequently. Observational studies that utilize computerized health records and electronic pharmacy databases, however, may avoid these limitations due to their ability to capture prescription/medication data on a regular basis. Moreover, results of studies that use electronic health records tend to be largely convergent with results of clinical trials, supporting the advantages of this study design for medication-related research. Large-scale studies involving networks of electronic databases could facilitate evidence development in this area.

- Regardless of the study design, analyses must consider time-varying effects when comparing results across studies. Duration of treatment may have an important influence on health outcomes. For HT, some risks tend to increase shortly after treatment initiation (e.g., venous thromboembolism, myocardial infarction) while other risks may be delayed (e.g., breast cancer). Conversely, some benefits may occur quickly (e.g., reduction in vasomotor symptoms), and others may require longer duration of treatment (reduction in osteoporotic fractures or slowing of atherogenesis in younger women). Comparisons across studies should account for duration of treatment. Clinical trials and observational studies of HT that initially appeared divergent showed similar results when analyses were stratified by duration of treatment (e.g., both the clinical trial and observational components of the WHI indicate a short-term increase in risk of CHD with HT followed by a declining risk with longer duration of treatment). Due to the high cost of clinical trials and generally short duration, information about long-term risks may rely heavily on observational sources. Thus, the *totality* of evidence from all available sources must be considered.

- Clinical trials have the advantage of minimizing confounding and selection biases through the process of randomization, which works particularly well when the sample size is large. Observational studies can reduce these biases by careful adjustment for lifestyle factors, disease-related risk factors, socioeconomic factors, and access to medical care. Although these biases have contributed to the discrepancies between observational studies and clinical trials, they appear to be less important than the methodologic factors addressed above or the biological differences in the populations studied. For example, HT results in observational studies and clinical trials are similar after accounting for differences in treatment duration (as discussed above) and differences in the age distribution of the study populations (as described below).

- Biological factors, particularly a woman's age, time since menopause, and underlying stage of atherosclerosis, may modulate her health outcomes on HT, particularly her risk of CHD. Estrogen is complex and has both favorable and adverse effects. Biological differences in study populations in observational studies and clinical trials may be primarily responsible for the discrepancies between these studies, although study design and methodologic factors have also contributed. Experimental studies in nonhuman primates also support a role of biological factors, such as time since menopause and underlying health of the vasculature, as modifying factors. Moreover, it is critically important to consider *absolute rates*, as well as *relative risks*, of health outcomes when evaluating the risk: benefit profile of a treatment in different populations. In the case of HT, the much lower *absolute rate* of cardiovascular disease (CVD) and other chronic diseases in younger women would suggest lower *attributable risks* in this population. Thus, the generalizability and applicability of findings to relevant clinical populations must be considered. The WHI was tremendously important in halting the growing practice of initiating HT in older women, and women at high risk of CHD, for the purpose of CVD prevention—this was demonstrated to be a harmful practice. However, the WHI could not provide conclusive answers about the risk–benefit profile of HT in recently menopausal women. Finally, the possibility of differences in health outcomes related to medication dose, formulation, and route of delivery warrants consideration and further study.
- Surrogate markers, such as intermediate biomarkers (lipoproteins, thrombotic and inflammatory markers), noninvasive imaging studies (coronary artery calcium measurements or carotid ultrasound, mammographic density studies) may provide important insights about the health effects of different HT formulations and dosages. However, due to the complexity of HT's effects and difficulty in predicting the net effect on risk, surrogate markers cannot substitute for the assessment of clinical events.

Conclusions

Observational studies, clinical trials, and basic research all have contributed critically important information to elucidate the health effects of HT and to inform decision making. Recent analyses have elucidated both methodological and biological explanations for the divergent findings and suggested avenues for additional research to advance evidence development. The primary lesson is that we should consider research findings in the context of the totality of available evidence and design studies to complement and extend the existing data. Importantly, observational studies should be designed to capture both short- and long-term risks and should have frequent updating of exposure variables of interest (electronic health records and pharmacy databases may be useful). Clinical trials must be adequately powered to assess clinically relevant subgroups and to address the possibility of a modulating effect of key clinical variables. Consideration of absolute risks in research presentation and interpretation is critically important. Finally, it may be helpful to incorporate intermediate and surrogate markers (such as from imaging studies) into research designs, although such markers can never fully replace clinical event ascertainment. For HT and CHD, the emerging evidence to support the "timing hypothesis" does *not* imply that recently menopausal women should be prescribed HT for cardiac protection; rather it suggests that healthcare providers should avoid initiating HT in older women who are distant from menopause but need not be unduly concerned about CHD risks when considering short-term treatment to relieve vasomotor symptoms in recently menopausal women. This new information should aid clinical practice, suggest avenues for future research, and improve the quality of medical care and clinical decision making.

DRUG-ELUTING CORONARY STENTS

Ashley B. Boam, M.S.B.E.
Andrew Farb, M.D.
Food and Drug Administration, Center for Devices and Radiological Health

Each year approximately one million patients in the United States undergo percutaneous coronary intervention (PCI) for the treatment of symptomatic coronary atherosclerosis, of which 80 percent undergo placement of a coronary stent as part of this procedure. It is estimated that 650,000 patients annually are treated with drug-eluting stents, which reduce the need for repeat procedures due to restenosis compared with bare metal stents. Currently available DES consist of a metal stent platform, which acts as a mechanical scaffold, with a polymer and drug mixture coated on the surface of the stent platform. The polymer controls the elution of the drug from the stent into the artery wall with the objective of reducing restenosis (in-stent tissue regrowth following implantation). The coated stent is mounted on a balloon catheter used to deploy the stent within a coronary atherosclerotic lesion (site of luminal narrowing).

Development of DES

Clinical restenosis after arterial balloon injury occurs as a result of luminal re-narrowing secondary to (1) development of a neointima (consisting of vascular smooth muscle cells with an extracellular soft tissue matrix) and (2) adventitial fibrosis-induced arterial constriction (negative remodeling). The semi-rigid scaffold afforded by metal stents prevents arterial constriction that occurs post-balloon angioplasty, so that restenosis occurs as a consequence of neointimal growth alone. Compared to balloon angioplasty, bare metal stents improve arterial patency rates via (1) a reduction in rates of acute vessel closure and recoil and (2) a modest reduction in long-term restenosis rates by preventing negative remodeling. Implanted bare metal stents are foreign bodies and present an early thrombosis risk. In human clinical use, this risk has been minimized by (1) deployment techniques that directly oppose the stent struts to the subjacent arterial wall and (2) the use of two adjunctive antiplatelet drugs (aspirin and clopidogrel) until the stent is covered by an endothelialized neointima.

Residual high restenosis rates after bare metal stenting in higher risk lesions combined with an understanding of the pathogenesis of restenosis lead to investigations of interventions aimed to inhibit neointimal growth. Success in inhibiting neointimal thickening was achieved via the local delivery of agents that specifically targeted the cell cycle; these agents inhibit cellular proliferation and have anti-inflammatory properties. Pre-clinical studies demonstrated that antimitogenic agents (such as sirolimus and paclitaxel) eluted over time from a polymer coating reduced in-stent stenosis at 28 days (Farb et al., 2001; Suzuki et al., 2001).

Regulation of DES

Coronary DES are regulated by the Food and Drug Administration (FDA) as combination products (FDA, 2008f) because they are comprised of two or more regulated components, i.e., a drug and a device. In response to a Request for Determination of jurisdiction, the FDA determined that the primary mode of action was that of the device component (the mechanical support of the metal stent), and primary review responsibilities were assigned to the Center for Devices and Radiological Health (CDRH), with substantial consultative review by the Center for Drug Evaluation and Research (CDER) (FDA, 2008d). Given this framework, when a manufacturer wishes to evaluate new DES, approval of an Investigational Device Exemption (IDE) by the FDA and approval of the investigational plan by local Institutional Review Boards (IRBs) are required prior to beginning clinical studies in the United States. Approval to market a DES in the United States requires approval of a premarket approval application (PMA) (FDA, 2008b).

Regulatory History

The first two DES to be approved for marketing in the United States were the CYPHER Sirolimus-Eluting Coronary Stent (Cordis Corporation, a Johnson & Johnson company, Miami Lakes, Florida) in April 2003 (FDA, 2008a) and the TAXUS Express[2] Paclitaxel-Eluting Coronary Stent (Boston Scientific, Natick, Massachusetts) in March 2004 (FDA, 2008e). The PMAs for these products included substantial laboratory testing and animal studies in addition to chemistry and manufacturing information. Pharmacokinetic (PK) assessments of drug elution were performed using in vitro methods, and in vivo PK studies were completed in animals and humans. DES were implanted in coronary arteries of animal models to evaluate device handling performance and histologic changes within arteries, myocardium, and other body organs. Both DES were evaluated in clinical trials that compared the DES to the identical bare metal (uncoated) stent in patients with symptomatic coronary artery disease undergoing PCI of a single lesion. In this patient population, both the CYPHER and TAXUS DES demonstrated clinically significant reductions in the incidence of repeat procedures needed to treat restenosis, without any apparent differences in the rates of death or myocardial infarction. This substantial improvement in effectiveness led to widespread adoption of these products, with DES used in up to 80 percent of PCI patients treated with stents. In anticipation of use of DES in a large number of patients, including use outside of the labeled indication, the FDA required both manufacturers to conduct postapproval studies in which 2,000 consecutive patients receiving the DES were enrolled into a single-arm registry study and followed for at least 1 year. The consecutive nature of these postapproval studies reduced the influence of selection bias but allowed for the enrollment of large numbers of "off-label" patients.

The Search for Potential Surrogate Endpoints

As rates of reintervention to treat restenosis fell from double to single digits, the size of a trial needed to show either non-inferiority or superiority of a new DES to one of the two approved DES grew rapidly in comparison to the initial trials in which superiority to a bare metal stent was the objective. Following approval and rapid clinical adoption of the first two DES, researchers turned their attention to the development of surrogate markers for effectiveness.

Angiographic evaluation of patients undergoing PCI has been a standard component of stent trials for many years. Such imaging studies provide insight into the mechanistic action of the stent by providing quantitative assessments of the amount of neointimal growth within the stent and the 5 mm margin proximal and distal to the stent. Angiographic end-points such as late lumen loss (the difference between minimal lumen diameter measured immediately post stent implantation and follow-up angiography, typically performed 9 months post stent implantation) and percent arterial diameter stenosis have been identified as potential surrogate markers for the clinical end-point of target lesion revascularization, or the need for reintervention to treat restenosis in the stented area (Mauri et al., 2005; Pocock et al., 2008). Imaging end-points are commonly measured as continuous variables, and this powerful discriminatory advantage can be utilized to design trials with sample sizes considerably smaller than typically needed for standard binary clinical end-points (e.g., target lesion or target vessel revascularization). Further, angiographic evaluations are objective measures evaluated by core laboratories, which helps to minimize potential bias.

Clinical Trials Utilizing Angiographic End-points

The third DES to be FDA-approved was the Endeavor Zotarolimus Drug-Eluting Coronary Stent (Medtronic, Santa Clara, California) (FDA, 2008c). The Endeavor stent was the first DES to incorporate a drug not previously approved for systemic use. Zotarolimus (Abbott Laboratories, Abbott Park, Illinois) was developed specifically for use on a DES; therefore, the DES manufacturer, Medtronic, provided safety information on the drug alone in addition to the stent-based drug delivery evaluation as performed for the CYPHER and TAXUS stents. The first major clinical study conducted by Medtronic was a randomized trial comparing Endeavor to the identical bare metal stent. This study was conducted outside of the United States as the manufacturer believed that a trial in which a DES was randomized to a bare metal stent could not be conducted in the United States due to the widespread adoption of the CYPHER stent by U.S. interventional cardiologists. A second study randomizing the Endeavor stent to the CYPHER stent was conducted in the United States, with a primary end-point based on angiographic evaluation. Finally, a third study was completed in the United States to evaluate the performance of the Endeavor stent versus the approved TAXUS stent. This third study utilized a clinical measure as the primary end-point, with a powered secondary end-point based on angiographic measurements. The Endeavor stent proved to have superior clinical performance (a composite of cardiac death, MI, and target vessel revascularization) in its comparison to the bare metal stent and to be non-inferior in clinical performance to the TAXUS stent. However, in both trials assessing angiographic outcomes, the Endeavor stent failed its non-inferiority comparison to both the CYPHER and TAXUS stents (see further discussion below regarding use of angiographic end-points). In the FDA's final evaluation, the strength of the clinical assessments and the absence of any safety concerns were found to outweigh the less favorable angiographic results, and the Endeavor stent was approved in February 2008.

Emergence of a Safety Concern

Following the approval of the first two coronary DES, data were presented at the American College of Cardiology Scientific Sessions in Atlanta, Georgia, in March 2006 and at the European Society of Cardiology Annual Meeting/World Congress of Cardiology Meeting in Barcelona, Spain, in September 2006 that suggested a small but significant increase in the rate of stent thrombosis associated with DES compared to bare metal stents, occurring after the first year of implantation. Such a finding was of significant concern to physicians, manufacturers, and the FDA, as stent thrombosis is associated with high rates of acute MI and mortality.

Stent thrombosis was a known safety concern that had been observed with use of bare metal stents prior to the introduction of DES. Experience with bare metal stents revealed that the appropriate use of dual oral anti-platelet medications (aspirin plus a thienopyridine such as clopidogrel[1]) minimized the occurrence of stent thrombosis (which was typically observed within the first 30 days post stenting) until an endothelial lining was regenerated over the stent surface. Based on the antiproliferative actions of the drugs released from DES, the recommended duration of dual antiplatelet therapy following DES implantation was extended to 3 to 6 months, in recognition that inhibition of restenosis may also inhibit re-endothelialization of injured arterial surfaces and prolong the window of risk for stent thrombosis. Several reports noted that premature discontinuation of clopidogrel was an independent risk factor for stent thrombosis (Iakovou et al., 2005; Kuchulakanti et al., 2006). Moreover, meta-analyses of available randomized trials of the CYPHER stent and the TAXUS stent showed a numerical increase in the rates of stent thrombosis for both DES compared to their respective bare metal stent controls after 1 year. Further, an ongoing risk of approximately 0.6 percent per year was reported in patients receiving DES in two large European institutions (Daemen et al., 2007). Such data questioned whether 3 to 6 months of clopidogrel was sufficient, and raised

---

[1] Plavix®, sanofi-aventis U.S. LLC/Bristol-Myers Squibb Company, Bridgewater, New Jersey.

the possibility that a longer administration may be prudent. However, other publications reported cases of stent thrombosis despite the continued use of clopidogrel (Airoldi et al., 2007; de la Torre-Hernandez et al., 2008). Finally, the risk of bleeding associated with extended use of clopidogrel (as reported in the CREDO [Steinhubl et al., 2002], CURE [Fox et al., 2004], and CHARISMA [Bhatt et al., 2006] studies) has not been well characterized in comparison to a presumed reduction in risk of stent thrombosis. While appropriate use of clopidogrel is certainly important, other issues observed in cases of DES thrombosis include lesion factors (e.g., arterial bifurcations and long lesions requiring overlapping stents), hypersensitivity reactions to the DES polymer coating, and stent strut malapposition to the underlying arterial wall (Finn et al., 2007; Virmani et al., 2004). Thus, the occurrence of stent thrombosis is multifactorial, and in some cases clopidogrel use may not influence stent thrombosis rates.

FDA convened an Advisory Panel meeting on December 7 and 8, 2006, in an effort to fully characterize the risks, timing, and incidence of DES thrombosis. Three topics were discussed by the experts on the panel, DES manufacturers, and clinical investigators: (1) the rates of stent thrombosis and associated clinical sequelae (death and MI) when DES are used in accordance with their labeled indications; (2) the rates of stent thrombosis and associated clinical sequelae (death and MI) when DES are used in a broader, more complex population of patients and lesions; and (3) the optimal duration of dual antiplatelet therapy in patients who receive DES. The Panel concluded that both the CYPHER and TAXUS DES are associated with a small increase in stent thrombosis compared to bare metal stents that emerges 1 year post stent implantation. However, based on the data available, this increased risk of stent thrombosis was not associated with an increased risk of death or MI compared to bare metal stents. The Panel also found that off-label use of DES is associated with an increased risk of stent thrombosis, death, or MI compared to on-label use; however, with more complex patients, an increased risk in adverse events is not unexpected. Data on off-label use are limited, and additional studies are needed to determine optimal treatment strategies for more complex patients. Finally, the Panel concluded that the optimal duration of antiplatelet therapy, specifically clopidogrel, is unknown and DES thrombosis may still occur despite continued therapy. However, it recommended that the labeling for both approved DES should include reference to the American College of Cardiology/America Hospital Assocation/Society for Cardiovascular Angiography and Interventions PCI Practice Guidelines, which recommend that patients receive aspirin indefinitely plus a minimum of 3 months (for CYPHER patients) or 6 months (for TAXUS patients) of clopidogrel, with therapy extended to 12 months in patients at a low risk of bleeding. More specific information about the meeting and the conclusions reached are available on the FDA's website.[2]

Lessons Learned

Experience from the development, review, and marketing of the first two DES has provided several important lessons. First, the application of knowledge gained from past devices, such as bare metal stents, is not always appropriate or predictive for DES. As noted above, while stent thrombosis was known to occur with bare metal stents, simply extending the duration of antiplatelet therapy until a point beyond when drug elution is presumably complete (and theoretically, arterial healing would be complete with re-establishment of a functional endothelial covering on the stent) does not appear to have been sufficient to eliminate the risk of DES thrombosis. Second, although the FDA anticipated that the overwhelming efficacy of DES in the prevention of restenosis would lead to extensive use of DES in higher risk patients and lesions beyond those studied for initial approval (which were reflected in the labeled indication), the extent of this off-label use was surprising. The "all-comers" postapproval studies conducted by the manufacturers of CYPHER and TAXUS indicated that approximately 60 percent of patients who received DES after FDA approval had indications for stenting beyond those in the labeled indication, including patients with multiple vessel disease, with disease in the left main artery or in a bifurcated artery, and those patients being treated for an acute MI. In this setting, the data previously collected to describe the safety profile of these stents were only applicable to 40 percent of the population actually receiving them, compelling the FDA and manufacturers to find reasonable approaches to development of additional data to understand the risks and benefits in treatment of patients treated with DES outside of their approved indication of use. Third, the postmarket experience gained with the CYPHER and TAXUS stents indicated a need for longer follow-up in postmarket studies. With the emergence of stent thrombosis events occurring after 1 year post implantation, longer studies are needed to understand whether these events continue to accrue at the same rate or at an increasing or decreasing frequency after the first year and to understand the impact of these events on the incidence of cardiac death and MI during this time period. Fourth, more recently, the clinical trials of the Endeavor stent have enhanced our understanding of the relationship of angiographic imaging measurements (such as late lumen loss) to clinical end-points (such as target lesion or target vessel revascular-

---

[2] FDA statements available at http://www.fda.gov/cdrh/news/091406.html and http://www. fda.gov/cdrh/news/010407.html. Panel summary and transcript available at http://www.fda. gov/ohrms/dockets/ac/cdrh06.html#circulatory.

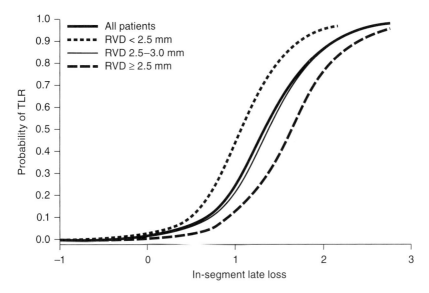

FIGURE 2-4 The relationship between late loss and TLR, evaluated using logistic regression.
SOURCE: Reprinted from the *Journal of the American College of Cardiology*, Vol 51, Pocock, SJ, et al., Angiographic surrogate endpoints in drug-eluting stent trials: A systematic evaluation based on individual patient data from 11 randomized, controlled trials. Pages 23-32. Copyright 2008, with permission from Elsevier.

ization [TLR or TVR, respectively]). As noted above, the Endeavor stent failed to meet non-inferiority for the angiographic endpoint comparing its late loss measurements to those of either CYPHER or TAXUS; however, a comparison of clinical measures (cardiac death, MI, and TVR) demonstrated that the Endeavor stent was non-inferior to the TAXUS stent. Why the apparent discrepancy? As observed in Figure 2-4, when the relationship between late loss and TLR is evaluated using logistic regression, the resulting model is curvilinear. In the case of the comparison of Endeavor to TAXUS, the observed late loss values (0.36 mm for Endeavor and 0.23 mm for TAXUS) are located on the flat portion of the late loss/TLR curve, a point at which a statistically significant difference in late loss between stents (or failure to achieve statistical non-inferiority) may not translate into important differences in a clinical end-point such as TLR.

Issues Needing Resolution

The issue of late stent thrombosis continues to be a critical issue for currently approved DES and the next generation of devices. Further study is needed to better define etiologies and their individual contributions to the overall risk of stent thrombosis. At present, there is no animal model that can predict stent thrombosis in patients, meaning that assessment of this clinically important event can only be conducted in human trials. Additionally, the FDA and the clinical community await further data to define the optimal duration of antiplatelet therapy that would appropriately balance a reduction in stent thrombosis with the risk of significant bleeding. Currently, the low event rates and the long term nature of the DES thrombosis question lead to the need for large trials of long duration. FDA currently requests that postmarket studies be designed and appropriately sized to define the incidence of stent thrombosis through at least 5 years of follow-up.

Patients who present with coronary artery disease and undergo stenting represent a heterogeneous population with diverse clinical features and atherosclerotic plaque morphology, which presents a challenge to manufacturers, investigators, and the FDA in the design of clinical studies. For certain patients, such as those with stable coronary artery disease involving discrete lesions in one or two coronary arteries, use of DES is the current standard of care, and as such, an approved DES can be used as a control. However, to evaluate DES in patients such as those who are treated in the course of an acute MI, or those with three-vessel disease, use of bare metal stents or coronary artery bypass graft surgery, respectively, may be an appropriate control. An efficient approach to study patients across this diverse population could lead to DES approval for extended indications, with more relevant clinical data available for physicians and patients weighing treatment options.

Issues for the Future

Looking ahead to development of new DES, a number of issues require consideration. With clinical event rates in the single digits and multiple DES on the market, manufacturers and investigators will face challenges in developing clinical trials that do not require ever-increasing sample sizes and that can be completed in a reasonable time period.

New technologies are also likely to pose additional issues for manufacturers and the FDA. By eliminating one or all of its components over time, degradable stent coatings and even fully degradable stents have the potential to reduce the risk of stent thrombosis compared to a permanent intra-arterial implant. However, standard test methods used for stents of durable materials will likely have to be altered and time periods for evaluation, such as in animal studies, lengthened to fully characterize the degradation process and the fate of the degradation products. Whether clinical studies will also require a longer follow-up duration, past the time of full degradation, to adequately assess safety and effectiveness remains to be determined. With the development of new stent platform designs and drug delivery mechanisms, future DES may elute more than one drug or be covered with biological substances such as cells or antibodies. Evaluation of novel DES, especially in the development of quality control measures, will require enhanced scientific methods and creativity on the part of the manufacturers and the FDA scientists tasked with assessment of these products.

Potential Solutions

Given the focus on safety concerns and the desire for clinical end-points, one might question whether angiographic studies still retain relevance. The FDA believes that these data remain important for several reasons. First, angiographic measurements provide mechanistic information about the performance of the stent. Second, because they enable comparative assessments of effectiveness in relatively small populations, angiographic end-points provide important information early in DES development when different drug doses or elution profiles are being considered. Such early studies may not only focus a manufacturer's efforts and resources on a DES candidate with a higher chance of success, they also may prevent ineffective stents from reaching large numbers of patients in a pivotal trial. Third, collection of intensive imaging assessments in early development may help to determine whether extended follow-up is necessary for degradable stents or durable stents with degradable coatings. In addition to angiography, other imaging modalities such as intravascular ultrasound (IVUS) provide important information on stent/arterial wall apposition and arterial remodeling.

As the FDA has moved to strengthen its available sources of information on products after they are approved for marketing, CDRH has also turned to the collection of postmarket information as a mechanism to augment premarket trial results, which by their nature are limited in scope and duration. As an example, an ideal safety end-point for a DES premarket trial would be a combination of cardiac death and MI; however, due to the low rates of these events, in a non-inferiority comparison to an approved DES that employs a clinically relevant non-inferiority margin, sample sizes would exceed 10,000. Therefore, the FDA recommends use of a composite that also contains an effectiveness measure (usually TLR) in premarket trials, but requests that a prespecified secondary hypothesis be established to compare rates of cardiac death and MI to the control, with a plan to collect additional data in postmarket studies to increase the precision of this comparison. Postmarket studies also allow for the evaluation of clinically significant adverse events that occur at very low rates, such as stent thrombosis. Such trials, especially if conducted as "all-comers" studies in which all consenting patients are entered, can enroll large numbers of patients rapidly, with extended follow-up to provide an improved assessment of the risk of stent thrombosis compared to relatively smaller and shorter premarket trials. In general, use of a combination of premarket trials and postmarket studies will provide the most efficient way to bring promising new products to market without compromising safety.

Postmarket studies also may offer a more efficient mechanism to gain certain expanded indications following initial marketing approval. The FDA is open to such an approach if hypotheses are established prospectively, appropriate performance goals or historical data can be identified to serve as controls, and the postmarket study is conducted under an IDE.

The lack of data to establish the optimal duration of dual antiplatelet therapy for patients receiving DES has left healthcare providers wondering how best to treat their patients, especially those who need to interrupt their therapy for an invasive surgical procedure. As noted above, however, given the low rates of stent thrombosis, to compare different durations of dual antiplatelet therapy would require studies of more than 10,000 patients for each individual DES. Based on available data, the FDA currently believes that this issue equally applies to all DES, which presents an opportunity to study this issue in DES as a class, rather than as separate products. With this in mind, as part of its Critical Path initiative,[3] the FDA is collaborating with device and drug manufacturers and academic physicians to develop a large study involving multiple DES in which clarity on this issue might finally be achieved.

In summary, a number of challenges face the FDA, manufacturers, and the clinical community in designing clinical trials to support marketing approval of future DES, in assuring that critical safety issues are answered, and in achieving these goals without stifling innovation. A mixture of premarket and postmarket data, thoughtful approaches to the design of clinical programs, and continued collaboration among manufacturers, healthcare providers, and the FDA will lead to potential solutions.

---

[3] More information available at http://www.fda.gov/oc/initiatives/criticalpath/.

BARIATRIC SURGERY

David R. Flum, M.D., M.P.H.
University of Washington

A Safer, Higher Quality, Learning Healthcare System in Surgery: The Role of Regional Collaboratives

One characteristic of a learning healthcare system is its capacity to generate the evidence needed to judge the effectiveness and cost-effectiveness of delivered care and to employ this evidence to deliver optimal care. Innovative surgical procedures and other invasive healthcare interventions represent a unique aspect of healthcare delivery that challenges a developing healthcare system. This review describes the challenges of evaluating interventions, the current state of evaluation of interventions and novel regional collaboratives that are more effectively evaluating the utility of procedures and should be an important component of our future healthcare system.

The Challenge of Evaluating Interventions

When considering the value of interventions the potential for harm caused by the intervention must be balanced by the harms relieved by addressing the condition. This is particularly the case with implantable devices, new procedures and techniques where there is no formalized process for training or postmarket surveillance of procedural harms. Since procedures are performed by individuals and often in nonstandardized fashion, the associated risk also may be considerably less predictable than the risk of more standardized interventions such as the administration of medications. Variation in outcome based on technical and technician factors is a well- established phenomenon, and variation in training, education, and practice is the hallmark of the surgical profession. For example, the adoption of new technologies into the operating room such as laparoscopic approaches to cholecystectomy, antireflux procedures and bariatric interventions did not follow rigorous animal testing or established training programs and at most hospitals required no proof of competency before introduction into practice. When first disseminated most practicing surgeons learned laparoscopy at weekend courses and then refined the skill in their patients. The surge in serious, common bile duct injury (CBDI) after the introduction of laparoscopic cholecystectomy (A prospective analysis of 1518 laparoscopic cholecystectomies. The Southern Surgeons Club, 1991) suggests in an extreme the potential of technician-related adverse outcome. In this case increasing rates of

CBDI (and variability in the occurrence of CBDI) were linked to surgeon inexperience and the inevitable outcome of a "technique in development" or the learning curve. Complicating issues of the learning curve is that there is no surveillance system for the detection of adverse outcomes. The regulatory environment places few limits on technologic innovation in the operating room and other areas where invasive treatments are performed. While pharmaceutical agents require rigorous pre- and sometimes post-market testing to demonstrate safety and efficacy, the regulatory burden for approval of new devices is much less stringent. For devices/procedures, regulatory systems focus on proof of concept rather than comparative effectiveness or even safety once the technology is no longer exclusively "in the hands" of experts. Furthermore, there is no regulatory requirement for innovative surgical interventions that do not involve a device but rather evolve from techniques and equipment already being used. Surgeons innovate on a daily basis using tools and techniques approved for other purposes with varying levels of success. Successful innovations are a staple of the profession and have undoubtedly resulted in improved procedures, but the failed innovations (and sometimes even the successful innovations) are neither systematically tracked nor reported to other surgeons. Moreover, industry stakeholders and thought leaders continually refine new techniques and devices making the study of any intervention a "moving target" and last year's research no longer applicable. Lastly, our healthcare culture includes doctors responding to marketing campaigns directed to patients and clinician-industry partnerships that make the control of new interventions and their evaluation deeply problematic.

Laparoscopic bariatric surgery—a set of interventions intended to help patients lose weight and address obesity-related comorbid conditions—are an example of a relatively newly developed procedure that demonstrates all of these pitfalls. While performed only occasionally in the early 1990s, by 2002 this was one of the fastest growing segments of the surgical marketplace. The growth was more than 10-fold in a decade (Santry et al., 2005) and laparoscopic roux-en-y gastric bypass is one of the most technically advanced and demanding. Training for these procedures was and remains highly variable; minimal credentialing requirements evolved only after the procedure grew in popularity, laparoscopic skills, techniques, and devices used for other operations were simply adapted to the bariatric field; and an entire field's experience grew through increasing practice. Absent a learning healthcare system, none of this growth or its expected outcomes was monitored in real time. Instead, scientific publications by the fields' experienced practitioners were taken to represent the community's experience with the procedures (Buchwald et al., 2004).

Effectiveness Versus Efficacy

A central problem in evaluating the value of interventions and devices is in distinguishing effectiveness (the extent to which it "works" in general practice) from efficacy (the extent to which it "works" in the controlled environment [i.e., among experts, research centers, trials, etc.]). It is very unusual for a new device or intervention to be tested in these real world environments, but effectiveness evaluations are really the only way to accommodate the varied training, experience, skill, and unselected populations that are found in the "average community." Case series predominate in the reporting of new devices and interventions, and these are most often the product of clinicians reporting their best results and journals more willing to publish studies with better outcomes and larger numbers of patients. This is a form of publication bias that is difficult to track but assuredly occurs. Even when consecutive cohort studies are considered they are most often the product of expert clinicians and referral centers. These doctors undoubtedly have learned how to select patients well and have developed nonintervention-related success strategies (i.e., post-procedural care, pre-procedural interventions like smoking cessation—subtle, nonreported exclusions) that may interact with the effects of the intervention. This form of selection bias (selected clinicians and selected patients) makes it very hard to estimate the anticipated effects of the procedure when applied in the general community. Though this efficacy versus effectiveness conundrum is critical when evaluating intended treatment effects, it may be even more important when considering unintended effects such as safety problems. Most studies of devices and interventions are aimed at demonstrating therapeutic effect and so are relatively underpowered to identify important procedure-related harms (i.e., laparoscopic cholecystectomy and bile duct injury). It may take many years for individual clinician case reports focused on efficacy to reveal a safety outcome of concern as the technique is diffusing. The healthcare community has occasionally anticipated such problems and controlled the diffusion of new techniques. One example is laparoscopic colon resection for cancer where the American Society of Colon and Rectal Surgeons (ASCRS) applied a virtual moratorium on this technique (The American Society of Colon and Rectal Surgeons, 1994) while several studies were being conducted to assess its safety. Perhaps learning from the bile duct injury experience, ASCRS applied professional "peer pressure" through its journals and meetings to essentially restrict the application of the technique until concerns about port site recurrence and other safety/efficacy outcomes could be resolved. Relying on professional societies to restrict the diffusion of new and emerging techniques and devices has by no means been the norm so it has fallen to evaluators of the healthcare system to assess a procedure's value after its introduction.

In bariatric surgery no such moratorium took hold and rapid diffusion among a group of laparoscopic surgeons with highly variable skillsets took place. There was the proliferation of many case series suggesting high levels of safety and efficacy (Buchwald et al., 2004), but equal reports from the media of high-profile adverse outcomes and deaths that stimulated some state agencies to close down bariatric programs and prompted radical responses from the academic and public health communities (Commonwealth of Massachusetts Betsy Lehman Center for Patient Safety and Medical Error Reduction Expert Panel on Weight Loss Surgery: Executive Report, 2005).

Population-Level Research

Usually the product of academic research projects, our current healthcare system employs several techniques to assess effectiveness and safety. Most of these strategies require a post-hoc approach that assesses the impact of interventions years after they have occurred. This is often accomplished by studying medical claims data that has been submitted to billing agencies, state or federal repositories. These claims include virtually no clinical data, rely on often crude codes to describe procedures, lack codes to match updated procedures and have limited outcome information beyond discharge disposition (alive, dead, skilled nursing facility, etc.). These datasets do not include interventions performed in the outpatient environment, most are cross-sectional and miss outcome (including death) after discharge, and the ones with more subtle coding schemes (CPT codes instead of ICD9 codes) are for limited populations (Medicaid, Medicare, individual insurers). The timeliness of the data is problematic (often available years after the events) as is the granularity and accuracy of the coding schemes for risk adjustment. Despite these considerable limitations, when used for specific purposes they can help inform the healthcare system about the impact of procedures in the real world—the average community, average patient, average clinicians—without concern of publication or selection bias. Our group has used a longitudinal dataset based on Washington State hospital discharge abstracts (CHARS) to demonstrate (1) higher than expected rates of bile duct injury when less experienced surgeons fail to use an intraoperative x-ray (cholangiogram) to confirm anatomy (Flum et al., 2001a), (2) serious injury with laparoscopic anti-reflux surgery (Flum et al., 2002), (3) recurrence rates after modern incisional hernia repairs (Flum et al., 2003), (4) unnecessary appendectomy despite the availability of better diagnostic testing (Flum et al., 2001b), and (5) perioperative deaths and complications after bariatric surgery (Flum and Dellinger, 2004). In each case, these rates were "higher than expected" because the expected was derived from case series provided mostly by highly experienced experts. These studies may be used to help frame a discussion about a procedures value through the context of effectiveness and can be important for insurance coverage decisions. For example, an evaluation showing relatively high perioperative mortality rates after bariatric surgery in a high-risk population—the Medicare disabled (Flum et al., 2005b)—was incorporated into a Centers for Medicare & Medicaid Services (CMS) coverage decision restricting the care of these patients to experienced centers. This was a public health policy intervention aimed at reducing procedural harm based on administrative data. Undoubtedly, our healthcare system "learns" from these research-based initiatives but the learning happens late, depends on interested investigators with narrow focus, and is at best uncoordinated.

Power of the Purchaser to Determine Effectiveness

Relying on the research community for these "after the fact" analyses, however, is a poor and not particularly sustainable way to build a safe, effective healthcare system. Large healthcare purchasers have been able to exert some positive influence in directing the system towards assessment of safety and effectiveness by crafting coverage decisions that generate evidence. On at least a few occasions, CMS has required that as a condition of coverage, patients be placed and followed on registry after novel interventions were introduced. Carotid stenting (Gray et al., 2007) and implantable defibrillators (Hammill et al., 2007) are two examples where this registry-based approach has undoubtedly limited the diffusion of the technique. For carotid stenting this registry approach has already identified a subgroup with a prohibitive risk for which stenting is not appropriate. More "coverage with registry" may be the single most effective way to determine the effectiveness of new interventions before their broad dissemination, but the lack of surveillance systems and reliable registry infrastructure may limit their development. Medicare's decision regarding bariatric surgery was like a "coverage on registry" approach in that it approved the procedures only at accredited centers and a component of accreditation is participation in a registry-like activity aimed at monitoring and improving outcomes.

A different approach to gathering real-world evidence using a randomized intervention was helpful in determining the true value of lung volume reduction surgery (LVRS) for patients with chronic obstructive pulmonary disease (COPD) (Fishman et al., 2003). After years of being touted as life-saving treatment compared to selected or historic nonoperative cohorts, CMS restricted its payments of the procedures to patients enrolled in a randomized trial. The study, though conducted at a limited number of centers, demonstrated that LVRS was effective for only a small subset of patients and was contraindicated in another. The study found that LVRS was not particularly cost effective, and taken together these findings have dramatically curtailed its use.

The LVRS example included safety, efficacy/effectiveness, and cost-effectiveness in a nearly real-time fashion to inform the system about the true value of LVRS, and it accelerated our understanding of its role in our healthcare system. That is the hallmark of a learning healthcare system but one that is hard to replicate.

Regional Collaboratives

Though perhaps ideal, the active evidence generation of the LVRS trial has not been repeated for other controversial procedures and devices. LVRS required tremendous political and administrative leadership, was quite controversial and expensive for both the National Institutes of Health (NIH) and CMS, and required academics with an interest in the topic to come together despite their opinions. For these reasons, such studies are not likely to be the mechanism for the future "learning healthcare system" to use and evaluate new procedures and devices contemporaneously. A novel approach to contemporaneous use/evaluation of new procedures is coming from regional clinical collaboratives aimed at improving healthcare delivery. These collaboratives acknowledge that the health system evaluations performed by academic researchers may not be the most effective way to correct the lapses they identify. Academics are rewarded for work that identifies outcome variation and lapses in quality through grants, media recognition, and promotions, but lack the incentive or the skillsets to be involved in the correction of these lapses. The latter is work that typically requires community engagement, is not well funded, and may take years to accomplish.

These collaboratives include larger groups of clinicians who are working in the field and taking it in their own hands to create the types of learning systems that will correct themselves and deliver more optimal care. They are often limited in scope and resources but can be very effective. In Kentucky (Shively et al., 2004) general surgeons organized in the late 1990s to gather data from their own cases, to define optimal care delivery for commonly performed procedures, and to create systems that accomplished their delivery. In New England, vascular surgeons from over 10 institutions have recently partnered in a peer-to-peer network called The Vascular Study Group of Northern New England[16] that is evaluating performance of certain novel vascular surgical procedures. In Washington State, surgeons from over 25 hospitals representing three-quarters of all the surgical care in the state have organized the Surgical Care and Outcomes Assessment Program (SCOAP) (Flum et al., 2005a).[4] These collaboratives represent a growing movement that may be the most effective way to track

---

[4] See www.surgicalCOAP.org.

the use of interventions and their outcomes while simultaneously working to improve their quality.

SCOAP is a regional collaborative improving the quality and safety of surgical care and delivering more appropriate and cost-effective care. SCOAP has two components—a surveillance system gathering data on process of care and outcome of consecutive procedures at all participating hospitals, and an active correction function that engages surgeons to correct lapses in care delivery. The surveillance system relies on information technology infrastructures of varying sophistication (from paper based to full electronic medical record [EMR]) and joins surgeons at hospitals from all over the state—in rural and urban environments and in hospitals big and small—in a data-sharing/feedback network. The corrective function of SCOAP works through education, peer support/pressure, and effective use of checklists. Now in its second year, SCOAP has been continuously assessing the processes and outcomes associated with emerging procedures (i.e., laparoscopic gastric bypass, endovascular procedures of the aorta, minimally invasive pediatric surgery, and many others) and helping clinicians redirect care when lapses have been identified. SCOAP allows for innovation on the surgeon level but engages innovating surgeons in a clinician-led management committee so the variables that account for innovation/variation are included in SCOAP data collection. In this way, new procedures and techniques are simultaneously used and evaluated, and a learning healthcare system can be driven toward better performance. For example, using SCOAP data and the SCOAP quality improvement (QI) platform, bariatric surgeons (like other general, colorectal, pediatric, and vascular surgeons) are tracking quarter by quarter for changes in outcome and helping direct local QI activities to improve care delivery.

Another program aiming to assess the impact of procedures is the National Surgical Quality Improvement Program (NSQIP). NSQIP is supported by the American College of Surgeons and measures morbidity and mortality from surgical care at nearly 200 hospitals across the United States. Other national initiatives to study procedural effectiveness come from specialty societies such as The Society for Thoracic Surgery (STS), American College of Cardiology, and the Association for Thoracic Surgery. Strengths of these programs are that participation has become a cultural norm and in some cases a requirement for procedural payment. But all of these national datasets function at the level of surveillance, and because they carry a heavy administrative burden may not change quickly to accommodate innovation particularly well. Only variably do these surveillance systems draw communities of clinicians together to respond to problems in performance, and they may not be as focused on creating the learning/improving aspects of the developing healthcare system. An interesting hybrid exists in Washington State where a regional collaborative called Clinical Outcomes

Assessment Program (COAP) (Maynard et al., 2003) has been working for a decade to draw all hospitals in the state that deliver cardiac care together in programs that respond to variation found through the STS data such as reducing the use of transfusions to make surgical care safer.

Barriers and Policy Opportunities for Creating a Learning Healthcare System

Regional activities like SCOAP face tremendous obstacles because they are both hard to develop and sustain. Linking clinicians and hospitals across regions requires a sense of community among these groups that may not exist, and in many geographic areas these relationships have been strained through competition and other forces. Reconnecting as a clinical community and developing trust and mutual interest requires genuine engagement, leveling of hierarchies, and some fence mending. There is also no financial incentive for the volunteered time, team building, and development work that are a component of these initiatives and better performance through collaborative work is not specifically reimbursed. In some regions, the public health importance of an activity like SCOAP may not be enough to overcome the lack of incentives and broken relationships and unless a large payer with dominance in the marketplace compels this activity it may not even be possible. When a large payer does step in, these payer-led programs usually become pay for performance (P4P) initiatives such as the Surgical Care Improvement Program (SCIP) (MedQIC, 2008). Because P4P involves reimbursement and by default "winners and losers," initiatives with heavy payer involvement focus on metrics that have the highest levels of evidence (and there are few procedure-based metrics that have high impact), require careful risk adjustment so that hospitals are not unfairly penalized (and there are not great risk-adjustment strategies), and come with a "top-down" feel that may not achieve the potential of peer-to-peer regional network. A variation on this theme that may work best has occurred in Michigan where a single payer aligned with clinical leaders at the University of Michigan and together they were able to build engagement across all hospitals and accomplish surveillance (using National Surgical Quality Improvement Program [NSQIP]) while hospitals benefited from millions of dollars worth of corporate investment and defrayed data collection costs (Birkmeyer et al., 2005). We have not found that other insurers in more plural markets have the willingness to commit to regional collaborative development on this level. Legislators also may want to compel this type of surveillance and QI activity, and while that may ensure that all hospitals participate and that at least certain metrics are measured, initiatives that come from legislative mandate have a punitive component. As a result, these may also fail to engage innovating clinicians in the most productive manner. Large healthcare providers and health maintenance organizations may be best suited to facilitate these activities. Because they both employ clinicians and insure patients, they have alignment of financial interest and direct oversight of care delivery that is unheard of in more fractured systems. These groups (i.e., Kaiser Permanente, Group Health Cooperative) usually have better information technology (IT) allowing surveillance without as much chart abstraction that is required at hospitals without EMRs. This linkage of financial accountability and IT systems effectively compels clinicians to participate in surveillance and correction, but will only affect the members of those care networks and has limited applicability to the broader healthcare system. For example, in Washington State, 88 percent of patients do not receive care in such a system.

There are several policy opportunities that would allow a regional collaborative to flourish and should be considered in the development of a more effective, learning healthcare system. The U.S. Department of Health and Human Services and the Agency for Healthcare Research and Quality have developed the Chartered Healthcare Value Exchange program (AHRQ, 2008) as an attempt to support regional quality improvement. While acute care has not been the focus of the program, including surgical/intervention care within its mandate and approving the ones (like SCOAP) that exist as test cases would clearly encourage the development of these systems to monitor and improve acute care. Medicare and other large insurers should consider preferential contracting to hospitals and clinicians that participate in such regional collaboratives as both demonstration projects and when considering "coverage with registry" decisions. This would obviate the need to recreate the wheel of valid and secure registries each time a new procedure was considered, would assure broad geographic application (i.e., not just major medical centers), and would assure that care delivered in these registries was being optimized by the engaged clinicians. Medicolegal protection of collaboratives such as SCOAP is also essential. SCOAP operates under the aegis of a state statute protecting these data from discovery (because they are being used for quality improvement), but not all states have such provisions, and the lack of such protection may be a barrier to further collaborative development. The limits of the current information technology infrastructure may be the greatest barrier to effective surveillance, and there are several congressional leaders working on this issue. We still appear to be many years away from the types of systems that would make monitoring of interventions with the "push of a button" a possibility at all hospitals across a region. For many years to come we will still rely on human abstraction of chart data, and while that will cost more, at least it should inform the design of the ultimately successful EMR. Lastly, a learning healthcare system has to recognize that it may not "get it right" the first time and that correcting lapses in care require both carrot and stick approaches. There are few carrots (i.e., financial incentives) for volunteering the time, energy and effort for clinicians and their hospitals to deliver optimal care. As outlined above, preferential contracting to SCOAP hospitals and surgeons, for example, would be the most effective carrot for their development but may limit their effectiveness if overly prescriptive. "Stick approaches" include public exposure of underperformance, and that is often a motivator for those who believe that all data from such collaboratives should be given to the public. It is well accepted that the public has a right to know how the health system is performing, and transparency of data will be a touchstone in developing our new, learning healthcare system. Complete transparency, however may not be compatible with the development of these voluntary, self-correcting collaboratives. We should recognize these nuances of transparency and acknowledge that a limited, "reporting" dataset that grows with time should be the aim while clinicians are working to understand and then improve using a more restricted "developmental" dataset. Only in this way will the healthcare system continue to innovate at the same time it evaluates and improves performance.

Summary

- Health system evaluation of the utility of new interventions, procedures, and devices is challenging because of differences in efficacy and effectiveness and in distinguishing the effects of the technology from the clinicians who apply the technology.
- The current system encourages innovation but has not effectively monitored safety/effectiveness or created ways to optimize interventions.
- A learning healthcare system should allow for the development/use of novel interventions while they are contemporaneously evaluated and then modified as needed to be maximally safe and effective.
- Common approaches to evaluate interventions are ineffective because they are not contemporaneous or sensitive enough (i.e., administrative database research) or because they are too costly and challenging to organize (large-scale randomized trials linked to coverage), but coverage on registry may be an effective tool especially if linked to regional collaboratives of engaged clinicians.
- Regional collaboratives that create a surveillance system assessing interventions and incorporating self-correction to improve performance offer the best elements of a learning healthcare system and should be encouraged.
- Policy opportunities to encourage regional collaboratives:
  — Medicare and other payer demonstration projects providing payer-based incentives for participating members and hospitals.

— Recognizing acute care delivery in current initiatives rewarding regional quality improvement (Chartered Healthcare Value Exchange).

— State-level protections of data from medicolegal exposure if used only for the purposes of quality improvement and recognizing the importance of reasonable, rather than complete, transparency of the data these collaboratives generate.

ANTIPSYCHOTIC THERAPEUTICS

Philip S. Wang, M.D., Dr.P.H., National Institute of Mental Health and Harvard Medical School; M. Alan Brookhart, Ph.D., Harvard Medical School; Soko Setoguchi, M.D., Dr.P.H., Harvard Medical School; Christine Ulbricht, B.A., National Institute of Mental Health; Sebastian Schneeweiss, M.D., Sc.D., Harvard Medical School

Abstract

Antipsychotic medications are now widely utilized by patients and account for a large proportion of pharmaceutical spending, particularly in public healthcare programs. In spite of this, there is a paucity of evidence on the clinical effectiveness of antipsychotic regimens to help guide clinical, purchasing, and policy decisions. Fortunately, there have been advances in the populations, databases, study designs, and analytic methods that investigators can employ to help ensure that antipsychotic medication use is clinically effective. Several studies are raised to illustrate the potential of these developments. Findings from the recently completed NIMH-sponsored comparative effectiveness trials of antipsychotic medications in patients with schizophrenia (the CATIE schizophrenia trial) and Alzheimer's dementia (the CATIE-AD trial) are described. An example of using clinical epidemiologic data and methods when trial data are not available—in this instance to determine if conventional and atypical antipsychotics share the same mortality risks in elderly patients—is also covered. Likewise, a study of the impact of limiting psychotropic prescriptions on patients with schizophrenia using quasi-experimental methods illustrates their utility when actual trials may not be feasible. Finally, simulation methods are raised as a means to answer questions concerning antipsychotic effectiveness when trials, clinical epidemiologic and even quasi-experimental studies may not be possible—in this case to shed light on the clinical effectiveness of a hypothetical strategy of using clozapine as a first-line antipsychotic agent.

Introduction

Both the Institute of Medicine's Roundtable on Value & Science-Driven Health Care and the Congressional Budget Office (2007) have raised the importance of research to improve the clinical effectiveness of medical treatments. Nowhere is the need for such research greater than in the case of antipsychotic medication regimens used to treat schizophrenia spectrum and other psychotic disorders. The remainder of this chapter provides a brief description of the reasons why this clinical effectiveness research is necessary, recent advances in the research armamentarium available to conduct such investigations, and examples of how these research designs and methods have been applied in studies of antipsychotic medication effectiveness.

Clinical Effectiveness Research on Antipsychotic Medications to Improve Practice and Inform Policy

Synthesis of the first antipsychotic medication, chlorpromazine, in 1954 launched the modern era of pharmacotherapy for schizophrenia as well as other mental disorders (Schatzberg and Nemeroff, 2006). Thereafter, numerous related "first-generation" neuroleptic drugs were developed that all blocked dopamine-2 receptors in the central nervous system. In the late 1980s, a newer "second-generation" of antipsychotic medications was developed that promised to improve upon the earlier, conventional drugs—hence their designation as "atypical" agents. While most atypicals are distinguishable only by their side effect profiles, one agent, clozapine, has been found to not only possess superior efficacy for treating refractory schizophrenia but also increases the risk for agranulocytosis (Kane et al., 1988).

In spite of a half-century of experience with antipsychotic medications, data on their clinical effectiveness are urgently needed for several reasons. First, in the absence of information on the effectiveness of agents—especially compared to available alternatives—practice decisions are often made on the basis of efficacy and safety data that may not represent the outcomes achievable in typical patients or circumstances. For example, earlier randomized controlled clinical trials suggested that the newer second-generation atypical antipsychotics were less likely than the older conventional neuroleptics to cause side effects such as extrapyramidal symptoms and were possibly more efficacious for the negative symptoms of schizophrenia (Leucht et al., 1999). On the basis of such data as well as their promotion as being safer and more tolerable, atypical use increased rapidly in the second half of the 1990s and soon accounted for the majority of antipsychotic use (Wang et al., 2000)—many years before findings from comparative effectiveness trials such as the NIMH CATIE study became available (Lieberman et al., 2005). When even RCT data do not exist, practice decisions are often made on the basis of anecdote or judgment. An analysis of a nationally generalizable sample of U.S. psychiatrists revealed that by the late 1990s over 1 in 6 patients with schizophrenia spectrum disorders were being given standing regimens of multiple concurrent antipsychotics, despite the lack of data on the effectiveness or safety of this practice (Wang et al., 2000). In fact, some emerging evidence suggests the polypharmacy regimen of clozapine plus risperidone may not be superior to clozapine alone (Honer et al., 2006).

In part because of rapid adoption and diffusion of new regimens before sufficient clinical effectiveness data are available, antipsychotic medication costs have increased dramatically especially in public programs such as Medicare and Medicaid. According to the Congressional Budget Office, federal spending on Medicare and Medicaid as a share of gross domestic product has tripled over the past 30 years, rising from 1.3 percent in 1975 to 4 percent in 2007; this spending is projected to continue increasing to 12 percent of gross domestic product (GDP) by 2050 under current policies (Congressional Budget Office, 2007). Spending on just atypicals comprises nearly 30 percent of total drug expenditures for some Medicaid programs (Polinski et al., 2007). Without clear data on the effectiveness and safety of antipsychotic regimens, public and private payers are left uncertain if such costs are justified. These challenges were evident in one recent analysis of Medicaid prior authorization policies, a frequently applied means by which insurers attempt to control drug costs (Polinski et al., 2007). In this analysis there appeared to be no consistent relationship between the application of prior authorization policies and overall spending on atypical antipsychotic medications, suggesting that Medicaid programs may not have sufficient data on their comparative effectiveness to know whether their use should be promoted or deterred. This study also suggested that a paucity of data may leave payers ill-equipped to respond to new challenges such as emerging drug safety issues or regulatory advisories. In April 2005, the Food and Drug Administration (FDA) issued an advisory describing increased mortality among elderly patients with dementia taking atypical antipsychotics. More than a year later, no state Medicaid program changed its prior authorization policy in response, again suggesting that insufficient clinical effectiveness data exist for policy makers to weigh risks and benefits from regimens and tailor their decisions accordingly (Polinski et al., 2007).

A final reason why new clinical effectiveness research is needed is that in spite of large healthcare expenditures, many people with schizophrenia and other forms of serious mental illness experience unmet needs for effective treatment and poor health outcomes. Studies of the general U.S. population have shown that the vast majority of people experiencing a serious psychotic disorder in the prior year fail to receive adequate care (Wang et al., 2002b). Examinations of geographic variation in health care spending and outcomes also suggest many of the treatments received are of poor quality and likely to be ineffective. For example, despite spending the greatest percentage of GDP on health care, there is little evidence that the United States achieves better outcomes; in fact, recent data from the World Health Organization's World Mental Health Survey indicate the rate of receiving effective treatment in the United States lags behind other developed nations (Wang et al., 2007).

Advances in Clinical Effectiveness Research

How can investigators answer the many remaining questions concerning the clinical effectiveness of antipsychotic medications, enhance practice, and inform policy as well as purchasing decisions? As importantly, how can valid answers—both externally as well as internally—be generated feasibly, quickly, and affordably? Fortunately, there have been recent advances in populations, databases, study designs, and analytic methods that have expanded the armamentarium investigators can draw upon.

New effectiveness trials—called practical clinical trials—can be used to explicitly answer the pressing questions faced by clinicians and decisions makers (March et al., 2005; Tunis et al., 2003). Practical clinical trials compare clinically relevant alternative regimens on a broad range of outcomes in typical patients. Recruiting representative and adequate numbers of such patients from diverse settings has been greatly assisted by establishing practice-based clinical trial networks. For example, building practice-based clinical trial networks in schizophrenia, depression, and bipolar disorder was essential for allowing NIMH to conduct the CATIE, STAR-D, and STEP-BD practical clinical trials (Lieberman et al., 2005; Sachs et al., 2007; Trivedi et al., 2006). Other advances in clinical trial methodology—such as new adaptive designs and cluster randomization (Glynn et al., 2007; Murphy et al., 2007) also have been crucial and offer great promise for conducting new clinical effectiveness research in the future.

Clearly many pressing questions will not be amenable to study through comparative effectiveness trials, either because such trials are not feasible, affordable, or in some cases ethical. For this reason, developments in clinical epidemiology and other clinical effectiveness research methodologies have been important. New study populations and data sources are available for descriptive and analytic studies of mental health treatments. Nationally representative resources include the American Psychiatric Association's Practice Research Network of psychiatrists and general population surveys such as the National Comorbidity Survey Replication (Wang et al.,

2000, 2005a). Available governmental administrative databases such as from Medicaid programs are often enriched with patients with psychiatric disorders due to the poverty and disability associated with mental illnesses; likewise, available HMO databases are an excellent resource for studying primary care, the most frequent setting for mental health treatments (Wang et al., 2002a). However, taking advantage of these resources for clinical effectiveness research has also required the development of new methodologies. For example, developing new analytic methods for observational studies that offer enhanced control for confounding, such as propensity scores and instrumental variable techniques, is crucial (Brookhart et al., 2007; Sturmer et al., 2007). Likewise, advances in the methodologies available for conducting quasi-experimental studies and simulation studies are critical (Gold et al., 1996; Schneeweiss et al., 2001).

Examples of Clinical Effectiveness Research on Antipsychotic Medications

The remainder of this article covers studies that illustrate how these developments in populations, databases, study designs, and analytic methods could be used to improve the clinical effectiveness of antipsychotic medications.

Comparative Effectiveness Trials of Antipsychotic Medications

The NIMH CATIE Schizophrenia Trial. As mentioned above, earlier randomized controlled efficacy trials had suggested that atypical agents might cause fewer extrapyramidal side effects and might possibly be better at treating negative symptoms than first-generation neuroleptics (Leucht et al., 1999). However, the largely industry-sponsored trials that were available presented an at times confusing view of the relative advantages and drawbacks of individual agents (Heres et al., 2006). Furthermore, head-to-head data on the comparative effectiveness of antipsychotic medications in real-world patient populations and typical practice conditions were lacking. For this reason, NIMH supported the Clinical Antipsychotic Trial of Intervention Effectiveness (CATIE) trials in schizophrenia. From the outset, the CATIE schizophrenia study was designed to be an effectiveness rather than an efficacy trial. It involved a large (1,460) number of patients with chronic schizophrenia drawn from 57 diverse practice sites in 24 states. Typical patients (e.g., those with comorbid conditions) and practice conditions (e.g., switching treatments and adjunctive medications) were included. Patients were randomized in Phase I to one of four atypical agents (olanzapine, quetiapine, risperidone, and ziprasidone) or an active comparator agent (the conventional drug perphenazine) and followed for 18 months. On the primary outcome of all-cause discontinuation, three-quarters of all patients were unable to remain on their treatments due to inefficacy or intolerable side effects (Lieberman et al., 2005). Olanzapine was the most effective antipsychotic but this superiority appeared to come at the price of greater weight gain and increases in glucose and lipids. The conventional antipsychotic, perphenazine, was comparable in efficacy to the remaining atypical agents although it was associated with more discontinuation due to extrapyramidal side effects. In a subsequent cost-effectiveness analysis, (Rosenheck et al., 2006) treatment with perphenazine was associated with 20–30 percent lower healthcare costs (largely due to lower drugs costs from available generics) and comparable effectiveness as the second-generation medications.

The NIMH CATIE Alzheimer's Dementia Trial. Antipsychotic medications are also prescribed to elderly patients with dementia to control behavioral disturbances. The frequency of neuroleptic prescribing led to federal legislation in the 1980s restricting such use (Schorr et al., 1994). However, the introduction of atypicals and some efficacy studies finding modest improvements in agitation with their use led to atypicals becoming the pharmacologic treatment of choice for behavioral disturbances in dementia patients (Alexopoulos et al., 2004; Jeste et al., 2005; Kindermann et al., 2002; Sink et al., 2005). One recent study estimated that one-quarter of Medicare beneficiaries in nursing homes are given atypical agents (Breisacher et al., 2005).

To shed light on the relative benefits and risks of such practices, NIMH also conducted a comparative effectiveness trial of atypical antipsychotic medications used in Alzheimer's dementia (CATIE-AD). Outpatients (421) were drawn from 42 practice sites and randomized to olanzapine, quetiapine, risperidone, or placebo and followed for up to 36 weeks. No differences were found between arms on the time to all-cause discontinuation. Although olanzapine and risperidone appeared to possess greater efficacy than quetiapine or placebo, these advantages were offset by more adverse effects (Schneider et al., 2006). In a cost-effectiveness analysis, there were no differences in effectiveness between active treatments or placebo, but there were significantly lower healthcare costs for patients assigned to placebo (Rosenheck et al., 2007).

Clinical Epidemiology Studies of Antipsychotic Effectiveness

Mortality Risks from Conventional versus Atypical Antipsychotics in the Elderly. Strengths of the CATIE trials—including their large number of typical patients drawn from diverse practice sites and observed over long follow-up periods—also contributed to high costs, in excess of $50 million. While there continues to be a pressing need for data on the comparative effectiveness of antipsychotic regimens, such costs, the time required for completion, and other challenges of conducting large practical clinical trials make it clear that additional means will be needed to answer urgent public health questions.

A study of the short-term mortality associated with conventional antipsychotic use by elderly patients illustrates how clinical epidemiology might be used when data from comparative effectiveness trials are not available or possible. In 2005, the FDA issued an advisory warning that the atypicals aripiprazole, olanzapine, quetiapine, and risperidone were associated with a 60–70 percent increased risk of death versus placebo in 17 short-term randomized placebo-controlled trials among elderly dementia patients (FDA, 2005). "Black box" warnings were added to the labels of all atypical antipsychotics describing these risks and advising that atypicals were not approved for behavioral symptoms from dementia in elderly patients. A meta-analysis by Schneider and colleagues (Schneider et al., 2005) of 15 short-term randomized controlled trials also found a statistically significant 54 percent increased relative risk of death and 1 percent absolute risk difference for atypical antipsychotics versus placebo.

Because of insufficient clinical trial data on the mortality associated with conventional antipsychotics in elderly dementia patients, the FDA did not include these agents in its advisory (FDA, 2005; Kuehn, 2005). For this reason, clinicians might have simply switched elderly patients to these older agents (Strong, 2005), particularly since their replacement by the newer drugs occurred relatively rapidly and recently (Dewa et al., 2002). However, based mainly on extrapolations from younger populations, some suggested that conventional antipsychotic medications could in theory pose risks equal to or greater than those of the newer drugs in older populations (Chan et al., 1999; Lawlor, 2004; Maixner et al., 1999; Tariot, 1999).

In a clinical epidemiologic study based upon data from the largest U.S. state pharmacy benefit program for the elderly, we found that those initiating conventional agents had a 37 percent greater dose-dependent risk of short-term mortality than those prescribed atypical antipsychotics (Wang et al., 2005b). These results were robust to alternative analytic methods to control for potential confounding, including multivariate Cox models, propensity-score adjustments, and an instrumental variable analysis employing the prescribing physician's preference for conventional or atypical antipsychotics as the instrument (Brookhart et al., 2007). In spite of confirmatory analyses in other populations and databases (Schneeweiss et al., 2007), the risk of unmeasured or unadjusted confounding cannot be completely excluded in clinical epidemiologic studies. For this reason, a meta-analysis of randomized trials among elderly with dementia that found the conventional agent, haloperidol, increased short-term mortality versus placebo by 107 percent (a risk numerically greater than that seen for atypical agents) provides some additional reassurance concerning the internal validity of these clinical epidemiologic findings (Schneider et al., 2005).

Quasi-Experimental Studies of Antipsychotic Effectiveness

Impact of Limiting Psychotropic Prescription Benefits on Patients with Schizophrenia. Quasi-experimental studies are another promising means for improving the effectiveness of antipsychotic regimens, particularly by informing the design of sound public policies. One illustrative example examined the impacts of imposing a three-prescription-per-month cap for psychotropic drugs on Medicaid beneficiaries with schizophrenia (Soumerai et al., 1994). Interrupted time series regression analyses were employed to examine changes in the rates of medication and other healthcare utilization—from a baseline 14-month period prior to the prescription cap's implementation, to the 11 months during its application, as well as to a 17-month period after the cap was discontinued. To control for background temporal trends in the use of psychotropic medications and other forms of health care, the investigators employed a comparison cohort from a state with no restrictions on drug reimbursement during the study periods.

Results from this study indicated that this form of limiting psychotropic prescription drug coverage significantly reduced antipsychotic medication consumption by 15 percent. Implementing the cap was also associated with a significant 57 percent increase in the frequency of visits to community mental health centers as well as a sharp increase in the use of emergency mental health services and partial hospitalizations. Use of antipsychotic and other psychotropic medications, as well as most mental health services, returned to their baseline levels after the psychotropic prescription cap policy was abandoned. An accompanying economic analysis indicated the increase in total mental healthcare costs per patient to Medicaid during the cap exceeded the savings in drug costs by a factor of 17.

Simulation Studies of Antipsychotic Effectiveness

The Cost-Effectiveness of Using Clozapine as a First-Line Versus Third-Line Antipsychotic. Clearly, clinical epidemiologic studies and quasi-experimental studies provide useful means for improving the effectiveness of antipsychotic medication practices and policies when comparative effectiveness trials may not be available, affordable, or feasible. However there also are many questions concerning the clinical effectiveness of antipsychotics that may not be answerable, even by clinical epidemiologic or quasi-experimental designs. This is especially true for hypothetical antipsychotic medication strategies or practices for which empirical data are absent. In such situations, simulation studies may be the only alternative available to shed light on the clinical effectiveness of regimens.

One such hypothetical regimen involves using the atypical clozapine as a first-line agent. Since its introduction in the late 1980s, clozapine has been restricted to only patients who have failed at least two trials of other antipsychotic medications because of concerns that its use as a first-line agent would lead to greater mortality, mainly through agranulocytosis. Another requirement initially imposed because of this risk was that patients have their white blood cell (WBC) counts checked weekly prior to receiving each week's prescription. Because of such requirements, clozapine has been underutilized even among treatment-resistant patients with schizophrenia (Conley and Buchanan, 1997).

However, since these restrictions on clozapine were imposed, additional evidence has emerged. A meta-analysis (Wahlbeck et al., 1999) and other RCT data (Lieberman et al., 2003) from treatment-sensitive as well as treatment-resistant patients, found that clozapine is significantly more likely than conventional antipsychotics to improve psychotic episodes and prevent relapse. Data from the Clozaril National Registry have shown that the incidence of agranulocytosis and fatality resulting from it are substantially lower than originally feared (Honigfeld et al., 1998). This has led to reductions in the requirements for WBC monitoring and costs associated with clozapine therapy. Clozapine has been shown to be relatively free of extrapyramidal side effects and may be a treatment for tardive dyskinesia (Lieberman et al., 1991). It also has been associated with lower rates of suicide attempts and completed suicides (Meltzer and Fatemi, 1995; Meltzer and Okayli, 1995; Meltzer et al., 2003; Walker et al., 1997). Finally, generic forms of clozapine have now become available, further lowering its cost.

Whether these potentially greater benefits as well as lower risks and costs for clozapine could justify its expanded use as a hypothetical first-line agent in treatment-sensitive patients remains a question for which empirical data are lacking. For that reason, we employed a simulation model to assess the effectiveness and costs of using clozapine as a potential first-line treatment for schizophrenia, relative to the current practice of restricting clozapine for only patients who have failed two trials of other antipsychotics (Wang et al., 2004). A Markov model was created based upon available RCTs and epidemiologic data and was used to track the clinical and economic outcomes of these two strategies in a hypothetical cohort of patients with schizophrenia undergoing an acute psychotic episode. Results of this simulation showed that using clozapine as a first agent would lead to modest gains in life expectancy as well as in quality-adjusted life expectancy, relative to restricting its use to patients who failed two other antipsychotics. The cost-effectiveness ratio of using clozapine first versus using clozapine third was $24,100 per quality-adjusted life year (QALY), well within conventional benchmarks used to determine whether healthcare interventions may be worth investing in. However, there is often great uncertainty with the inputs in such simulation models. For this reason, it was reassuring that in both one-way and probabilistic sensitivity analyses, the base-case findings from this simulation study were robust to a wide variety of assumptions.

Conclusions

Throughout the IOM Roundtable on Value & Science-Driven Health Care workshop on Redesigning the Clinical Effectiveness Research Paradigm, the breadth, depth, and pressing nature of needs for new clinical effectiveness research on medical treatments was evident. As this chapter illustrates, the need for such research on antipsychotic medications is no exception. Such research is critical to enhance practice, inform policy and purchasing decisions, and ultimately improve the health outcomes experienced by extremely vulnerable populations like those with psychotic disorders. Advances in the armamentarium available to conduct such research provide some grounds for optimism that these needs can be met in the future.

CANCER SCREENING

Peter B. Bach, M.D., M.A.P.P.
Memorial Sloan-Kettering Cancer Center

New Cancer Screening Tests: Challenges for Evidence

In the context of clinical medicine or typical practice, clinical disease usually "presents." That is, patients arrive with symptoms or signs—fever and night sweats with a cough, or a fractured limb—and thus the "afflicted population" is constituted of those individuals presenting with frank manifestations of their condition. However, a strong argument can be made for looking for preclinical conditions; in other words, the patient who should receive a vaccination against pneumonia before he/she develops fever and night sweats, or a patient who is at risk for falls before he/she breaks a limb. This is what screening is intended to do—essentially scan an unaffected population to look for people who are at risk for developing some condition. The underlying general rationale of screening is that we can decrease morbidity and mortality and other negative outcomes by looking for patients with preclinical conditions, as the interventions at that point reduce future negative health outcomes.

One could argue that screening is in fact the dominant activity in much of primary care. For example, testing for serum glucose levels in patients to look for diabetes in asymptomatic individuals—largely those without polyuria, polydypsia, or any other presentation of diabetes. In such cases, blood tests are ordered for patients who feel fine in order to scan for relevant preclinical conditions. Similarly, the pap smear looks primarily for predisease, such as dysplastic cells in the epithelium; it also looks for invasive and noninvasive cancers. A third example is that of the electrocardiogram (EKG). Included in the "Welcome to Medicare" visit, for example, an EKG performed in a patient without cardiac symptoms not only looks for a number of cardiac defects, including conduction abnormalities, but also screens for undiagnosed or silent coronary disease. Fundamentally, such screens look for a precondition in a patient who has no symptoms or "clinical presentation."

Screening encompasses a large range of today's medical activities. At one end are basic screening questions that physicians are to ask their patients. Such questions range from inquiries about gun ownership in the home and the presence of a swimming pool to questions about a family history of cancer. They all fall under the rubric of screening, in that they provide an avenue through which clinicians can gauge the risk for someone being shot in the home or drowning in the swimming pool or develop cancer—all with an expectation that those risks can be altered once they are known about.

At the other end are several different kinds of tests. Radiologic surveys, such as whole body computed tomography (CT) scans or magnetic resonance angiography of the cerebral circulation in a patient with no history of cerebral ischemia are one kind. Genetic profiles are another. In oncology, the test for the BRCA mutations has become increasingly popular, despite genuine uncertainty regarding the extent to which its presence predicts the development of either breast or ovarian cancer (Begg et al., 2008).

Value from Screening: Case Finding, Surrogate Markers, End-point Alteration

To determine the value of screening tests is difficult, whether the test is a questionnaire or an expensive diagnostic test being used off-label for screening. The problem begins with finding agreement on the intent of the screening evaluation: Is it intended to merely detect individuals at risk (i.e., find "cases"), or is its value predicated on its ability to alter the natural history of the condition that is being screened (i.e., "end-point alteration"). To be certain, screening tests are often evaluated purely for their ability to find cases, or individuals with preclinical disease. For example, the way one evaluates different questionnaires to screen for alcoholism is to determine how frequently, when applying this test, researchers are likely to find people who are alcoholics. While such information is vitally important to the process of care, it provides very little evidence that screening patients for alcoholism helps the patient, or is a good use of medical resources. What one aims to do, however, is to identify an individual at excess risk of health consequences of alcohol use, such as liver failure, then intervene to decrease the amount drunk and hence the risk of these complication. Finding people who are alcoholics (i.e., "case finding") does not ensure that the risk of liver failure is reduced.

Because case finding does not necessarily alter the end-point, screening tests are often evaluated for their ability to lead to an action—usually some kind of active prevention—that should then mitigate the risk of the actual end-point. This makes the "action" a surrogate marker of benefit. In the example of alcohol use, a surrogate marker of benefit might be that people found to have alcoholism through screening are fairly likely to enroll in Alcoholics Anonymous when their physician, who screened them, recommends it.

But, it has to be appreciated that enrollment in Alcoholics Anonymous is still a surrogate for a health benefit achieved by screening patients for alcoholism and then referring them to the program. To truly know if one of these screening evaluation yields a benefit, its use would have to be linked to reductions in liver failure or other alcohol-related complications. Enrollment in Alcoholics Anonymous is just a predictor (of uncertain correlation) with the benefit. In truth, one does not know whether or not the questionnaire detected alcoholics who really are as likely to develop liver failure and other complications as alcoholics who enroll in Alcoholics Anonymous after some other event, such as a traffic accident.

So, the most relevant approach to evaluating a screening test is precisely the same as the manner in which any medical intervention should be evaluated: Determine whether or not the intervention alters the clinical outcome. The ideal way to do this is by determining whether or not the use of the screen decreases, for instance, the frequency of the complication. In the case of alcoholism screening, the end-point would be the occurrence of a medical or social complication of alcoholism. In cancer screening, death due to the disease is typically the end-point of interest. Because the net effect of the screen, the actions taken as a result of the screen, and the end-point are assessed together, a comparator is needed, and so some sort of comparative study of screened and unscreened individuals must be run. In cancer screening trials, for example, determining if a screened subject's risk of dying of cancer is reduced relative to a scenario where they had not been screened is the goal—most often achieved by a randomized comparative trial. Comparators can come from a variety of other sources, however, such as a parallel or historical population, but for screening approaches, the randomized comparator is the least fraught with bias.

Even though there is an established gold standard for the evaluation of screening tests, there is no guarantee that such comparative trials, be they randomized or historic, are done before screening tests are adopted. For instance, the PSA test for prostate cancer has yet to be evaluated in a randomized trial where it can be determined if screening with PSA, finding prostate cancer through screening, and treating it reduces the risk a screened man will die of prostate cancer (there is one such study—the PLCO—ongoing).

Take the more dynamic example of lung cancer screening. The Princeton Longevity Center, for instance, advertises lung cancer screening. Its website includes some statements of fact about the lung cancer mortality rates in the United States. The website also cites, correctly, mortality rates from different cancers. It also quotes a prominent advocate of CT screening stating that "the current 5-year survival rate for lung cancer is only 14 percent, but that could soar to 80 percent if all smokers received annual CT exams and early treatment." Beneath all this the website states that lung scans are recommended for cigarettes or cigar smokers, those with a history of tuberculosis or pneumonia, and for nonsmokers with exposure to second-hand smoke or exposure to asbestos or radon—in other words, a relatively large fraction of the adult population (www.theplc.net). The site notably omits the fact that lung cancer screening has been evaluated by numerous organizations, and not one recommends it (Table 2-7).

Why might this website promote CT screening while recommending bodies do not? The answer lies in the continuum of possible evaluations of screening. In lung cancer screening, particularly given the risks and costs, the appropriate end-point for benefit evaluation is disease-specific mortality and the appropriate comparator is an un-screened group. The randomized studies are still ongoing. Meanwhile, advocates of screening are accepting case finding and other weak surrogates of benefit, such as disease-specific survival of cases, as evidence of benefit.

The data on case finding are impressive, as are the surrogate measures of benefit. Several high-quality studies for instance have demonstrated that CT scanning identifies numerous small foci of lung cancer in smokers, averaging 1–2 percent of CT screenings (Swensen et al., 2003). In the pilot study of the National Lung Screening Trial, nearly half of all lung cancers found through screening were early stage (Gohagan et al., 2005). Most of these cancers are conventionally considered to be highly treatable: so-called "resectable" cancers that practitioners in cancer care would like to encounter more often than they typically do.

Several studies also have demonstrated an impressive surrogate end-point—excellent survival after treatment of small cancers found by CT screening (Henschke, 2007). These studies have suggested that disease-specific survival is above 80 percent at 5 years for individuals with early stage cancer found by CT. This contrasts to a 15 percent 5-year survival probability in epidemiologic or cancer registry data, where more than 75 percent of cancers found are advanced and therefore incurable. So,

TABLE 2-7 Recommendations for Low-Dose CT (LDCT) Scans by Leading Medical Organizations

Recommending Body	Recommendation
National Cancer Institute (www.cancer. gov/cancertopics/pdq/screening/lung/ healthprofessional)	The evidence is inadequate to determine whether screening reduces mortality from lung cancer. On the basis of solid evidence, screening would lead to false-positive results and unnecessary invasive diagnostic procedures and treatments.
American Cancer Society (Smith RA, Cokkinides V, Eyre HJ. American Cancer Society guidelines for early detection of cancer, 2005. CA Cancer J Clin 2005; 55:31-44)	Lung cancer screening is not a routine practice for the general public or even for people who are at increased risk, such as smokers.
U.S. Preventive Services Task Force (www. ahrq.gov/clinic/uspstf/uspslung.htm)	The evidence is insufficient to recommend for or against screening asymptomatic individuals for lung cancer with LDCT, chest x-ray, sputum cytology, or a combination of these tests.
Canadian Coordination Office for Health Technology Assessment (www.cadth. ca/media/pdf/213_ct_cetap_e.pdf)	Evidence does not exist to suggest that detecting early-stage lung cancer reduces mortality.
American College of Chest Physicians	Not recommended outside of well-designed clinical trial.
Society of Thoracic Radiology (Aberle D, Gamsu, Henschke C, et al. A consensus statement of the Society of Thoracic Radiology: screening for lung cancer with helical computed tomography. J Thorac Imaging 2001; 16:65-68)	Mass screening for lung cancer is not currently advocated. Suitable subjects who wish to participate should be encouraged to do so in controlled trials so that the value of CT screening can be ascertained as soon as possible.

NOTE: Modified and reprinted with permission from Copyright Clearance Center, Copyright © 2007.
SOURCE: Bach, P. B., G. A. Silvestri, M. Hanger, and J. R. Jett. 2007b. Screening for lung cancer: American College of Chest Physicians evidence-based clinical practice guidelines (2nd edition). *Chest* 132(3 Suppl):69S-77S.

these studies are good news, but they are nonetheless focusing on case finding and surrogate measures of benefit.

My colleagues and I published a paper in 2007 that examined the interrelationship between case finding, surrogate end-points of stage distribution and case survival, and an actual measure of screening's benefits: the extent to which it alters disease-specific mortality. Our findings emphasize just how misleading the intermediate measures of benefit can be. The paper, which was the first comparative assessment of CT screening for lung cancer, used a computer simulation model to estimate what would have happened in the absence of screening among 3,000 individuals who were screened (Bach et al., 2007a). The model's predictions come from multi-variable models based on data from a large randomized trial conducted by the National Cancer Institute (NCI), and had hundreds of thousands of person-years and more than a thousand events. The predictors are age, smoking status (duration and intensity), and asbestos exposure. We validated these models in several studies before undertaking this analysis (Bach and Begg, 2006; Bach et al., 2003, 2004; Cronin et al., 2006). The validations demonstrated that the models predict within a few percentage points (worst case, plus or minus 8 percent) the number of events that would occur in current and former smokers in the relevant age over time in the absence of screening.

In the study, we documented that the prior assessments that had been done were correct—we revalidated that screening populations with CT locates a large proportion of early-stage cancers—in our case, 65 percent of cancer detected were early stage. We also reaffirmed that screen-detected cases have an excellent survival rate. When we considered only the early cancers, the survival rate was 94 percent. These are clearly spectacular outcomes, and they match all of the prior studies. The results were rather different, however, when we looked at end-points that screening is intended to affect—there was neither a reduction in advanced cancers nor in deaths from lung cancer. We found no evidence that CT screening intercepted early cases before they became advanced, and we did not find that screening and early treatment led to a reduction in deaths from lung cancer.

Figure 2-5 shows one of these results. The x-axis represents years, the solid lines are the observed counts, and the dotted lines are the models' predictions. There is a marked increase in the number of lung cancer diagnoses relative to what would have been seen absent screening. But, there was no "stage shift" or substitution—the same number of advanced cancers were encountered as would have been seen in the absence of screening.

Of particular importance in this analysis is that the risk ratio for cases found by screening relative to what would occur in the absence of screening has continued to diverge over time, exceeding 2.5 in each year of follow-up. The overall risk ratio is about 3.2. This result can only be explained if screening is finding cancers that otherwise would not have appeared clinically, and so this is one of the fallacies of case finding as a metric of benefit: Screening tests can find cases that are not precursors of serious disease, and thus finding these cases cannot benefit the patient.

While occurrence of advanced cancer is a legitimate end-point, lung cancer death is the health outcome of greatest importance. Figure 2-6

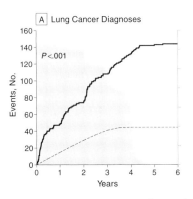
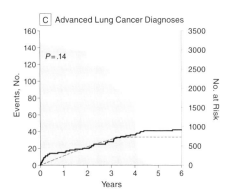

FIGURE 2-5 Lung cancer data indicating that a large increase in findings of cases through screening (A) did not lead to a reduction in advanced cancer diagnoses (C).
SOURCE: Bach, P. B., J. R. Jett, U. Pastorino, M. S. Tockman, S. J. Swensen, et al. 2007. Computed tomography screening and lung cancer outcomes. *Journal of the American Medical Association* 297(9):953-961. Copyright © 2007 American Medical Association. All rights reserved.

compares the number of lung cancer resections of early-stage cancers performed in this population relative to what was expected in the absence of screening. There was a 10-fold increase resulting from screening. These additional treatments are reasonably considered the action that should result in benefit. Thus, in a paradigm where screening is evaluated purely

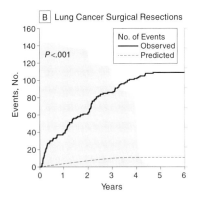
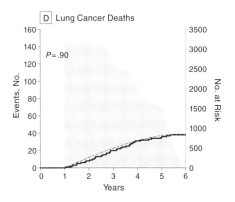

FIGURE 2-6 Treatment of early lung cancer cases (B) not averting death (D).
SOURCE: Bach, P. B., J. R. Jett, U. Pastorino, M. S. Tockman, S. J. Swensen, et al. 2007. Computed tomography screening and lung cancer outcomes. *Journal of the American Medical Association* 297(9):953-961. Copyright © 2007 American Medical Association. All rights reserved.

through surrogates, a finding that an increased number of patients were treated could be construed as a marker of screening's benefits. Yet, in this same population, as can be seen in the figure, there was no reduction in the number of lung cancer deaths relative to what was predicted. The counts of predicted and observed deaths were essentially perfectly matched, at 38.8 predicted and 38.0 observed. So, even though there is clearly an uptick in the action that should lead to benefit, there is no evidence that added action results in better outcomes for the screened population.

We derive several concluding observations about screening. First, the paradoxical reality of surrogate end-points is that they are readily available but can be misleading. Simply stated, screening often picks up pseudodisease, disease that is often too quickly characterized as "early" or "curable," rather than clinically unimportant or benign. In point of fact, lung cancer screening provides something of a textbook example, in that as one begins to look for conditions and apply tests that are imperfect or that rely on what might be characterized as amplifying weak and potentially uncertain signals, one will stumble upon abnormalities that have no clinical future. This appears to be happening in lung cancer screening to a very significant extent. There are similar examples where cancer screening has led to upticks in case finding, but the extent to which this leads to appropriate action that reduces disease-specific mortality is uncertain. In each case, as you begin to look, you find much more disease than you would expect, and more than can frankly progress to cause clinical conditions or death.

In other words, to evaluate screening methods, appropriate comparators are needed because they are illuminating, while surrogate end-points such as case finding are deceptive. To obtain an appropriate comparator, randomized controlled trials are the gold standard. But, alternatives, such as historical controls, parallel controls, or modeled controls (as in our example), can also be informative.

Doing comparative studies for screening tests is hard, however. In the case of lung cancer screening, the fact that there is broad equipoise made it possible for the NCI to launch a multicenter randomized trial comparing CT screening to chest-X-ray screening, and for several European countries to launch trials comparing CT to no screening. But even in lung screening, there has been resistance to the trial by pro-screening groups, and widespread advertising of CT screening as "proven" even though the trial is ongoing. In general terms, randomized trials will not always be done, and so it is important to construct approaches to the evaluation of screening tests that are sufficiently valid in the absence of randomization. As we showed in our study, which took advantage of the relatively unique linkage between lung cancer risk and reportable risk factors, we were able to assess the impact of CT screening without randomization to some extent, and at least from that we could determine that there would at best be substantial trade-offs between harms and benefits if screening were undertaken.

The evaluation of neuroblastoma screening and of the Pap smear were assessed using comparisons between population mortality rates due to the disease between those who were and were not screened (using either historical or parallel populations)—something only achievable when widespread screening has already been adopted. In each case, the results were convincing. More commonly, there will be neither a feasible mechanism for randomizing patients nor sufficient adoption to gauge changes in population mortality rates. In these situations, single arm registry–based trials are conceivably a reasonable way to assess the consequences of screening. Such an approach could work as long as the expected rates of death from the disease are known in advance, and the entire population of screened individuals are followed successfully, to ascertain the rates. Other problems include the reality that only a handful of conditions lend themselves well to determining "expected rates," and that few screening tests can really be disentangled from the cascade of events that follow them to a sufficient extent to determine whether or not the finding of additional cases through screening was responsible for the benefits or harms that occurred.

Whether or not payment policy or regulation can enhance learning about screening technologies prior to their wide adoption is also a challenging question. Payers will find that mandating registry participation or enrollment in a trial will promote the ire of screening advocates, who are particularly skilled at mobilizing advocacy groups. Moreover, many unproven screening tests are affordable to some, even though the procedures and tests they trigger can add up to great expense. For instance, phone calls to the various I-ELCAP lung cancer screening sites demonstrated that most of the centers ask for $400 to $500 for a single screening test, so individuals with high net worth will obtain these tests without reimbursement.

For most patients, such tests are out of reach financially, and so restriction of payment, or requirements for coverage with evidence development (CED) may be an effective way of ensuring that screening tests are assessed using appropriate endpoints at the time they are being introduced. For instance, CMS recently announced a proposed national coverage of computed tomography coronary arteriography under CED—the design of the assessment has not been articulated, but the notion that coverage of the technology may be coupled to an evaluation of it is very promising.

Regulatory routes are also something that could be considered, but policies would need to change. For instance, the FDA could hold screening assays and tests to a standard of demonstrated benefit, rather than the current lower standards. At best such an approach could limit the introduction of new tests that have no current usages until the right assessments are done. However, this may constitute too high a bar to introduction for the makers of many of these tests, and thus may stifle enthusiasm for pursuing innovation in prediction and prognostication—an undesirable consequence. Moreover, many of the current screening approaches, such as CT screening of the lung, merely involve the off-label use of an approved device. In this case, the CT scanner is already approved for diagnosis, and the FDA's ability to limit its use off label is essentially nonexistent. Organized medicine could play a more active role too, emphasizing the importance of following preventive services guidelines when offering screening examinations. But, there are bound to be outliers who are compelled by indirect measures of benefit, no matter what organized bodies conclude about the evidence.

In summary, evaluating screening tests is challenging, and surrogates such as case finding rates are deceptive and always biased in favor of the screening test. It is worth establishing paths for screening tests to be evaluated in a consistent manner before they are widely adopted. Doing so will be difficult. The desire to believe in the paradigm of early detection is strong. But, judicious use of coverage and payment, particularly towards the goal of generating population-based longitudinal data on outcomes among screened groups, compared to a relevant unscreened population, is an avenue that can and should be actively pursued.

REFERENCES

AHRQ (Agency for Healthcare Research and Quality). 2008. *Chartered Value Exchanges: Local Networks with National Standards.* http://www.ahrq.gov/qual/value/local networks.htm (accessed February 19, 2008).

Airoldi, F., A. Colombo, N. Morici, A. Latib, J. Cosgrave, L. Buellesfeld, E. Bonizzoni, M. Carlino, U. Gerckens, C. Godino, G. Melzi, I. Michev, M. Montorfano, G. M. Sangiorgi, A. Qasim, A. Chieffo, C. Briguori, and E. Grube. 2007. Incidence and predictors of drug-eluting stent thrombosis during and after discontinuation of thienopyridine treatment. *Circulation* 116(7):745-754.

Alexopoulos, G. S., J. Streim, D. Carpenter, and J. P. Docherty. 2004. Using antipsychotic agents in older patients. *Journal of Clinical Psychiatry* 65(Supl 2):5-99; discussion 100-102; quiz 103-104.

The American Society of Colon and Rectal Surgeons. 1994. Approved statement on laparoscopic colectomy. *Diseases of the Colon & Rectum* 37:8-12.

Anderson, G. L., M. Limacher, A. R. Assaf, T. Bassford, S. A. Beresford, H. Black, D. Bonds, R. Brunner, R. Brzyski, B. Caan, R. Chlebowski, D. Curb, M. Gass, J. Hays, G. Heiss, S. Hendrix, B. V. Howard, J. Hsia, A. Hubbell, R. Jackson, K. C. Johnson, H. Judd, J. M. Kotchen, L. Kuller, A. Z. LaCroix, D. Lane, R. D. Langer, N. Lasser, C. E. Lewis, J. Manson, K. Margolis, J. Ockene, M. J. O'Sullivan, L. Phillips, R. L. Prentice, C. Ritenbaugh, J. Robbins, J. E. Rossouw, G. Sarto, M. L. Stefanick, L. Van Horn, J. Wactawski-Wende, R. Wallace, and S. Wassertheil-Smoller. 2004. Effects of conjugated equine estrogen in postmenopausal women with hysterectomy: The women's health initiative randomized controlled trial. *Journal of the American Medical Association* 291(14):1701-1712.

Angerer, P., S. Stork, W. Kothny, P. Schmitt, and C. von Schacky. 2001. Effect of oral post-menopausal hormone replacement on progression of atherosclerosis: A randomized, controlled trial. *Arteriosclerosis, Thrombosis, and Vascular Biology* 21(2):262-268.

Bach, P. B., and C. B. Begg. 2006. Further validation of lung cancer mortality model. *Chest.* Published online, March 18, 2005. No longer accessible.

Bach, P. B., M. W. Kattan, M. D. Thornquist, M. G. Kris, R. C. Tate, M. J. Barnett, L. J. Hsieh, and C. B. Begg. 2003. Variations in lung cancer risk among smokers. *Journal of the National Cancer Institute* 95(6):470-478.

Bach, P. B., E. B. Elkin, U. Pastorino, M. W. Kattan, A. I. Mushlin, C. B. Begg, and D. M. Parkin. 2004. Benchmarking lung cancer mortality rates in current and former smokers. *Chest* 126(6):1742-1749.

Bach, P. B., J. R. Jett, U. Pastorino, M. S. Tockman, S. J. Swensen, and C. B. Begg. 2007a. Computed tomography screening and lung cancer outcomes. *Journal of the American Medical Association* 297(9):953-961.

Bach, P. B., G. A. Silvestri, M. Hanger, and J. R. Jett. 2007b. Screening for lung cancer: ACCP evidence-based clinical practice guidelines (2nd edition). *Chest* 132(3 Suppl):69S-77S.

Begg, C. B., R. W. Haile, A. Borg, K. E. Malone, P. Concannon, D. C. Thomas, B. Langholz, L. Bernstein, J. H. Olsen, C. F. Lynch, H. Anton-Culver, M. Capanu, X. Liang, A. J. Hummer, C. Sima, and J. L. Bernstein. 2008. Variation of breast cancer risk among BRCA1/2 carriers. *Journal of the American Medical Association* 299(2):194-201.

Bhatt, D. L., K. A. Fox, W. Hacke, P. B. Berger, H. R. Black, W. E. Boden, P. Cacoub, E. A. Cohen, M. A. Creager, J. D. Easton, M. D. Flather, S. M. Haffner, C. W. Hamm, G. J. Hankey, S. C. Johnston, K. H. Mak, J. L. Mas, G. Montalescot, T. A. Pearson, P. G. Steg, S. R. Steinhubl, M. A. Weber, D. M. Brennan, L. Fabry-Ribaudo, J. Booth, and E. J. Topol. 2006. Clopidogrel and aspirin versus aspirin alone for the prevention of athero-thrombotic events. *New England Journal of Medicine* 354(16):1706-1717.

Birkmeyer, N. J., D. Share, D. A. Campbell, Jr., R. L. Prager, M. Moscucci, and J. D. Birkmeyer. 2005. Partnering with payers to improve surgical quality: The Michigan plan. *Surgery* 138(5):815-820.

Breisacher, B., R. Limcangco, and L. Simoni-Wastila. 2005. The quality of antipsychotic drug prescribing in nursing homes. *Archives of Internal Medicine* 165:1280-1285.

Brookhart, M. A., J. A. Rassen, P. S. Wang, C. Dormuth, H. Mogun, and S. Schneeweiss. 2007. Evaluating the validity of an instrumental variable study of neuroleptics: Can between-physician differences in prescribing patterns be used to estimate treatment effects? *Medical Care* 45(10 Suppl 2):S116-S122.

Brownley, K. A., A. L. Hinderliter, S. G. West, K. M. Grewen, J. F. Steege, S. S. Girdler, and K. C. Light. 2004. Cardiovascular effects of 6 months of hormone replacement therapy versus placebo: Differences associated with years since menopause. *American Journal of Obstetrics and Gynecology* 190(4):1052-1058.

Buchwald, H., Y. Avidor, E. Braunwald, M. D. Jensen, W. Pories, K. Fahrbach, and K. Schoelles. 2004. Bariatric surgery: A systematic review and meta-analysis. *Journal of the American Medical Association* 292(14):1724-1737.

Chan, Y. C., S. F. Pariser, and G. Neufeld. 1999. Atypical antipsychotics in older adults. *Pharmacotherapy* 19(7):811-822.

Commonwealth of Massachusetts Betsy Lehman Center for Patient Safety and Medical Error Reduction Expert Panel on Weight Loss Surgery: Executive report. 2005. *Obesity Research* 13(2):205-226.

Congressional Budget Office. 2007. *Research on the comparative effectiveness of medical treatments: Issues and options for an expanded federal role.* Washington, DC: Congress of the United States.

Conley, R. R., and R. W. Buchanan. 1997. Evaluation of treatment-resistant schizophrenia. *Schizophrenia Bulletin* 23(4):663-674.

Cronin, K., M. H. Gail, Z. Zou, P. B. Bach, J. Virtamo, and D. Albanes. 2006. Validation of a model of lung cancer risk prediction among smokers. *Journal of the National Cancer Institute* 98:1-4.

Daemen, J., P. Wenaweser, K. Tsuchida, L. Abrecht, S. Vaina, C. Morger, N. Kukreja, P. Juni, G. Sianos, G. Hellige, R. T. van Domburg, O. M. Hess, E. Boersma, B. Meier, S. Windecker, and P. W. Serruys. 2007. Early and late coronary stent thrombosis of sirolimus-eluting and paclitaxel-eluting stents in routine clinical practice: Data from a large two-institutional cohort study. *Lancet* 369(9562):667-678.

de la Torre-Hernandez, J. M., F. Alfonso, F. Hernandez, J. Elizaga, M. Sanmartin, E. Pinar, I. Lozano, J. M. Vazquez, J. Botas, A. P. de Prado, J. M. Hernandez, J. Sanchis, J. M. Nodar, A. Gomez-Jaume, M. Larman, J. A. Diarte, J. Rodriguez-Collado, J. R. Rumoroso, J. R. Lopez-Minguez, and J. Mauri. 2008. Drug-eluting stent thrombosis: Results from the multicenter spanish registry estrofa (estudio espanol sobre trombosis de stents farmaco-activos). *Journal of the American College of Cardiology* 51(10):986-990.

Dewa, C. S., G. Remington, N. Herrmann, J. Fearnley, and P. Goering. 2002. How much are atypical antipsychotic agents being used, and do they reach the populations who need them? A Canadian experience. *Clinical Therapeutics* 24(9):1466-1476.

Estrogen and progestogen use in peri- and postmenopausal women: March 2007 position statement of the North American Menopause Society. 2007. *Menopause* 14(2):168-182.

Ettinger, B., G. D. Friedman, T. Bush, and C. P. Quesenberry, Jr. 1996. Reduced mortality associated with long-term postmenopausal estrogen therapy. *Obstetrics and Gynecology* 87(1):6-12.

Executive summary. Hormone therapy. 2004. *American Journal of Obstetrics and Gynecology* 104(4 Supl):1S-4S.

Farb, A., P. F. Heller, S. Shroff, L. Cheng, F. D. Kolodgie, A. J. Carter, D. S. Scott, J. Froehlich, and R. Virmani. 2001. Pathological analysis of local delivery of paclitaxel via a polymer-coated stent. *Circulation* 104(4):473-479.

FDA (Food and Drug Administration). 2005. *FDA Public Health Advisory: Deaths with Antipsychotics in Elderly Patients with Behavioral Disturbances.* http://www.fda.gov/cder/drug/advisory/antipsychotics.htm (accessed April 15, 2005).

———. 2008a. *Center for Devices and Radiological Health: CYPHER™ Sirolimus-eluting Coronary Stent on RAPTOR® Over-the-wire Delivery System or RAPTORRAIL® Rapid Exchange Delivery System–p020026.* http://www.fda.gov/cdrh/pdf2/P020026.html (accessed May 20, 2008).

———. 2008b. *Center for Devices and Radiological Health: Device Advice.* http://www.fda.gov/cdrh/devadvice/ (accessed May 20, 2008).

———. 2008c. *Endeavor® Zotarolimus-eluting Coronary Stent on the Over-the-wire (OTW), Rapid Exchange (RX), or Multi Exchange II (MX2) Stent Delivery Systems–p060033.* http://www.fda.gov/cdrh/pdf6/P060033.html (accessed May 20, 2008).

———. 2008d. *Jurisdictional update: Drug-eluting Cardiovascular Stents.* http://www.fda.gov/oc/combination/stents.html (accessed May 20, 2008).

———. 2008e. *TAXUS™ Express 2™ Paclitaxel-eluting Coronary Stent System (Monorail and Over-the-wire)–p030025 Name.* http://www.fda.gov/cdrh/pdf3/P030025.html (accessed May 20, 2008).

———. 2008f. Title 21: Chapter 1—food and drugs, subchapter a—general, part 3—product jurisdiction. In *Code of Federal Regulations.* Washington, DC: Food and Drug Administration, Department of Health and Human Services.

Finn, A. V., G. Nakazawa, M. Joner, F. D. Kolodgie, E. K. Mont, H. K. Gold, and R. Virmani. 2007. Vascular responses to drug eluting stents: Importance of delayed healing. *Arteriosclerosis, Thrombosis, and Vascular Biology* 27(7):1500-1510.

Fishman, A., F. Martinez, K. Naunheim, S. Piantadosi, R. Wise, A. Ries, G. Weinmann, and D. E. Wood. 2003. A randomized trial comparing lung-volume-reduction surgery with medical therapy for severe emphysema. *New England Journal of Medicine* 348(21):2059-2073.

Flum, D. R., and E. P. Dellinger. 2004. Impact of gastric bypass operation on survival: A population-based analysis. *Journal of the American College of Surgeons* 199(4):543-551.

Flum, D. R., T. Koepsell, P. Heagerty, M. Sinanan, and E. P. Dellinger. 2001a. Common bile duct injury during laparoscopic cholecystectomy and the use of intraoperative cholangiography: Adverse outcome or preventable error? *Archives of Surgery* 136(11):1287-1292.

Flum, D. R., A. Morris, T. Koepsell, and E. P. Dellinger. 2001b. Has misdiagnosis of appendicitis decreased over time? A population-based analysis. *Journal of the American Medical Association* 286(14):1748-1753.

Flum, D. R., T. Koepsell, P. Heagerty, and C. A. Pellegrini. 2002. The nationwide frequency of major adverse outcomes in antireflux surgery and the role of surgeon experience, 1992-1997. *Journal of the American College of Surgeons* 195(5):611-618.

Flum, D. R., K. Horvath, and T. Koepsell. 2003. Have outcomes of incisional hernia repair improved with time? A population-based analysis. *Annals of Surgery* 237(1):129-135.

Flum, D. R., N. Fisher, J. Thompson, M. Marcus-Smith, M. Florence, and C. A. Pellegrini. 2005a. Washington state's approach to variability in surgical processes/outcomes: Surgical clinical outcomes assessment program (SCOAP). *Surgery* 138(5):821-828.

Flum, D. R., L. Salem, J. A. Elrod, E. P. Dellinger, A. Cheadle, and L. Chan. 2005b. Early mortality among medicare beneficiaries undergoing bariatric surgical procedures. *Journal of the American Medical Association* 294(15):1903-1908.

Fox, K. A., S. R. Mehta, R. Peters, F. Zhao, N. Lakkis, B. J. Gersh, and S. Yusuf. 2004. Benefits and risks of the combination of clopidogrel and aspirin in patients undergoing surgical revascularization for non-st-elevation acute coronary syndrome: The clopidogrel in unstable angina to prevent recurrent ischemic events (cure) trial. *Circulation* 110(10):1202-1208.

Glynn, R. J., M. A. Brookhart, M. Stedman, J. Avorn, and D. H. Solomon. 2007. Design of cluster-randomized trials of quality improvement interventions aimed at medical care providers. *Medical Care* 45(10 Supl 2):S38-S43.

Gohagan, J. K., P. M. Marcus, R. M. Fagerstrom, P. F. Pinsky, B. S. Kramer, P. C. Prorok, S. Ascher, W. Bailey, B. Brewer, T. Church, D. Engelhard, M. Ford, M. Fouad, M. Freedman, E. Gelmann, D. Gierada, W. Hocking, S. Inampudi, B. Irons, C. C. Johnson, A. Jones, G. Kucera, P. Kvale, K. Lappe, W. Manor, A. Moore, H. Nath, S. Neff, M. Oken, M. Plunkett, H. Price, D. Reding, T. Riley, M. Schwartz, D. Spizarny, R. Yoffie, and C. Zylak. 2005. Final results of the lung screening study, a randomized feasibility study of spiral CT versus chest x-ray screening for lung cancer. *Lung Cancer* 47(1):9-15.

Gold, M., J. Siegel, L. Russell, and M. Weinstein, eds. 1996. *Cost-effectiveness in Health and Medicine.* New York: Oxford University Press.

Grady, D., D. Herrington, V. Bittner, R. Blumenthal, M. Davidson, M. Hlatky, J. Hsia, S. Hulley, A. Herd, S. Khan, L. K. Newby, D. Waters, E. Vittinghoff, and N. Wenger. 2002. Cardiovascular disease outcomes during 6.8 years of hormone therapy: Heart and estrogen/progestin replacement study follow-up (HERS II). *Journal of the American Medical Association* 288(1):49-57.

Gray, W. A., J. S. Yadav, P. Verta, A. Scicli, R. Fairman, M. Wholey, L. N. Hopkins, R. Atkinson, R. Raabe, S. Barnwell, and R. Green. 2007. The capture registry: Predictors of outcomes in carotid artery stenting with embolic protection for high surgical risk patients in the early post-approval setting. *Catheterization and Cardiovascular Interventions* 70(7):1025-1033.

Grodstein, F., and M. Stampfer. 2002. The epidemiology of postmenopausal hormone therapy and cardiovascular disease. In *Thrombosis and Thromboembolism*, edited by S. Z. Goldhaber and P. M. Ridker. New York: Marcel Dekker. Pp. 67-78.

Grodstein, F., J. E. Manson, G. A. Colditz, W. C. Willett, F. E. Speizer, and M. J. Stampfer. 2000. A prospective, observational study of postmenopausal hormone therapy and primary prevention of cardiovascular disease. *Annals of Internal Medicine* 133(12):933-941.

Grodstein, F., T. B. Clarkson, and J. E. Manson. 2003. Understanding the divergent data on postmenopausal hormone therapy. *New England Journal of Medicine* 348(7):645-650.

Grodstein, F., J. E. Manson, and M. J. Stampfer. 2006. Hormone therapy and coronary heart disease: The role of time since menopause and age at hormone initiation. *Journal Women's Health (Larchmt)* 15(1):35-44.

Hammill, S. C., L. W. Stevenson, A. H. Kadish, M. S. Kremers, P. Heidenreich, B. D. Lindsay, M. J. Mirro, M. J. Radford, Y. Wang, C. M. Lang, J. C. Harder, and R. G. Brindis. 2007. Review of the registry's first year, data collected, and future plans. *Heart Rhythm* 4(9):1260-1263.

Harman, S. M., E. A. Brinton, M. Cedars, R. Lobo, J. E. Manson, G. R. Merriam, V. M. Miller, F. Naftolin, and N. Santoro. 2005. KEEPS: The Kronos Early Estrogen Prevention Study. *Climacteric* 8(1):3-12.

Hecht, H. S., M. J. Budoff, D. S. Berman, J. Ehrlich, and J. A. Rumberger. 2006. Coronary artery calcium scanning: Clinical paradigms for cardiac risk assessment and treatment. *American Heart Journal* 151(6):1139-1146.

Heckbert, S. R., R. C. Kaplan, N. S. Weiss, B. M. Psaty, D. Lin, C. D. Furberg, J. R. Starr, G. D. Anderson, and A. Z. LaCroix. 2001. Risk of recurrent coronary events in relation to use and recent initiation of postmenopausal hormone therapy. *Archives of Internal Medicine* 161(14):1709-1713.

Hemminki, E., and K. McPherson. 1997. Impact of postmenopausal hormone therapy on cardiovascular events and cancer: Pooled data from clinical trials. *British Medical Journal* 315(7101):149-153.

Henschke, C. I. 2007. Survival of patients with clinical stage I lung cancer diagnosed by computed tomography screening for lung cancer. *Clinical Cancer Research* 13(17):4949-4950.

Heres, S., J. Davis, K. Maino, E. Jetzinger, W. Kissling, and S. Leucht. 2006. Why olanzapine beats risperidone, risperidone beats quetiapine, and quetiapine beats olanzapine: An exploratory analysis of head-to-head comparison studies of second-generation antipsychotics. *American Journal of Psychiatry* 163(2):185-194.

Herrington, D. M., D. M. Reboussin, K. B. Brosnihan, P. C. Sharp, S. A. Shumaker, T. E. Snyder, C. D. Furberg, G. J. Kowalchuk, T. D. Stuckey, W. J. Rogers, D. H. Givens, and D. Waters. 2000. Effects of estrogen replacement on the progression of coronary-artery atherosclerosis. *New England Journal of Medicine* 343(8):522-529.

Hodis, H. N. 2007. *Early versus Late Intervention Trial with Estrogen (ELITE) Website.* http://clinicaltrials.gov/show/NCT00114517 (accessed May 20, 2008).

Hodis, H. N., W. J. Mack, R. A. Lobo, D. Shoupe, A. Sevanian, P. R. Mahrer, R. H. Selzer, C. R. Liu Cr, C. H. Liu Ch, and S. P. Azen. 2001. Estrogen in the prevention of atherosclerosis. A randomized, double-blind, placebo-controlled trial. *Annals of Internal Medicine* 135(11):939-953.

Hodis, H. N., W. J. Mack, S. P. Azen, R. A. Lobo, D. Shoupe, P. R. Mahrer, D. P. Faxon, L. Cashin-Hemphill, M. E. Sanmarco, W. J. French, T. L. Shook, T. D. Gaarder, A. O. Mehra, R. Rabbani, A. Sevanian, A. B. Shil, M. Torres, K. H. Vogelbach, and R. H. Selzer. 2003. Hormone therapy and the progression of coronary-artery atherosclerosis in postmenopausal women. *New England Journal of Medicine* 349(6):535-545.

Honer, W. G., A. E. Thornton, E. Y. Chen, R. C. Chan, J. O. Wong, A. Bergmann, P. Falkai, E. Pomarol-Clotet, P. J. McKenna, E. Stip, R. Williams, G. W. MacEwan, K. Wasan, and R. Procyshyn. 2006. Clozapine alone versus clozapine and risperidone with refractory schizophrenia. *New England Journal of Medicine* 354(5):472-482.

Honigfeld, G., F. Arellano, J. Sethi, A. Bianchini, and J. Schein. 1998. Reducing clozapine-related morbidity and mortality: 5 years of experience with the clozaril national registry. *Journal of Clinical Psychiatry* 59(Supl 3):3-7.

Hormone therapy for the prevention of chronic conditions in postmenopausal women: Recommendations from the U.S. Preventive Services Task Force. 2005. *Annals of Internal Medicine* 142(10):855-860.

Hsia, J., M. H. Criqui, D. M. Herrington, J. E. Manson, L. Wu, S. R. Heckbert, M. Allison, M. M. McDermott, J. Robinson, and K. Masaki. 2006. Conjugated equine estrogens and peripheral arterial disease risk: The Women's Health Initiative. *American Heart Journal* 152(1):170-176.

Hulley, S., D. Grady, T. Bush, C. Furberg, D. Herrington, B. Riggs, and E. Vittinghoff. 1998. Randomized trial of estrogen plus progestin for secondary prevention of coronary heart disease in postmenopausal women. Heart and estrogen/progestin replacement study (HERS) research group. *Journal of the American Medical Association* 280(7):605-613.

Iakovou, I., T. Schmidt, E. Bonizzoni, L. Ge, G. M. Sangiorgi, G. Stankovic, F. Airoldi, A. Chieffo, M. Montorfano, M. Carlino, I. Michev, N. Corvaja, C. Briguori, U. Gerckens, E. Grube, and A. Colombo. 2005. Incidence, predictors, and outcome of thrombosis after successful implantation of drug-eluting stents. *Journal of the American Medical Association* 293(17):2126-2130.

Jeste, D., J. Sable, and C. Salzman. 2005. Treatment of late-life disordered behavior, agitation, and psychosis. In *Clinical Geriatric Psychopharmacology*. 4th ed., edited by C. Salzman. Philadelphia, PA: Lippincott, Williams & Wilkins. Pp. 129-195.

Kane, J., G. Honigfeld, J. Singer, and H. Meltzer. 1988. Clozapine for the treatment-resistant schizophrenic. A double-blind comparison with chlorpromazine. *Archives of General Psychiatry* 45(9):789-796.

Kindermann, S. S., C. R. Dolder, A. Bailey, I. R. Katz, and D. V. Jeste. 2002. Pharmacological treatment of psychosis and agitation in elderly patients with dementia: Four decades of experience. *Drugs Aging* 19(4):257-276.

Kuchulakanti, P. K., W. W. Chu, R. Torguson, P. Ohlmann, S. W. Rha, L. C. Clavijo, S. W. Kim, A. Bui, N. Gevorkian, Z. Xue, K. Smith, J. Fournadjieva, W. O. Suddath, L. F. Satler, A. D. Pichard, K. M. Kent, and R. Waksman. 2006. Correlates and long-term outcomes of angiographically proven stent thrombosis with sirolimus- and paclitaxel-eluting stents. *Circulation* 113(8):1108-1113.

Kuehn, B. M. 2005. FDA warns antipsychotic drugs may be risky for elderly. *Journal of the American Medical Association* 293(20):2462.

Lawlor, B. A. 2004. Behavioral and psychological symptoms in dementia: The role of atypical antipsychotics. *Journal of Clinical Psychiatry* 65(Supl 11):5-10.

Lemaitre, R. N., N. S. Weiss, N. L. Smith, B. M. Psaty, T. Lumley, E. B. Larson, and S. R. Heckbert. 2006. Esterified estrogen and conjugated equine estrogen and the risk of incident myocardial infarction and stroke. *Archives of Internal Medicine* 166(4):399-404.

Leucht, S., G. Pitschel-Walz, D. Abraham, and W. Kissling. 1999. Efficacy and extrapyramidal side-effects of the new antipsychotics olanzapine, quetiapine, risperidone, and sertindole compared to conventional antipsychotics and placebo. A meta-analysis of randomized controlled trials. *Schizophrenia Research* 35(1):51-68.

Lieberman, J. A., B. L. Saltz, C. A. Johns, S. Pollack, M. Borenstein, and J. Kane. 1991. The effects of clozapine on tardive dyskinesia. *British Journal of Psychiatry* 158:503-510.

Lieberman, J. A., M. Phillips, H. Gu, S. Stroup, P. Zhang, L. Kong, Z. Ji, G. Koch, and R. M. Hamer. 2003. Atypical and conventional antipsychotic drugs in treatment-naive first-episode schizophrenia: A 52-week randomized trial of clozapine vs chlorpromazine. *Neuropsychopharmacology* 28(5):995-1003.

Lieberman, J. A., T. S. Stroup, J. P. McEvoy, M. S. Swartz, R. A. Rosenheck, D. O. Perkins, R. S. Keefe, S. M. Davis, C. E. Davis, B. D. Lebowitz, J. Severe, and J. K. Hsiao. 2005. Effectiveness of antipsychotic drugs in patients with chronic schizophrenia. *New England Journal of Medicine* 353(12):1209-1223.

Lobo, R. A. 2004. Evaluation of cardiovascular event rates with hormone therapy in healthy, early postmenopausal women: Results from 2 large clinical trials. *Archives of Internal Medicine* 164(5):482-484.

Maixner, S. M., A. M. Mellow, and R. Tandon. 1999. The efficacy, safety, and tolerability of antipsychotics in the elderly. *Journal of Clinical Psychiatry* 60(Supl 8):29-41.

Manson, J. E., and S. S. Bassuk. 2007a. *Hot Flashes, Hormones and Your Health.* New York: McGraw-Hill.

———. 2007b. Invited commentary: Hormone therapy and risk of coronary heart disease why renew the focus on the early years of menopause? *American Journal of Epidemiology* 166(5):511-517.

Manson, J. E., J. Hsia, K. C. Johnson, J. E. Rossouw, A. R. Assaf, N. L. Lasser, M. Trevisan, H. R. Black, S. R. Heckbert, R. Detrano, O. L. Strickland, N. D. Wong, J. R. Crouse, E. Stein, and M. Cushman. 2003. Estrogen plus progestin and the risk of coronary heart disease. *New England Journal of Medicine* 349(6):523-534.

Manson, J. E., S. S. Bassuk, S. M. Harman, E. A. Brinton, M. I. Cedars, R. Lobo, G. R. Merriam, V. M. Miller, F. Naftolin, and N. Santoro. 2006. Postmenopausal hormone therapy: New questions and the case for new clinical trials. *Menopause* 13(1):139-147.

Manson, J. E., M. A. Allison, J. E. Rossouw, J. J. Carr, R. D. Langer, J. Hsia, L. H. Kuller, B. B. Cochrane, J. R. Hunt, S. E. Ludlam, M. B. Pettinger, M. Gass, K. L. Margolis, L. Nathan, J. K. Ockene, R. L. Prentice, J. Robbins, and M. L. Stefanick. 2007. Estrogen therapy and coronary-artery calcification. *New England Journal of Medicine* 356(25):2591-2602.

March, J. S., S. G. Silva, S. Compton, M. Shapiro, R. Califf, and R. Krishnan. 2005. The case for practical clinical trials in psychiatry. *American Journal of Psychiatry* 162(5): 836-846.

Mauri, L., E. J. Orav, and R. E. Kuntz. 2005. Late loss in lumen diameter and binary restenosis for drug-eluting stent comparison. *Circulation* 111(25):3435-3442.

Maynard, C., J. R. Goss, D. J. Malenka, and M. Reisman. 2003. Adjusting for patient differences in predicting hospital mortality for percutaneous coronary interventions in the clinical outcomes assessment program. *American Heart Journal* 145(4):658-664.

MedQIC. 2008. *SCIP Project Information.* http://www.medqic.org/scip (accessed February 19, 2008).

Meltzer, H., and H. Fatemi. 1995. Suicide in schizophrenia: The effect of clozapine. *Clinical Neuro-pharmacology* 18:S18-S24.

Meltzer, H. Y., and G. Okayli. 1995. Reduction of suicidality during clozapine treatment of neuroleptic-resistant schizophrenia: Impact on risk-benefit assessment. *American Journal of Psychiatry* 152(2):183-190.

Meltzer, H. Y., L. Alphs, A. I. Green, A. C. Altamura, R. Anand, A. Bertoldi, M. Bourgeois, G. Chouinard, M. Z. Islam, J. Kane, R. Krishnan, J. P. Lindenmayer, and S. Potkin. 2003. Clozapine treatment for suicidality in schizophrenia: International suicide prevention trial (intersept). *Archives of Geneneral Psychiatry* 60(1):82-91.

Mendelsohn, M. E., and R. H. Karas. 2005. Molecular and cellular basis of cardiovascular gender differences. *Science* 308(5728):1583-1587.

Michels, K. B., and J. E. Manson. 2003. Postmenopausal hormone therapy: A reversal of fortune. *Circulation* 107(14):1830-1833.

Mikkola, T. S., and T. B. Clarkson. 2002. Estrogen replacement therapy, atherosclerosis, and vascular function. *Cardiovascular Research* 53(3):605-619.

Mosca, L., C. L. Banka, E. J. Benjamin, K. Berra, C. Bushnell, R. J. Dolor, T. G. Ganiats, A. S. Gomes, H. L. Gornik, C. Gracia, M. Gulati, C. K. Haan, D. R. Judelson, N. Keenan, E. Kelepouris, E. D. Michos, L. K. Newby, S. Oparil, P. Ouyang, M. C. Oz, D. Petitti, V. W. Pinn, R. F. Redberg, R. Scott, K. Sherif, S. C. Smith, Jr., G. Sopko, R. H. Steinhorn, N. J. Stone, K. A. Taubert, B. A. Todd, E. Urbina, and N. K. Wenger. 2007. Evidence-based guidelines for cardiovascular disease prevention in women: 2007 update. *Circulation* 115(11):1481-1501.

Murphy, S. A., D. W. Oslin, A. J. Rush, and J. Zhu. 2007. Methodological challenges in constructing effective treatment sequences for chronic psychiatric disorders. *Neuropsychopharmacology* 32(2):257-262.

Pocock, S. J., A. J. Lansky, R. Mehran, J. J. Popma, M. P. Fahy, Y. Na, G. Dangas, J. W. Moses, T. Pucelikova, D. E. Kandzari, S. G. Ellis, M. B. Leon, and G. W. Stone. 2008. Angiographic surrogate end points in drug-eluting stent trials: A systematic evaluation based on individual patient data from 11 randomized, controlled trials. *Journal of the American College of Cardiology* 51(1):23-32.

Polinski, J. M., P. S. Wang, and M. A. Fischer. 2007. Medicaid's prior authorization program and access to atypical antipsychotic medications. *Health Affairs (Millwood)* 26(3): 750-760.

Prentice, R. L., R. D. Langer, M. L. Stefanick, B. V. Howard, M. Pettinger, G. L. Anderson, D. Barad, J. D. Curb, J. Kotchen, L. Kuller, M. Limacher, and J. Wactawski-Wende. 2006. Combined analysis of Women's Health Initiative observational and clinical trial data on postmenopausal hormone treatment and cardiovascular disease. *American Journal of Epidemiology* 163(7):589-599.

A prospective analysis of 1518 laparoscopic cholecystectomies. The Southern Surgeons Club. 1991. *New England Journal of Medicine* 324(16):1073-1078.

Roberts, T. G., Jr., and B. A. Chabner. 2004. Beyond fast track for drug approvals. *New England Journal of Medicine* 351(5):501-505.

Rosenheck, R. A., D. L. Leslie, J. Sindelar, E. A. Miller, H. Lin, T. S. Stroup, J. McEvoy, S. M. Davis, R. S. Keefe, M. Swartz, D. O. Perkins, J. K. Hsiao, and J. Lieberman. 2006. Cost-effectiveness of second-generation antipsychotics and perphenazine in a randomized trial of treatment for chronic schizophrenia. *American Journal of Psychiatry* 163(12):2080-2089.

Rosenheck, R. A., D. L. Leslie, J. L. Sindelar, E. A. Miller, P. N. Tariot, K. S. Dagerman, S. M. Davis, B. D. Lebowitz, P. Rabins, J. K. Hsiao, J. A. Lieberman, and L. S. Schneider. 2007. Cost-benefit analysis of second-generation antipsychotics and placebo in a randomized trial of the treatment of psychosis and aggression in alzheimer disease. *Archives of General Psychiatry* 64(11):1259-1268.

Rossouw, J. E., G. L. Anderson, R. L. Prentice, A. Z. LaCroix, C. Kooperberg, M. L. Stefanick, R. D. Jackson, S. A. Beresford, B. V. Howard, K. C. Johnson, J. M. Kotchen, and J. Ockene. 2002. Risks and benefits of estrogen plus progestin in healthy postmenopausal women: Principal results from the Women's Health Initiative randomized controlled trial. *Journal of the American Medical Association* 288(3):321-333.

Rossouw, J. E., R. L. Prentice, J. E. Manson, L. Wu, D. Barad, V. M. Barnabei, M. Ko, A. Z. LaCroix, K. L. Margolis, and M. L. Stefanick. 2007. Postmenopausal hormone therapy and risk of cardiovascular disease by age and years since menopause. *Journal of the American Medical Association* 297(13):1465-1477.

Sachs, G. S., A. A. Nierenberg, J. R. Calabrese, L. B. Marangell, S. R. Wisniewski, L. Gyulai, E. S. Friedman, C. L. Bowden, M. D. Fossey, M. J. Ostacher, T. A. Ketter, J. Patel, P. Hauser, D. Rapport, J. M. Martinez, M. H. Allen, D. J. Miklowitz, M. W. Otto, E. B. Dennehy, and M. E. Thase. 2007. Effectiveness of adjunctive antidepressant treatment for bipolar depression. *New England Journal of Medicine* 356(17):1711-1722.

Salpeter, S. R., J. M. Walsh, E. Greyber, T. M. Ormiston, and E. E. Salpeter. 2004. Mortality associated with hormone replacement therapy in younger and older women: A meta-analysis. *Journal of General Internal Medicine* 19(7):791-804.

Salpeter, S. R., J. M. Walsh, E. Greyber, and E. E. Salpeter. 2006. Brief report: Coronary heart disease events associated with hormone therapy in younger and older women. A meta-analysis. *Journal of General Internal Medicine* 21(4):363-366.

Santry, H. P., D. L. Gillen, and D. S. Lauderdale. 2005. Trends in bariatric surgical procedures. *Journal of the American Medical Association* 294(15):1909-1917.

Schatzberg, A. F., and C. B. Nemeroff. 2006. *Essentials of Clinical Psychopharmacology*. 2nd ed. Arlington, VA: American Psychiatric Publishing, Inc.

Schneeweiss, S., M. Maclure, A. M. Walker, P. Grootendorst, and S. B. Soumerai. 2001. On the evaluation of drug benefits policy changes with longitudinal claims data: The policy maker's versus the clinician's perspective. *Health Policy* 55(2):97-109.

Schneeweiss, S., S. Setoguchi, A. Brookhart, C. Dormuth, and P. S. Wang. 2007. Risk of death associated with the use of conventional versus atypical antipsychotic drugs among elderly patients. *Canadian Medical Association Journal* 176(5):627-632.

Schneider, L. S., K. S. Dagerman, and P. Insel. 2005. Risk of death with atypical antipsychotic drug treatment for dementia: Meta-analysis of randomized placebo-controlled trials. *Journal of the American Medical Association* 294(15):1934-1943.

Schneider, L. S., P. N. Tariot, K. S. Dagerman, S. M. Davis, J. K. Hsiao, M. S. Ismail, B. D. Lebowitz, C. G. Lyketsos, J. M. Ryan, T. S. Stroup, D. L. Sultzer, D. Weintraub, and J. A. Lieberman. 2006. Effectiveness of atypical antipsychotic drugs in patients with Alzheimer's disease. *New England Journal of Medicine* 355(15):1525-1538.

Schorr, R., R. Fought, and W. Ray. 1994. Changes in antipsychotic drug use in nursing homes during implementation of the OBRA-87 regulations. *Journal of the American Medical Association* 271:358-362.

Shively, E. H., M. J. Heine, R. H. Schell, J. N. Sharpe, R. N. Garrison, S. R. Vallance, K. J. DeSimone, and H. C. Polk, Jr. 2004. Practicing surgeons lead in quality care, safety, and cost control. *Annals of Surgery* 239(6):752-760; discussion 760-752.

Sink, K. M., K. F. Holden, and K. Yaffe. 2005. Pharmacological treatment of neuropsychiatric symptoms of dementia: A review of the evidence. *Journal of the American Medical Association* 293(5):596-608.

Soumerai, S. B., T. J. McLaughlin, D. Ross-Degnan, C. S. Casteris, and P. Bollini. 1994. Effects of a limit on medicaid drug-reimbursement benefits on the use of psychotropic agents and acute mental health services by patients with schizophrenia. *New England Journal of Medicine* 331(10):650-655.

Steinhubl, S. R., P. B. Berger, J. T. Mann, 3rd, E. T. Fry, A. DeLago, C. Wilmer, and E. J. Topol. 2002. Early and sustained dual oral antiplatelet therapy following percutaneous coronary intervention: A randomized controlled trial. *Journal of the American Medical Association* 288(19):2411-2420.

Strong, C. 2005. Antipsychotic use in elderly patients with dementia prompts new FDA warning. *Neuropsychiatry Review* 6:1-17.

Sturmer, T., R. J. Glynn, K. J. Rothman, J. Avorn, and S. Schneeweiss. 2007. Adjustments for unmeasured confounders in pharmacoepidemiologic database studies using external information. *Medical Care* 45(10 Supl 2):S158-S165.

Suzuki, T., G. Kopia, S. Hayashi, L. R. Bailey, G. Llanos, R. Wilensky, B. D. Klugherz, G. Papandreou, P. Narayan, M. B. Leon, A. C. Yeung, F. Tio, P. S. Tsao, R. Falotico, and A. J. Carter. 2001. Stent-based delivery of sirolimus reduces neointimal formation in a porcine coronary model. *Circulation* 104(10):1188-1193.

Swensen, S. J., J. R. Jett, T. E. Hartman, D. E. Midthun, J. A. Sloan, A. M. Sykes, G. L. Aughenbaugh, and M. A. Clemens. 2003. Lung cancer screening with CT: Mayo clinic experience. *Radiology* 226(3):756-761.

Tariot, P. N. 1999. The older patient: The ongoing challenge of efficacy and tolerability. *Journal of Clinical Psychiatry* 60(Supl 23):29-33.

Trivedi, M. H., M. Fava, S. R. Wisniewski, M. E. Thase, F. Quitkin, D. Warden, L. Ritz, A. A. Nierenberg, B. D. Lebowitz, M. M. Biggs, J. F. Luther, K. Shores-Wilson, and A. J. Rush. 2006. Medication augmentation after the failure of SSRIS for depression. *New England Journal of Medicine* 354(12):1243-1252.

Tunis, S. R., D. B. Stryer, and C. M. Clancy. 2003. Practical clinical trials: Increasing the value of clinical research for decision making in clinical and health policy. *Journal of the American Medical Association* 290(12):1624-1632.

Virmani, R., G. Guagliumi, A. Farb, G. Musumeci, N. Grieco, T. Motta, L. Mihalcsik, M. Tespili, O. Valsecchi, and F. D. Kolodgie. 2004. Localized hypersensitivity and late coronary thrombosis secondary to a sirolimus-eluting stent: Should we be cautious? *Circulation* 109(6):701-705.

Wahlbeck, K., M. Cheine, A. Essali, and C. Adams. 1999. Evidence of clozapine's effectiveness in schizophrenia: A systematic review and meta-analysis of randomized trials. *American Journal of Psychiatry* 156(7):990-999.

Walker, A. M., L. L. Lanza, F. Arellano, and K. J. Rothman. 1997. Mortality in current and former users of clozapine. *Epidemiology* 8(6):671-677.

Wang, P. S., J. C. West, T. Tanielian, and H. A. Pincus. 2000. Recent patterns and predictors of antipsychotic medication regimens used to treat schizophrenia and other psychotic disorders. *Schizophrenia Bulletin* 26(2):451-457.

Wang, P., A. Walker, and J. Avorn. 2002a. The pharmacoepidemiology of psychiatric medications. In *Textbook in Psychiatric Epidemiology*. 2nd ed., edited by M. T. Twang and M. Tohen. New York: John Wiley & Sons, Inc. Pp. 181-194.

Wang, P. S., O. Demler, and R. C. Kessler. 2002b. Adequacy of treatment for serious mental illness in the United States. *American Journal of Public Health* 92(1):92-98.

Wang, P. S., D. A. Ganz, J. S. Benner, R. J. Glynn, and J. Avorn. 2004. Should clozapine continue to be restricted to third-line status for schizophrenia?: A decision-analytic model. *Jounal of Mental Health Policy and Economics* 7(2):77-85.

Wang, P. S., M. Lane, M. Olfson, H. A. Pincus, K. B. Wells, and R. C. Kessler. 2005a. Twelve-month use of mental health services in the United States: Results from the national comorbidity survey replication. *Archives of General Psychiatry* 62(6):629-640.

Wang, P. S., S. Schneeweiss, J. Avorn, M. A. Fischer, H. Mogun, D. H. Solomon, and M. A. Brookhart. 2005b. Risk of death in elderly users of conventional vs. atypical antipsychotic medications. *New England Journal of Medicine* 353(22):2335-2341.

Wang, P. S., S. Aguilar-Gaxiola, J. Alonso, M. C. Angermeyer, G. Borges, E. J. Bromet, R. Bruffaerts, G. de Girolamo, R. de Graaf, O. Gureje, J. M. Haro, E. G. Karam, R. C. Kessler, V. Kovess, M. C. Lane, S. Lee, D. Levinson, Y. Ono, M. Petukhova, J. Posada-Villa, S. Seedat, and J. E. Wells. 2007. Use of mental health services for anxiety, mood, and substance disorders in 17 countries in the WHO world mental health surveys. *Lancet* 370(9590):841-850.

Waters, D. D., E. L. Alderman, J. Hsia, B. V. Howard, F. R. Cobb, W. J. Rogers, P. Ouyang, P. Thompson, J. C. Tardif, L. Higginson, V. Bittner, M. Steffes, D. J. Gordon, M. Proschan, N. Younes, and J. I. Verter. 2002. Effects of hormone replacement therapy and antioxidant vitamin supplements on coronary atherosclerosis in postmenopausal women: A randomized controlled trial. *Journal of the American Medical Association* 288(19):2432-2440.

Wathen, C. N., D. S. Feig, J. W. Feightner, B. L. Abramson, and A. M. Cheung. 2004. Hormone replacement therapy for the primary prevention of chronic diseases: Recommendation statement from the Canadian Task Force on Preventive Health Care. *Canadian Medical Association Journal* 170(10):1535-1537.

3

Taking Advantage of
New Tools and Techniques

INTRODUCTION

As with virtually every scientific endeavor, clinical effectiveness research can be improved and expedited through innovation. In this case, innovation means the better use of existing tools and techniques as well as the development of entirely new methods and approaches. Understanding these emerging tools and techniques is critical to the discussion of improvements to the clinical effectiveness research paradigm. Better tools and enhanced techniques are fundamental building blocks in redesigning the clinical effectiveness paradigm, and new methods and strategies for evidence development are needed to use these tools to capture and analyze the increasingly complex information and data generated. In turn, better evidence will lead to stronger clinical and policy decisions and set the stage for further research.

Opportunities provided by developments in health information technology are reviewed in Chapter 4. In this chapter we review innovative uses of existing research tools as well as emerging methods and techniques. Part of the reform needed to enhance clinical effectiveness research is a more widespread understanding of different research tools and techniques, including greater clarity about what each can offer the overall research enterprise, both alone and in synergy with other approaches. A further need is broad, substantive support for ongoing development of new approaches and applications of existing tools and techniques that researchers believe may offer more benefits. As noted in Chapter 1, greater attention is needed to understand which approach is best suited for which situation and under what circumstances.

The papers included in this chapter offer observations on improvements needed in the design and interpretation of intervention trials; methods that take better advantage of system-level data; possible improvements in analytic tools, sample size, data quality, organization, and processing; and novel techniques that researchers are beginning to use in conjunction with new information, models, and tools.

Citing models from Duke University, The Society of Thoracic Surgeons (STS), and the Food and Drug Administration's (FDA's) Critical Path Clinical Trials Transformation Initiative, Robert M. Califf from Duke University discusses opportunities to improve the efficiency of clinical trials and to reduce their exorbitant costs. Innovations in the structure, strategy, conduct, analysis, and reporting of trials promise to make them less expensive, faster, more inclusive, and more responsive to important questions. Particular attention is needed to identify regulations that improve clinical trial quality and eliminate practices that increase costs without an equal return in value. Finally, establishing "envelopes of creativity" in which innovation is encouraged and supported is essential to maximizing the appropriate use of this methodology.

Confounding is often the biggest issue in effectiveness analyses of large databases. Innovative analytic tools are needed to make the best use of large clinical and administrative databases. Sebastian Schneeweiss from Harvard Medical School observes that instrumental variable analysis is an underused, but promising, approach for effectiveness analyses. Recent developments of note include approaches that exploit the concepts of proxy variables using high-dimensional propensity scores and provider variation in prescribing preference using instrumental variable analysis.

Rejecting any suggestion that "one trial = all trials," Donald A. Berry from the University of Texas M.D. Anderson Cancer Center makes the case that adaptive and, particularly, Bayesian approaches lend themselves well to synthesizing and combining sources of information, such as meta-analyses, and provide means of modeling and assessing sources of uncertainty appropriately. Therefore, Berry asserts, they are ideally suited for experimental trial design.

Mark S. Roberts of the University of Pittsburgh, representing Archimedes Inc. at the workshop, suggests that physiology-based simulation and predictive models, such as an eponymous model developed at Archimedes, have the potential to augment and enhance knowledge gained from randomized controlled trials (RCTs) and can be used to fill "gaps" that are difficult or impractical to answer using clinical trial methods. Of particular relevance is the potential for these models to perform virtual comparative effectiveness trials.

This chapter concludes with a discussion of the dramatic expansion of information on genetic variation related to common, complex disease and the potential of these insights to improve clinical care. Teri A. Manolio of the National Human Genome Research Institute reviews recent findings from genomewide association studies that will enable examination of inherited genetic variability at an unprecedented level of resolution. She proposes opportunities to better capture and use these data to understand clinical effectiveness.

INNOVATIVE APPROACHES TO CLINICAL TRIALS

Robert M. Califf, M.D.
Vice Chancellor for Clinical Research
Duke University

As we enter the era in which we hope that "learning health systems" (IOM, 2001) will be the norm, the evolution of randomized controlled trials required to meet the tremendous need for high-quality knowledge about diagnostic and therapeutic interventions has emerged as a critical issue. All too often, discussion about medical evidence gravitates toward a comparison of randomized controlled trials and studies based on observational data, rather than toward a serious examination of ways to improve the operational methods of both approaches. My own experience in assessing the relative merits of RCTs versus observational studies dates back more than 25 years (Califf and Rosati, 1981), and recent discussions on this topic remind me of conversations I had as a medical student in 1977 with Eugene Anson Stead, Jr., M.D., the former chair of the Department of Medicine at Duke University. Dr. Stead founded the Duke Cardiovascular Disease Database, which eventually evolved into the Duke Clinical Research Institute; he is credited with helping change cardiovascular medicine from a discipline largely based on anecdotal observation to one based on clinical evidence. Dr. Stead, who was significantly ahead of his time, introduced us to a device not yet in common use—the computer—and urged us to record outcomes data on all of our patients. Further, he stressed that simply collecting information on acute, hospital-based practice was not sufficient; instead, we should add to this computerized collection throughout our patients' lives.

I firmly believe that this approach—building human systems that take advantage of the power of modern informatics—is the key to improving both RCTs and observational studies. Within the domain of clinical trials, an informatics-based approach holds promise both for pragmatic trials in broad populations, as well as in proof-of-concept (POC) trials intended to elucidate complex biological effects in small groups of people.

In 1988, our research group published a paper in which we concluded that well-designed and carefully executed observational studies could provide research data that were comparable in quality to those provided by

RCTs (Hlatky et al., 1988). We have learned much since then, a point recently driven home during rounds in the Duke Coronary Care Unit (CCU). Time after time, we were faced with decisions that, had there had been a trial with an inception time for enrollment that coincided with the time point when we needed to make that clinical decision, the trial would likely have provided invaluable information for our CCU deliberations.

While observational studies can provide useful knowledge, they are inadequate for detecting modest differences in effects between treatments (Peto et al., 1995), because without a common inception point and randomization to equally distribute known and unknown confounding factors, the risk of an invalid answer is substantial (DeMets and Califf, 2002a, 2002b). Innovation in clinical trials, in my view, is mostly concerned with performing them in optimal fashion, so that more knowledge is created more efficiently.

How Can We Foster Quality in Clinical Trials?

The most urgently needed innovation in implementing clinical trials is a more intelligent approach to defining and producing quality. Since randomization is such a powerful tool for creating a basis to compare alternatives from a common inception point, we should abandon the assumption that the common critiques of RCTs stem from unalterable rules governing the conduct of such trials. Clinical trials are not required of their nature to be expensive, slow, noninclusive, and irrelevant to measurement of outcomes that matter to patients and medical decision makers. While innovative statistical methods have provided exciting additions to our capabilities, the main source of innovation in trials must be a focus on the fundamental "blocking and tackling" of clinical trials.

A Structural Framework for Clinical Trials

We have published a model, shown in simplified form in Figure 3-1, which integrates quantitative measurements of quality and performance into the development cycle of existing and future therapeutics (Califf et al., 2002). Such a model can serve as a basic approach to the development of reliable knowledge about medical care that is necessary but not sufficient for those wishing to provide the best possible care for their patients. Currently, it takes too long to complete this cycle, but if we had continuous, practice-based registries and the ability to randomize within those registries, we could see in real time which patients were included and excluded from trials. Further, upon completing the study, we could then measure the uptake of the results of the trial in practice. Such an approach provides a

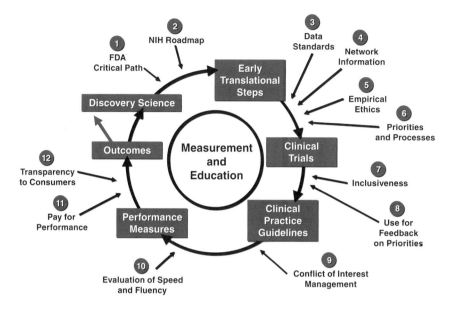

FIGURE 3-1 Innovation in clinical trials: relevance of evidence system.
SOURCE: Copyrighted and published by Project HOPE/Health Affairs as Califf, R. M., R. A. Harrington, L. K. Madre, E. D. Peterson, D. Roth, and K. A. Schulman. 2007. Curbing the cardiovascular disease epidemic: Aligning industry, government, payers, and academics. *Health Affairs (Millwood)* 26(1):62-74. The published article is archived and available online at www.healthaffairs.org.

system wherein everyone contributes to the registry and the results of trials are fed back into the registry in a rapid cycle.

We have invested considerable efforts in evaluating the details of the system for generating clinical evidence from the perspective of cardiovascular medicine, where there is a long history of applying scientific discoveries to large clinical trials, which in turn inform clinical practice. Figure 3-1 summarizes the complex interplay of relevant factors. If we assume that scientific discoveries are evaluated through proper clinical trials, clinical practice guidelines and performance indicators can be devised and continuous evaluation through registries can measure improved outcomes as the system itself improves. In this context, there are at least a dozen major factors that must be iteratively improved in order for this system to work more efficiently and at lower cost (Califf et al., 2007).

A specific model of this approach has been implemented by STS (Ferguson et al., 2000). Over time, STS has developed a clinical practice

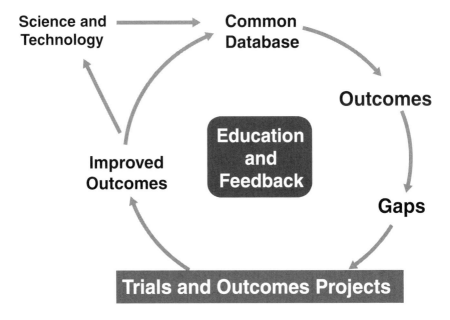

FIGURE 3-2 The Society of Thoracic Surgeons evidence system model.
SOURCE: Derived from Ferguson, T. B., et al. 2000. The STS national database: Current changes and challenges for the new millennium. Committee to establish a national database in cardiothoracic surgery, The Society of Thoracic Surgeons. *The Annals of Thoracic Surgery* 69(3):680-691.

database that is used for quality reporting, and, increasingly, for continuously analyzing operative issues and techniques (Figure 3-2). The STS model also allows randomized trials to be conducted within the database.

The most significant aspects of this model lie in its constantly evolving, continuously updated information base and its methods of engaging practitioners in this system by providing continuous education and feedback. Many have assumed that we must wait on fully functional electronic health records (EHRs) for such a system to work. However, we need not wait for some putatively ideal EHR to emerge. Current EHRs have serious shortcomings from the perspective of clinical researchers, since these records must be optimized for individual provider–patient transactions. Consequently, they are significantly *sub*optimal with respect to coded data with common vocabulary—an essential feature for the kind of clinical research enterprise we envision. This deficit severely hobbles researchers seeking to evaluate aggregated patient information in order to draw inferential conclusions about treatment effects or quality of care. While we await the

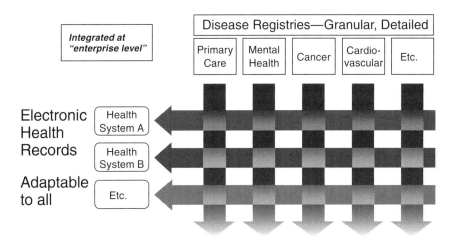

FIGURE 3-3 Fundamental informatics infrastructure—matrix organizational structure.

resolution of issues regarding EHR functionality, the best approach will be to construct a matrix between the EHR and continuous professional-based registries (disease registries) that measure clinical interactions in a much more refined and structured fashion (Figure 3-3). Such a system would allow us to perform five or six times as many trials as can now be done for the same amount of money; even better, such trials would be more relevant to clinical practice. As part of our Clinical and Translational Sciences Award (CTSA) cooperative agreement with the National Institutes of Health (NIH), we are presently working on such a county-wide matrix in Durham County, North Carolina (Michener et al., 2008).

New Strategies for Incorporating Scientific Evidence into Clinical Practice

New efficiencies can be gained through applying innovative informatics-based approaches to the broad pragmatic trials discussed above; however, we also must develop more creative methods of rapidly translating new scientific findings into early human studies. The basis for such POC clinical trials lies in applying an intervention to elucidate whether an intended biological pathway is affected, while simultaneously monitoring for unanticipated effects on unintended biological pathways ("off-target effects"). This process includes acquiring a preliminary indication of dose–response relationships and of whether unintended pathways are also being perturbed (again, while providing a basic understanding of dose–response relationships). POC studies are performed to advance purely scientific understanding or to inform a decision about whether to proceed to the next stage of clinical investigation. We used to limit ourselves by thinking that we could only perform POC studies in one institution at a time, but we now know that we can perform exactly the same trials, with the same standard operating procedures and the same information systems in India and Singapore, as well as in North Carolina. The basis for this broadened capability, as in pragmatic clinical trials, is the building of clinical research networks that enable common protocols, data structures, and sharing of information across institutions. This broadening of scope affords the ability to rethink the scale, both physical and temporal, for POC clinical trials. The wide variation in costs in these different environments also deserves careful consideration by U.S. researchers.

New Approaches to Old Problems: Conducting Pragmatic Clinical Trials

When considering strategies for fostering innovation in clinical trials, several key points must be borne in mind. The most important is that there exists, particularly in the United States, an entrenched notion that each clinical trial, regardless of circumstances or aims, must be done under precisely the same set of rules, usually codified in the form of standard operating procedures (SOPs). Upon reflection, it is patently obvious that this is not (or should not be) the case; further, acting on this false assumption is impairing the overall efficiency of clinical trials. Instead, the conduct of trials should be tailored to the type of question asked by the trial, and to the circumstances of practice and patient enrollment for which the trial will best be able to answer that question. We need to cultivate environments where creative thought about the pragmatic implementation of clinical trials is encouraged and rewarded ("envelopes of innovation"), and given the existing barriers to changes in trial conduct, financial incentives may be required in order to encourage researchers and clinicians to "break the mold" of entrenched attitudes and practices.

What is the definition of a high-quality clinical trial? It is one that provides a reliable answer to the question that the trial intended to answer. Seeking "perfection" in excess of this goal creates enormous costs while at the same time paradoxically reducing the actual quality of the trial by distracting research staff from their primary mission. Obviously, in the context of a trial evaluating a new molecular entity or device for the first time in humans, there are compelling reasons to measure as much as possible about the subjects and their response to the intervention, account for all details, and ensure that the intensity of data collection is at a very high level. Pragmatic clinical trials, however, require focused data collection in large numbers of subjects; they also take place in the clinical setting where their usual medical interactions are occurring, thereby limiting the scope of detail for the data that can be collected on each subject. To cite a modified Institute of Medicine definition of quality, "high quality with regard to procedural, recording and analytic errors is reached when the conclusion is no different than if all of these elements had been without error" (Davis, 1999).

Efficacy trials are designed to determine whether a technology (a drug, device, biologic, well-defined behavioral intervention, or decision support algorithm) has a beneficial effect in a specific clinical context. Such investigation requires carefully controlled entry criteria and precise protocols for intervention. Comparisons are often made with a placebo or a less relevant comparator (these types of studies are not sufficiently informative for clinical decision making because they do not measure the balance of risk and benefit over a clinically relevant period of time). Efficacy trials— which speak to the fundamental question, "can the treatment work?"—still require a relatively high level of rigor, because they are intended to establish the effect of an intervention on a specific end-point in a carefully selected population.

In contrast, pragmatic clinical trials determine the balance of risk and benefit in "real world" practice; i.e., "Should this intervention be used in practice compared with relevant alternatives?" (Tunis et al., 2003). The population of such a study is allowed to be "messy" in order to simulate the actual conditions of clinical practice; operational procedures for the trial are designed with these decisions in mind. The comparator is pertinent to choices that patients, doctors, and health systems will face, and outcomes typically are death, clinical events, or quality of life. Relative cost is important and the duration of follow-up must be relevant to the duration that will be recommended for the intervention in practice.

When considering pragmatic clinical trials, I would argue we actually do *not* want professional clinical trialists or outstanding practitioners in the field to dominate our pool of investigators. Rather, we want to incorporate real-world conditions by recruiting typical practitioners who practice the way they usually do, with an element of randomization added to the system to provide, at minimum, an inception time and a decision point from which to begin the comparison. A series of papers recently have been published that present a detailed summary of the principles of pragmatic clinical trials (Armitage et al., 2008; Baigent et al., 2008; Cook et al., 2008; Duley et al., 2008; Eisenstein et al., 2008; Granger et al., 2008; Yusuf et al., 2008).

The Importance of Finding Balance in Assessing Data Quality

If we examine the quality of clinical trials from an evidence-based perspective we might emerge with a very different system (Yusuf, 2004). We know, for example, that an on-site monitor almost never detects fraud, largely because if someone is clever enough to think they can get away with

TABLE 3-1 Taxonomy of Clinical Errors

Error Type	Monitoring Method
Design error	Peer review, regulatory review, trial committee oversight
Procedural error	Training and mentoring during site visits; simulation technology
Recording error	
Random	Central statistical monitoring; focused site monitoring based on performance metrics
Fraud	Central statistical monitoring; focused site monitoring based on unusual data patterns
Analytical error	Peer review, trial committees, independent analysis

fraud, that person is likely to be adroit at hiding the signs of their deception from inspectors. A better way to detect fraud is through statistical process control, performed from a central location. For example, a common indicator of fraudulent data is that the data appear to be "too perfect." If data appear ideal in a clinical trial, they are unlikely to be valid: That is not the way that human beings behave. Table 3-1 summarizes monitoring methods to find error in clinical trials that take advantage of a complete perspective on the design, conduct, and analysis of trials.

Recent work sheds light on how to take advantage of natural units of practice (Mazor et al., 2007). It makes sense, for example, to randomize clusters of practices rather than individuals when a policy is being evaluated (versus treating an individual). Several studies that have followed this approach were conducted as embedded experiments within ongoing registries; the capacity to feed information back immediately within the registry resulted in improvements in practice. Although the system is not perfect, there is no question that it makes possible the rapid improvement of practice and allows us to perform trials and answer questions with randomization in that setting.

Disruptive Technologies and Resistance to Change

All this, however, suggests the question: If we are identifying more efficient ways to do clinical trials, why are they not being implemented? The problem is embedded in the issue of disruptive technology—initiating a new way of doing a clinical trial is disruptive to the old way. Such disruption upsets an industry that has become oriented, both financially and philosophically, toward doing things in the accustomed manner. In less highly regulated areas of society, technologies develop in parallel and the "winners" are chosen by the marketplace. Such economic Darwinian selection causes companies that remain wedded to old methods to go out of business when their market is captured by an innovator who offers a disruptive technology that works better. In most markets, technology and organizational innovation drive cost and quality improvement. Providing protection for innovation that will allow those factors to play out naturally in the context of medical research might lead to improved research practices, thereby generating more high-quality evidence and, eventually, improving outcomes.

In our strictly regulated industry, however, regulators bear the mantle of authority, and the risk that applying new methods will result in lower quality is not easily tolerated. This in turn creates a decided barrier to innovation, given the extraordinarily high stakes. There is a question that is always raised in such discussions: If you do human trials less expensively and more efficiently, can you prove that you are not hurting patient safety?

What effect is all of this having? A major impact is cost: Many recent cardiovascular clinical outcomes trials have cost more than $350 million dollars to perform. In large part this expense reflects procedures and protocols that are essentially unnecessary and unproductive, but required nonetheless according to the prevailing interpretation of regulations governing clinical trials by the pharmaceutical and device companies and the global regulatory community.

Costing out the consequences of the current regulatory regime can yield staggering results. As one small example, a drug already on the market evidenced a side effect that is commonly seen in the disease for which it is prescribed. The manufacturer believed that it was required to ship by overnight express the adverse event report to all 2,000 investigators, with instructions that the investigators review it carefully, classify it, and send it to their respective IRBs for further review and classification. The cost of that exercise for a single event that contributed no new knowledge about the risk and benefit balance of the drug was estimated at $450,000.

Starting a trial in the United States can cost $14,000 per site before the first patient is enrolled simply because of current regulations and procedures governing trial initiation, including IRB evaluation and contracting. A Cooperative Study Group funded by the National Cancer Institute recently published an analysis demonstrating that a *minimum* of more than 481 discrete processing steps are required for an average Phase II or Phase III cancer protocol to be developed and shepherded through various approval processes (Dilts et al., 2008). This results in a delay of more than 2 years from the time a protocol is developed until patient enrollment can begin, and means that "the steps required to develop and activate a clinical trial may require as much or more time than the actual completion of a trial."

We must ask: Do the benefits conferred by documenting pre-study evaluation visits or pill counts really outweigh the costs of collecting such data, for example? Do we need 800 different IRBs reviewing protocols for large multicenter trials, or could we enact studies using central IRBs or collaborative agreements among institutional IRBs? Is all the monitoring and safety reporting that we do really necessary (or even helpful)?

Transforming Clinical Trials

All is not dire, however. One promising new initiative is the FDA Critical Path Initiative (public/private partnership [PPP]): the Clinical Trials Transformation Initiative (CTTI), which is intended to map ways to better trials (www.trialstransformation.org). A collaboration among the FDA, industry, academia, patient advocates, and nonacademic clinical researchers, CTTI is designed to conduct empirical studies that will provide evidence to support redesign of the overall framework of clinical trials and to eliminate practices that increase costs but provide no additional value. The explicit mission of CTTI is to identify practices that through adoption will increase the quality and efficiency of clinical trials.

Another model that we could adapt from the business world is the concept of establishing "envelopes of creativity." In short, we need to create spaces within organizations where people can innovate with a certain degree of creative freedom, and where financial incentives reward this creativity. Pediatric clinical trials offer a good example of this approach. Twenty years ago, clinical trials were rarely undertaken in children; many companies argued that they simply could not be done. Pediatricians led the charge to point out that the end result of such an attitude was a shocking lack of knowledge about the risks and benefits of drugs and devices in children. Congress was persuaded to require pediatric clinical trials and grant patent extensions for companies that performed appropriate trials in children (Benjamin et al., 2006). The result was a significant increase in the number of pediatric trials and a corresponding growth in knowledge about the effects of therapeutics in children (Li et al., 2007).

Conclusions

If we all agree that clinical research must be improved in order to provide society with answers to critical questions about medical technologies and best practices, a significant transformation is needed in the way we conduct the clinical trials that provide us with the most reliable medical evidence. We need not assume that trials must be expensive, slow, noninclusive, and irrelevant to the measurement of important outcomes that matter most to patients and clinicians. Instead, smarter trials will become an integral part of practice in learning health systems as they are embedded into the information systems that form the basis for clinical practice; over time, these trials will increasingly provide the foundation for integrating modern genomics and molecular medicine into the framework of clinical care.

INNOVATIVE ANALYTIC TOOLS FOR LARGE CLINICAL AND ADMINISTRATIVE DATABASES

Sebastian Schneeweiss, M.D., Sc.D.
Harvard Medical School
BWH DEcIDE Research Center on Comparative Effectiveness Research

Instrumental Variable Analyses for Comparative Effectiveness Research Using Clinical and Administrative Databases

Physicians and insurers need to weigh the effectiveness of new drugs against existing therapeutics in routine care to make decisions about treatment and formularies. Because FDA approval of most new drugs requires demonstrating efficacy and safety against placebo, there is limited interest by manufacturers in conducting such head-to-head trials. Comparative effectiveness research seeks to provide head-to-head comparisons of treatment outcomes in routine care. Because healthcare utilization databases record drug use and selected health outcomes for large populations in a timely way and reflect routine care, they may be the preferred data source for comparative effectiveness research.

Confounding caused by selective prescribing based on indication, severity, and prognosis threatens validity of nonrandomized database studies that often have limited details on clinical information. Several recent developments may bring the field closer to acceptable validity, including approaches that exploit the concepts of proxy variables using high-dimensional propensity scores and exploiting provider variation in prescribing preference using instrumental variable analysis. The paper provides a brief overview of those two approaches and discusses their strengths, weaknesses, and future developments.

Very briefly, what is confounding? Patient factors become confounders ("C" in Figure 3-4) if they are associated with treatment choice and are also independent predictors of the outcome. When researchers are interested in the causal effect of a treatment on an outcome, factors that are independently predicting the study outcome, such as severity of the underlying condition, prognosis, co-morbidity, are at the same time also driving the treatment decision. Once these two conditions are fulfilled, you have a confounding situation and you get biased results. In large-claims database

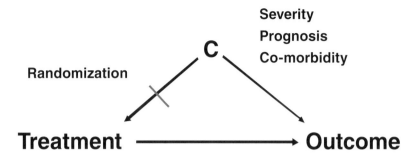

FIGURE 3-4 Explanation of confounding factors in comparative effectiveness research.

analyses, confounding is one of the biggest issues in comparative effectiveness research. Randomization breaks this association between patient factors and treatment assignment. In Figure 3-1, once you break one of the two arms of the tent, then you no longer have confounding.

We have a large continuum of comparative effectiveness research, within which some questions are heavily confounded by design while others are not; the separation is usually by unintended treatment effects and intended treatment effects. An example is in the use of selective Cox-2 inhibitors (coxibs) and cardiac events. In 1999 and 2000 when coxibs were first marketed, nobody was thinking that independent cardiovascular risk factors would influence the decision of whether to treat with the coxibs or nonselective nonsteroidal anti-inflammatory drugs (nsNSAIDs), so there was no association. Consequently there is very little potential for confounding studying unintended cardiovascular outcomes. However, when we studied coxib use and the reduction in gastric toxicity, a heavily marketed advantage of coxibs, risk factors for future gastroinstinal (GI) events drive the decision to use coxibs; consideration of GI symptoms, although often quite subtle and likely not recorded in databases, are nevertheless driving the treatment decision and may therefore cause confounding.

As Figure 3-5 suggests, epidemiologists have a whole toolbox of techniques to control confounding by measured factors (Schneeweiss, 2006). But what about the unmeasured confounders, such as the subtle GI symptoms that are not recorded in claims data, but nevertheless are driving the treatment decision?

We can sample a subpopulation and collect more detailed data there, but what options are there when such a subsampling to measure clinical details is not a possible or practical? One of the strategies is to use instrumental variables. An instrumental variable (IV) is an unconfounded substitute for the actual treatment. In this approach, instead of model-

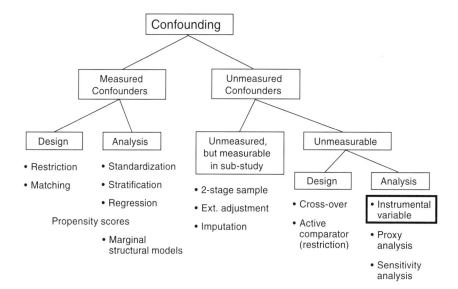

FIGURE 3-5 Dealing with unmeasured confounding factors in claims data analyses.
SOURCE: Schneeweiss, S. 2006. Sensitivity analysis and external adjustment for unmeasured confounders in epidemiologic database studies of therapeutics. *Pharmacoepidemiology and Drug Safety* 15:291-303. Reprinted with permission from Wiley-Blackwell, Copyright © 2006.

ing treatment and outcome, researchers model the instrument—which is unrelated to patient characteristics and therefore unconfounded—and then rescale the estimate for the correlation between the instrumental variable and the actual treatment.

One of the key assumptions is that the instrumental variable is not associated with either the measured or unmeasured confounders and is not related to the outcome directly other than through the actual treatment. This is necessary for instrumental variables to produce valid results. Consequently, in working with such instruments, researchers have to identify a sort of quasi-random treatment assignment in the real world. For the sake of this paper, two are readily identifiable:

Interruption in Medical Practice

This quasi-random treatment assignment can be caused by sudden and massive interruptions of treatment patterns, for example by regulatory changes. An example might be the FDA aprotinin advisory that reduced the medication's use by 50 percent—a massive shift. For the same patient candidates for aprotinin, a cardiac surgeon would likely choose a different course of treatment before and after the advisory. A similar example is found in the evolution of the coronary stents; a patient coming for a percutaneous procedure on one day might be treated with a bare metal stent but a year later, after the rapid adoption of drug-eluting stents that same patient might be given a drug-coated stent.

Strong Treatment Preference

Several papers have contributed to our understanding of this valuable instrument for evaluating the comparative effectiveness of therapeutics, which considers such instruments as the distance to specialist, geographic area, physician prescribing preference, and hospital formularies (Brookhart et al., 2006; McClellan et al., 1994; Stukel et al., 2007). A valid preference-based instrument would be the observation of a quasi-random treatment choice mechanism, for example, some hospitals have certain drugs on formulary and others don't, but patients do not elect to go to one hospital versus another based on whether or not a particular medication is on formulary.

Figure 3-6 presents an example focused on the use of coxibs and nsNSAIDs, with GI complications as the causal relationship, and physician preference to prescribed coxibs versus nonselective NSAIDs (Schneeweiss et al., 2006). This nightmare for everyone writing treatment guidelines might be the dream of an epidemiologist: The same patients get treated differently by different physicians; some physicians always prescribe coxibs and some physicians never prescribe coxibs to patients that need pain therapy (Schneeweiss et al., 2005; Solomon et al., 2003).

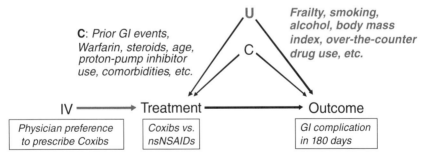

FIGURE 3-6 IV estimation of the association between NSAIDs and GI complication. SOURCE: Adapted by permission from Macmillan Publishers, Ltd. *Clinical Pharmacology & Therapeutics* 82:143-156, Copyright © 2007.

Some confounders such as the use of steroids and other medications can be measured with information that we can draw from claims data. However, there will remain unmeasured confounders—for example, body mass index, and the use of over-the-counter drugs. Such information is usually not available in claims data, leading one to ask what happens when one compares the conventional multivariate-adjusted analysis to an instrumental variable based on physician preference. Data not shown here indicate that the risk difference estimates for GI complications for coxibs in a conventional multivariate analysis is around 0, meaning "no association." What we would expect, of course, is a protective effect. When we did the instrumental variable analysis on coxibs and reduced GI toxicity (not shown), we see a negative risk difference, indicating a protective effect of the coxibs as compared to nsNSAIDs. This is an example where the confounding is strong and the confounding factor is either not measured in claims data or is measured only to a small extent.

Let us consider three core assumptions about instrumental variables (Angrist, 1996). One assumption is that the instrument is related to the actual exposure—otherwise it can't be an instrument—and is a strong predictor of treatment. The assumption is that physician prescribing preference strongly predicts future choices of treatments. This assumption is empirically testable. In comparison with IV analyses from economics, the strength of the physician prescribing preference IV is greater than most but not all published examples (Rassen, 2008).

A second assumption is that the instrument should not be associated with any measured or unmeasured patient care characteristics. To prove such an assumption—a more difficult exercise than proving the first assumption—one must consider the extent to which one achieves balance in the measured covariates between the two treatment groups. This involves summarizing all of the measurable individual covariants into a summary metric called the Mahalanobis distance that considers the covariance between individual patient factors. In this case the physician preference for a variety of instrument definitions has led to substantial reduction in imbalance among observed patient characteristics (Rassen, 2008). The hope is that when improvement in balance in the measured covariates can be achieved by the instrument, there will be a corresponding improvement in the unmeasured covariates. This is different from the balance achieved by propensity score matching that is limited to the measured patient characteristics and their correlates (Seeger et al., 2005).

A third assumption is that there should be no direct relationship with outcome other than through actual treatment. It can be attempted to empirically test this assumption in the case of the treatment preference instrument through what is colloquially called the "good doc/bad doc" model, which suggests that treatment preference may be correlated with other physician characteristics that relate to better outcomes. For example, some physicians who generally practice medicine better might have a preference for coxibs versus other NSAIDs. This creates a physician-level correlation and therefore introduces confounding. To test this assumption, other quality of care measures, such as prescribing long-acting benzodiazepines, or problematic tricyclic antidepressant prescribing could be assessed in a study of the effectiveness of antipsychotics. The result was that among general practitioners there was no quality of prescribing and thus a reduced chance of violations of this third assumption (Brookhart et al., 2007).

Another example used regional variation in heart catheterization rates in patients with acute myocardial infarctions as an instrument (Stukel et al., 2007). As seen in Figure 3-7, patients in this study were arranged by quintile of regional cardiac catheterization rates. In the first quintile, 43 percent of patients received a heart catheter; in the highest quintile group, 65 percent received heart catheterization.

One could argue that there shouldn't be anything different between these populations because patients did not select their residence according to whether their regional cardiac catheterization rate is high. If this argument holds than there are some patients not receiving catheterization who would receive catheterization if they happened to live in another region. Thus there is quasi-random treatment assignment for these patients.

Looking at the effect estimates in Figure 3-7 we find that the protective effect of heart catheterization in patients with acute myocardial infarction

	Quintile (Range) of Regional Cardiac Catheterization Rate, %				
	1 (29.2-48.1)	2 (48.2-53.0)	3 (53.1-56.3)	4 (56.4-60.2)	5 (60.3-82.3)
No. of patients	24,872	24,184	24,718	24,063	24,287
Cardiac catheterization rate	42.8	50.6	54.7	58.0	65.0
Mean predicted 1-year mortality (AMI severity)*	26.1	26.0	25.5	25.3	24.6

Decrease in effect size with better adjustment for measured and unmeasured confounders:

Risk-Adjustment Method	Absolute Mortality Difference (Δ) (SE)	
1-Year mortality		RD
Unadjusted	−0.244 (0.002)	
Multiple linear regression†	−0.162 (0.002)	
Instrumental variable, adjusted‡	−0.054 (0.015)	

FIGURE 3-7 Regional variation in cardiac catheterization and risk of death.
SOURCE: *Journal of the American Medical Association* 297(3):278-285. Copyright © 2007 American Medical Association. All rights reserved.

Variable	*Reference group: males. †Reference group: 65–74 y.	Estimated odds ratio (95 per cent CI)			
		Logistic regression		GMM IVA	
Beta-blocker use within 30 days	0.68	(0.60–0.77)	0.23	(0.04–1.09)	
Sex*	0.69	(0.64–0.74)	0.70	(0.65–0.75)	
Age group†					
75–84 y	1.33	(1.23–1.45)	1.32	(1.21–1.44)	
≥85 y	1.85	(1.68–2.04)	1.81	(1.64–2.01)	
Contraindication	1.27	(1.17–1.37)	1.26	(1.17–1.36)	
Polanczyk co-morbidity score	1.10	(1.09–1.12)	1.10	(1.09–1.12)	

FIGURE 3-8 Time as an instrumental variable.
SOURCE: Johnston, K. M., P. Gustafson, A. R. Levy, and P. Grootendorst. 2008. Use of instrumental variables in the analysis of generalized linear models in the presence of unmeasured confounding with applications to epidemiological research. *Statistics in Medicine* 27(9):1539-1556. Reproduced with permission of John Wiley & Sons, Ltd.

in an unadjusted analysis of 24 less deaths per year per 100 patients reduces in the multivariate-adjusted regression to only 16 deaths prevented; and with the instrumental variable regression, only 5.

One final example (Figure 3-8) uses time as an instrumental variable. The question here concerns the use of beta-blocker after heart failure hospitalization and 1-year mortality, and whether beta-blocker use is correlated with reduced mortality. After some landmark trials had been published, beta-blocker use in patients with heart failure increased substantially. The investigators defined the binary instrument either before or after this increased use of beta-blocker. As the figure shows, the estimated odds ratio using standard logistic regression was 0.68, whereas the instrumental variable ratio was 0.23—without suggesting which is "right," we see that there is a considerable difference between the two estimates.

The most frequently mentioned limitation of instrumental variables is that two critical assumptions are not testable but assumptions must be argued using context knowledge. Several empirical tests were suggested to partially evaluate IV assumptions using empirical data, but ultimately we cannot fully prove that assumptions are fully valid. However, readers may be reminded that conventional regression analyses are based on assumptions, including that the model is specified correctly, i.e., that all confounders are measured and included in the model, an assumption that is inherently untestable. The lower statistical efficiency as a consequence of the two-stage estimation process is another limitations. In large databases with tens of thousands of people exposed to drug therapy that is usually a minor issue.

Comparative effectiveness research should routinely explore whether a valid instrument variable is identifiable in settings where important confounders remain unmeasured. One should search for random components in the treatment choice process, which will sometimes lead to a valid instrument. We have found that the physician prescribing preference instrument is worth considering in many situations of drug effectiveness research. We have further recommended that instrumental variable analyses should be secondary to conventional regression modeling until we better understand the qualities of preference-based instruments and how to best empirically test IV assumptions. We further suggest to perform sensitivity analyses to assess how much violation of IV assumptions may change the primary effect estimate (Brookhart, 2007).

In conclusion, instrumental variable analyses are currently underutilized but very promising approaches for comparative effectiveness research using nonrandomized data. Instrumental variable analyses can lead to substantial improvements, particularly in situations with strong unmeasured confounding. The prospect of reducing residual confounding comes at the price of somewhat untestable assumptions for valid estimation. Plenty of research is ahead, particularly developing better methods to empirically assess the validity of IV assumptions and systematic screens for instrument candidates.

ADAPTIVE AND BAYESIAN APPROACHES TO STUDY DESIGN

Donald A. Berry, Ph.D.
Head, Division of Quantitative Sciences
Professor and Frank T. McGraw Memorial Chair for Cancer Research
Chairman, Department of Biostatistics
The University of Texas M.D. Anderson Cancer Center

Modern clinical studies are subject to the most rigorous of scientific standards. In particular, modern research relies heavily on the randomized clinical study that was introduced by A. Bradford Hill in the 1940s (MRC Streptomycin in Tuberculosis Studies Committee, 1948). Applying randomization in a clinical research setting was an enormous advance and it revolutionized the notion of treatment comparisons. For a variety of reasons, mostly coincidence, the RCT became tied to the frequentist approach to statistical inference. In this approach the inferential unit is the study itself, and the conventional measure of inference is the level of statistical significance. In the early days of the RCT the sample size was fixed in advance. Over time, preplanned interim analyses were incorporated to allow for stopping the study early for sufficiently conclusive results.

Randomization will continue to be important in clinical research. However, randomization is difficult and expensive to effect, and there are legitimate ways of learning without randomizing. Moreover, learning can take place at any time during a study and not just when accrual is stopped and sufficient follow-up information obtained. The goal of this chapter is to describe an approach to clinical study design that improves on randomization in two ways. One way is to make RCTs more flexible, with data accrues during the study used to guide the study's course. The other improvement is incorporating different sources of information to enable better conclusions about comparative effectiveness. Both use the Bayesian approach to statistics (Berry, 1996, 2006). This approach is ideal for both purposes. As regards the first, Bayes rule provides a formalism for updating knowledge with each new piece of information that is obtained, with updates occurring at any time. As regards the second, the Bayesian approach is inherently synthetic. Its principal measures of inference are the probabilities of hypotheses based on the totality of information available at the time.

Précis for Frequentist Statistics

Historically, the standard statistical measures used in clinical research have been frequentist. Frequentist conclusions are tailored to and driven by the study's design. Probability calculations are restricted to the so-called "sample space," the set of outcomes possible for the design used. To make these calculations requires the assumption that a particular mechanism that produces the observation. An especially important assumption is that the experimental treatment being evaluated is ineffective, the "null hypothesis." Other hypotheses can be assumed as well, including that the experimental treatment has a particular specified advantage.

The most familiar frequentist inferential measure is the "p-value," or observed statistical significance level. This is the probability of observations in the sample space as extreme or more extreme than the results actually observed, calculated assuming the null hypothesis. To make this calculation requires finding the probabilities (under the null hypothesis) of results that are potentially observable. It also requires ordering the possible results of the experiment so that "more extreme results" can be identified to enable adding probabilities over these results.

An important frequentist calculation made in advance of a study is its statistical power. This is the probability of achieving statistical significance in the study (defined as having a p-value of 0.05 or smaller) when the truth is that the experimental treatment has some particular benefit.

In all of the above calculations the design must be completely described in advance for otherwise the probabilities in the sample space and even the sample space itself will be unknown. And the study must be complete, having followed the design as specified in advance. The mathematics are easiest when the sample size is fixed and treatment assignments do not depend on the interim results. But frequentist measures can be calculated (perhaps only via simulation) for any prospective design, however complicated. One potential stumbling block in a complicated study is identifying an ordering of the study results. There is no natural way of ordering study results in the frequentist approach when the study has a complicated design. For example, there is no good frequentist approach to answer questions such as, "Given the current results of the study, how much credibility should I place in the null hypothesis as opposed to competing hypotheses?" That makes it difficult to alter the course of the study on the basis of those results.

Précis for Bayesian Statistics

There are many publications describing the Bayesian approach—for example, Berry (2006) and Spiegelhlater (2004). I will give a brief description here, highlighting some points of special importance in clinical study design. In the Bayesian approach, anything which is unknown—including hypotheses—has a probability. So the null hypothesis has a probability. And this probability can be calculated at any time: at the end of the study, during the study, and at the beginning of the study. The last of these is called a "prior probability." Probabilities calculated during or after a study are based on whatever results are available at the time and are called "posterior probabilities." For example, a Bayesian can always answer the question in the previous paragraph by giving the current (posterior) probability of the null hypothesis.

The Bayesian approach has a characteristic that is very important in designing clinical studies: It enables calculating probabilities of future observations based on previous observations. Frequentists can calculate probabilities of future observations only by assuming particular hypotheses. In the Bayesian approach predictive probabilities do not require assuming a particular hypothesis because these probabilities are averages with respect to the current posterior probabilities of the various hypotheses.

The online learning aspect of the Bayesian approach makes it ideal for building adaptive designs. If a study's design is developed as the study is being conducted, which is possible in the Bayesian approach, it is impossible to calculate the study's false-positive rate. This is why I insist on building designs prospectively. It is more work because one must consider many possibilities that will not arise in the actual trial: "What would I want to do if the data after 40 patients are as follows: . . .?" The various "operating characteristics" of any prospective study design, including its false-positive rate, can be calculated. Except in the simplest of adaptive designs, such calculation will require simulation.

Clinical Studies with Adaptive Designs

Clinical studies, including RCTs, are usually static in the sense that sample size and treatment assignment are fixed in advance. Results observed during the study are not used to guide the study's course. There are exceptions. One is a two-stage Phase II cancer trial in which stopping is possible after the first stage if the results are either very promising or very discouraging. Also, Phase III and Phase IV trial designs usually prescribe interim analyses for early stopping in case one treatment arm is performing much better than the other. However, these methods are crude and they are limited in the design modifications that are possible. In particular, interim analyses are allowed at only a small number of epochs, limiting ability to adjust course in mid-study. In addition, traditional early stopping criteria in late phase studies are so conservative that few of them stop early in practice.

The simplicity of studies that have static designs makes them appealing inferential tools. But such studies are costly, in both time and resources. Late-phase clinical trials tend to be large. Large clinical trials are expensive, which increases the cost of health care. And large studies use patient resources that might be used more effectively for other investigations. Moreover, large sample size means exposing many patients to a treatment that may be ineffective and perhaps even harmful. Despite being large, static studies too often reach their full accrual goal and prescribed patient follow-up time only to conclude that the scientific goal was not achieved.

A more flexible approach is to use the information that accrues in a study to modify its subsequent course. Such designs are *adaptive* in that modifications depend on the interim results. Among the modifications possible are stopping the study early, changing eligibility criteria, expanding accrual (by adding additional clinical sites), extending accrual beyond the study's original sample size if its conclusion is still not clear, dropping or adding arms (including combinations of other arms) or doses, switching from one clinical phase to another, and shifting focus to subsets of the patient populations (such as responders). Combinations of these are possible. For example, one might learn that an arm performs poorly in one subset of patients and so that arm is dropped within that subset but it continues otherwise. Adaptive designs also include unbalanced randomization (more patients assigned to some of the treatment arms than others based on interim results of the study) where the degree of imbalance depends on the accumulating data. For example, arms that will provide more information or that are performing better than other arms can be weighted more heavily in the randomization. Adaptations are considered in the light of accumulating information concerning the hypotheses in question.

Consider two examples. First is a circumstance that occurs commonly in drug studies. Patient accrual and follow-up end without a clear conclusion—the results are neither clearly positive nor clearly negative. For example, the statistical significance level for the primary end-point may be slightly larger than the targeted 5 percent. The company has to carry out another study. A flexible approach in the original study would include the possibility of continuing to accrue patients depending on the results available at the time of the targeted end of accrual. (The overall false-positive rate is affected by such analyses but the final significance levels can be adjusted accordingly.) Allowing for the possibility of extending accrual may increase the study's sample size. A modest increase in average sample size buys a substantial increase in statistical power. This favorable trade-off is because accrual is extended only when the available information indicates that such an extension is worthwhile. Most importantly, the possibility of extending accrual minimizes the chance of having to carry out an additional study when the drug is in fact effective. Moreover, any increase in average sample size can be more than compensated by incorporating frequent interim analyses with the possibility of stopping for futility (that is, if the results on the experimental agent are not sufficiently promising).

A more extreme example of flexibility has the explicit goal of treating patients in the study as effectively as possible, while learning rapidly about relative therapeutic benefits. Patients are assigned with higher probabilities to therapies that are performing better. Such designs are attractive to patients and so can lead to increased participation in clinical studies. And they lead to rapid learning about better performing therapies. Inferior treatments are dropped from consideration early (Giles et al., 2003). Logistics are more complicated because study databases must be updated as soon as results become available; such updating includes information about early end-points that may be related to the primary long-term end-points.

Adaptations are not limited to the data accumulating in the study in question. Information that is reported from other studies also may be used in affecting a study's course.

Using Multifarious Sources of Information

The Bayesian approach is inherently synthetic. Inferences use all available sources of information. Appropriately combining these sources is seldom easy. Populations may be different. Protocols may be different. Some sources may be clinical trials while others are databases accumulated in clinical practice.

Because the Bayesian approach is tailored to combining information, it is increasingly used in meta-analyses (Stangl, 2000). But it can be used in much more complicated settings as well. One of the most complicated is the following. Breast cancer mortality in the United States started to drop in about 1990, decreasing by about 24 percent over the decade 1990–2000.

Possible explanations included mammographic screening and adjuvant treatment with tamoxifen and chemotherapy. The National Cancer Institute funded seven groups to sort out the issue, with the goal of proportionally attributing the decrease to these explanations (Berry et al., 2005).

One of the seven groups took a simulation-based Bayesian approach (Berry et al., 2006). We used relevant empirical information from 1975 to 2000, including the use of screening mammography (schedules such as annual, biennial, haphazard) by the woman's age and year, the characteristics of tumors detected by screening (and which screen) and symptomatically (including interval cancers), the use of tamoxifen by disease stage and the woman's age (and the tumor's hormone-receptor status), the use of polychemotherapy by disease stage and age, and the survival benefits of tamoxifen and chemotherapy by disease stage, age, and hormone-receptor status. We did not have longitudinal information on any set of women and so we had to piece together the effects of the various factors.

As in Bayesian modeling more generally, the important unknown parameters (benefits of treatment, survival after breast cancer depending on method of detection, background incidence of cancer [no screening] over time) had prior probability distributions. For example, for the survival benefit of tamoxifen for women with hormone-receptor positive tumors we based the prior distribution on the Oxford Overview of randomized trials, but with much greater standard deviation than that from the Overview to account for the possibility that tamoxifen used in clinical practice might not have the same benefit as in clinical trials. We generated many thousands of cohorts of 2 million U.S. women having the age distribution of U.S. women in 1975. We accounted for emigration and immigration. For each simulation we selected a particular value from each of the various prior distributions. For example, for one cohort we might have chosen a 20 percent reduction in the risk of breast cancer death when using tamoxifen. We assigned non-breast-cancer survival times to each woman consistent with the overall survival pattern of the actual U.S. population. Women in each simulation got breast cancer with probabilities according to their ages and their use of screening, again consistent with the actual U.S. population. Their cancers had characteristics depending on age and method of detection. Their treatment depended on their tumors' characteristics and was consistent with the mores of the day. We generated breast cancer survival ages for women who were diagnosed with the disease, and these women were recorded as dying of breast cancer if these ages were younger than their non-breast-cancer survival.

For each simulation we tabulated over 1975–2000 the incidence of breast cancer by stage and breast cancer mortality. If these matched the actual U.S. population statistics sufficiently well then we "accepted" the values of the parameters for that simulation into the posterior distribution of the parameters. Most simulations did not match actual mortality. But some did. We simulated enough cohorts to form reasonable conclusions about the posterior distributions.

One set of conclusions in this example was the relative contributions of screening and treatment to the observed decrease in mortality. Another was that despite having access to the various sources of data, our conclusions about the relative contributions of screening and treatment were uncertain. The Bayesian approach allowed for quantifying this uncertainty. The six non-Bayesian models provided point estimates of the relative contributions. Interestingly, these point estimates were consistent with the uncertainty concluded by the Bayesian model.

Still another conclusion from the Bayesian model was that the benefits of tamoxifen and chemotherapy in clinical practice are similar to the benefits seen in the clinical trials. Again, there is some uncertainty in this statement. Although the means of the posterior distributions of these parameters were very similar to the means of the corresponding prior distributions, the posterior standard deviations were not much smaller than the prior distributions.

Conclusion

Statistical philosophy and methodology has contributed in important ways to medical research. The standard approaches are rigorous and not very flexible. Such a tack has been critical to establishing medicine as a science. But having achieved a high plateau, we must move even higher. In this chapter I have suggested some ways that medical research can be more flexible and yet maintain scientific rigor. Bayesian thinking and methodology can help in synthesizing information from various sources and in building more efficient designs. Efficiencies include smaller sample sizes, usually, but also greater accuracy in comparing treatment effectiveness.

SIMULATION AND PREDICTIVE MODELING

Mark S. Roberts, M.D., M.P.P.,
University of Pittsburgh
David M. Eddy, M.D., Ph.D.,
Archimedes, Inc.

Randomized clinical trials have substantial advantages in isolating and testing the effect of an intervention. However, RCTs have weaknesses and limitations, including problems with generalizability, duration, and costs. Physiology-based models, such as the Archimedes model, have the potential to augment and enhance knowledge gained from clinical trials and can be used to fill in "gaps" that are difficult or impractical to answer using clinical trial methods.

Physiology-based models are mechanistic in nature and model disease processes at a biological level rather than through statistical relationships between observed data and outcomes. When properly constructed, they replicate the results of the studies used to build them, not only in terms of outcomes but also in terms of the changes in biomarkers and clinical findings as well. A unique characteristic of a properly constructed physiology-based model is its ability to predict the results of studies and trials that have not been used in the model's construction, a process that provides very strong validation of its predictions.

This paper will describe the Archimedes model as an example of a physiology-based model and will propose uses for such models. The methods for representing and calibrating the mechanistic processes will be described, and comparisons of simulated trials to actual clinical trials as a method of validation will be presented. Multiple uses of the Archimedes model to enhance and extend existing clinical trials as well as to conduct virtual comparative effectiveness trials also will be discussed.

Strengths and Weakness of Randomized Controlled Trials

The main strength of randomized controlled trials is that the random assignment to treatment and control group renders those groups equivalent and eliminates bias by indication, resulting in intervention and control groups that are balanced in known and unknown parameters. At the same time, strictly controlled protocols isolate the specific effect of the intervention.

The weaknesses of RCTs are well known. They often represent a narrow spectrum of disease, are conducted in specialized, highly controlled environments, and are expensive. Patients and physicians must agree to participate, which produces a selection bias that limits generalizability to other populations. They often require a large number of patients and follow-up times so long that the trial results might be eclipsed by the pace of technologic change. This is true, for example, in HIV disease, in which antiretroviral resistance patterns are rapidly and constantly changing, and the number of HIV drugs is rapidly expanding. Finally, RCTs usually represent efficacy, not effectiveness, as they are typically conducted in tightly controlled settings in which care processes have high levels of compliance and protocol adherence.

Physiology-Based Models

The use of physiology-based or mechanistic models as an adjunct or alternative to RCTs has been increasing in several different fields. Although only recently used in medicine, there are some interesting examples of this in sepsis (Day et al., 2006; Reynolds et al., 2006; Vodovotz et al., 2004), in critical care and injury (Clermont et al., 2004b; Saka et al., 2007), in the acquisition of antiretroviral resistance in HIV disease (Braithwaite et al., 2006, 2008), and in the Archimedes model, which currently includes car-diovascular and metabolic diseases (Eddy and Schlessinger, 2003a; Heikes et al., 2007; Sherwin et al., 2004).

Physiology-based models seek to represent the underlying biology of the disease. They are continuous in time and generally model the physi-ological processes that create the data observed in the world: They do not simply model the relationship between observed variables and outcomes statistically. Physiology-based models can represent many different levels of detail, from physiologic variables and biomarkers that create disease through anatomy, symptoms, behaviors, all the way up through interactions with health systems, utilization, and costs.

The Archimedes model is designed to represent actual biological rela-tionships and is best illustrated visually in a similar manner to how these relationships are presented in a standard textbook of physiology, with physiological parameters and their relationships described with influence-diagrams at multiple levels of detail from whole organ relationships to processes that occur within organs to those within cells, etc. Similarly, every virtual individual in the Archimedes model has a virtual heart with four virtual chambers, a virtual circulatory system that has a virtual blood pres-sure and responds to virtual changes in cardiovascular dynamics. The vir-tual individual has a virtual liver that produces virtual glucose, a virtual gut that absorbs virtual nutrients, a virtual pancreas with virtual beta cells that make virtual insulin, and virtual muscle mass and virtual fat cell mass that utilizes glucose as a function of the amount of virtual insulin available.

Figure 3-9 shows a small portion of the model, but illustrates the types of variables and relationships that are in the Archimedes model. The figure resembles the "bubble diagrams" from physiology texts, and in this particu-lar example, represents some of the factors that affect diabetes and other metabolic conditions. In the figure, every oval represents a characteristic, biological parameter, condition, test, intervention, symptom, or other type of clinically important variable. Some of the relationships are trivial and obvious as, for example, is the relationship between height and weight that defines the body mass index (BMI) with a simple functional form. Most of the functions are substantially more complicated and are typically rep-resented as differential equations that relate the instantaneous change in a particular physiological parameter to the level and change of many other variables. The equations that are contained in the Archimedes model relate the various physiological variables to each other and to specific outcomes, such as the development of diabetes and heart disease. The functional

183

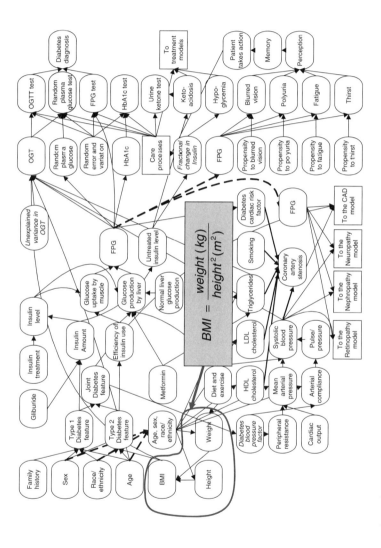

FIGURE 3-9 Physiological factors affecting development of diabetes. BMI is shown as one such variable, composed of the components height and weight through the indicated equation.
SOURCE: Copyright © 2003 American Diabetes Association. From *Diabetes Care*, Vol. 26, 2003; 3093-3101. Modified with permission from the American Diabetes Association.

form of the equations and the coefficients on the terms of the equations are derived from and calibrated with data from a wide variety of empirical sources, ranging from studies of basic biology to large longitudinal trials and datasets. A more complete description of the Archimedes model and its development is available elsewhere (Eddy and Schlessinger, 2003a; Schlessinger and Eddy, 2002).

Validation of a Physiology-Based Model

One of the most important steps in the building and use of a model is validation. Confidence in a model's predictions is necessary if models are to be used for clinical and health policy decisions. In general, model validation starts with demonstrating that the model can replicate the results of the trials and studies that were used to develop and calibrate the model. This is called a "dependent" validation. This method of validation is used in both biological and statistical models. However, perhaps the most appropriate "gold standard" of validation is the ability to replicate the results of multiple actual clinical trials that have not been used to build or modify the model. This is called an "independent" validation. A clinical trial enrolls real people, administers real treatments (usually by randomizing them to specific therapies), and records real outcomes a specified time later. The Archimedes model can replicate that process by enrolling virtual people with the exact characteristics of their counterparts in real clinical trials and randomly assign them to virtual treatments that represent the real treatments used in the trial, record virtual outcomes using the same definitions and methods used in the trials, and then compare the results of the virtual trial to those of the real trial. Data available from separate Phase I or Phase II trials can be used to estimate the effects of the intervention on the relevant biomarkers. The Archimedes model has been validated by successfully replicating more than 50 major clinical trials. About half of these validations have been independent.

An example of a dependent validation is provided in Figure 3-10, which compares the actual results from the UK Prospective Diabetes Study (UKPDS) to the simulated results calculated by replicating the trial in Archimedes. Although technically a dependent validation, it is important to note that the models results shown in Figure 3-10 were not "fitted" to the results of the trial. Rather, data from the trial were used to fit only two equations: the rate of progression of insulin resistance in untreated diabetes and the effect of insulin resistance on progression of plaque in coronary arteries. Simulation of the trial involved scores of other equations that were not touched by any data from the trial. Thus even though dependent, this validation tests large parts of the model.

Prospective and independent validations also have been conducted.

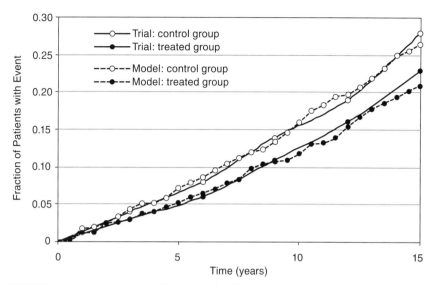

FIGURE 3-10 Retrospective (dependent) validation: Simulated UKPDS trial comparing real trial results (fatal and nonfatal myocardial infarction) to a simulated version of the trial using the Archimedes model.
SOURCE: Copyright © 2003 American Diabetes Association. From *Diabetes Care*, Vol. 26, 2003; 3102-3110. Modified with permission from the American Diabetes Association.

Figure 3-11 shows the results of a validation that was both prospective and independent. It predicted the results of the Collaborative Atorvastatin Diabetes Study (CARDS), which tested the ability of a lipid-lowering medication to reduce cardiovascular events in patients with diabetes. The figure shows the actual trial result for both the intervention and control arm (solid lines) and the predictions of the Archimedes model (dotted lines). In this validation, the model's results were sent in sealed envelopes to the ADA and the study investigators prior to the release of the study's results.

The results for 18 clinical trials have been published. Figure 3-12 compares the results of 74 simulated trials in diabetes, lipid control, and cardiovascular disease, and graphs the actual relative risk found from a trial and the results calculated by the Archimedes model. Because the ability to replicate the results from each arm is considered a validation of the model, this graph represents many more validations than the simple number of clinical trials. The correlation coefficient of the actual and predicted results is $r = 0.99$.

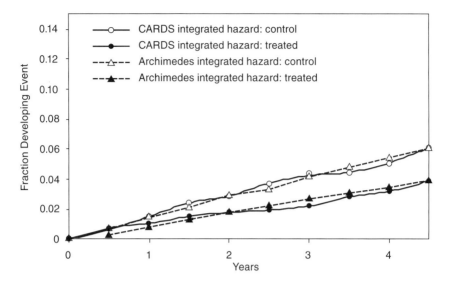

FIGURE 3-11 Prospective and independent validation of the CARDS trial comparing real trial results to results predicted by the Archimedes model.
SOURCE: Derived from Mount Hood Modeling Group. 2007. Computer modeling of diabetes and its complications: A report on the fourth mount hood challenge meeting. *Diabetes Care* 30(6):1638-1646. Modified with permission from the American Diabetes Association.

Applications of Physiology-Based Models

There are several ways that physiology-based prediction models can be used to enhance clinical trials. One is to help identify and set priorities for new trials. Another is to facilitate the design of new trials. For example, as the validations described above have shown the Archimedes model can be used to estimate the rates of outcomes in control groups and the expected magnitude of the effects of treatments. This information can then be used to help calculate sample sizes, and the durations required to detect outcomes with specified powers. Another use of physiology-based models is to extend clinical trials to estimate long-term outcomes. If a model has successfully calculated the outcomes in the trial of interest over the duration of the trial, and if it has successfully calculated the important biomarkers and clinical outcomes in a variety of other trials that involve similar populations and interventions, then there is good reason to believe its projections for the outcomes of trial over a longer follow-up period will be accurate. At the least, such a trial-validated application is the best available method for estimating longer term outcomes. Related roles of well-validated physiology-

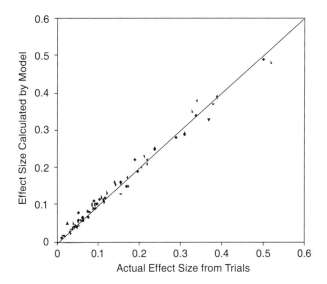

FIGURE 3-12 Comparison of Archimedes model and multiple trials. The x-axis represents the size of the effect measured in the actual trial; the y-axis is the size of the effect in the simulated version of the trial in Archimedes.
SOURCE: Copyright © 2003 American Diabetes Association. From *Diabetes Care*, Vol. 26, 2003; 3102-3110. Modified with permission from the American Diabetes Association. Modified from Eddy and Schlessinger, 2003a.

based models are to extend a trial's results to other outcomes that were not examined in the original trial, such as logistic or economic outcomes, and to examine the results for subpopulations.

Physiology-based models can also be used to customize the results of atrial to different settings. For example, a model that has been demonstrated to be accurate in predicting the results of the original trial and related trials can be used to address such issues as settings that have different levels of performance and compliance, and settings that have different background protocols and/or cost structures. For example, a common complaint of clinical trials is that they represent efficacy, the effect of a medication or intervention in tightly controlled, highly specialized environments. However, the effectiveness of these therapies in real-world conditions may be quite different, because of different levels of adherence to the intervention or differences in the quality of baseline care. The model also can study variations in the background rates of healthcare practices seen in different settings. For example, if we are testing a medication for decreasing cardiovascular risk in diabetic patients, but happen to be concerned about a setting in which patients seen in emergency rooms have a very small chance of being treated with thrombolytic, the overall effect on cardiovascular outcomes will be different than would be seen in a setting in which the use of thrombolytics is very high. These types of processes can be included large-scale physiologic-based models but are virtually impossible to incorporate in regression based and Markov models.

Physiology-based models also can be used for analyzing the comparative effectiveness of different treatments for a condition. Suppose there are trials of Medication A versus placebo and of Medication B versus placebo but no trials directly comparing Medication A versus Medication B. Rather than conduct a new trial that compares A versus B, which could be extremely expensive and take years (by which time new medications will invariably have been introduced), physiology-based models that have successfully predicted the two original trials can provide the best currently available estimate of what a real trial of A versus B would be likely to show. This information can then be used to understand the potential value of a new trial of A versus B, to plan a new trial if it is deemed to be desirable, and to recommend what practices should be followed while waiting for the trials results.

The development and calibration of physiology-based models require good data for each of the elements it includes. A model like Archimedes would not have been possible without large-scale cross-sectional and longitudinal datasets such as National Health and Nutrition Examiniation Survey, Framingham, and Atherosclerosis Risk in Communities. A model like Archimedes also rests on clinical trials for understanding the natural progression of diseases and the effects of treatments, for both dependent and independent validations. Data for physiology-based models are most useful if they contain data on demographics (e.g., age, gender, ethnicity); past medical history, family history, physical findings; biomarkers; signs and symptoms; and outcomes. The volume and quality of data of these types can be expected to increase as the use of electronic medical records spreads.

The key to all of these applications is that if a model is to be used to predict, plan, extend, or help fill the gaps between clinical trials, it must prove its ability to reproduce and predict the results of many real clinical trials, using only data available at the start of the trial, and not using any results from the trial to build or modify the model to fit the results of new trials. It is very easy to build models that fit the results of any particular trial, using regression models, Markov models, or other non-physiology-based approaches. It also is easy to build simple models that fit data from multiple disparate sources if each of the sources addresses a different part of the model (e.g., one study of incidence, another of progression, a third of the effect of a treatment on one outcome, and a fourth of the effect of a treatment on a different outcome). This type of validation by itself provides little evidence about the model's ability to predict the results of a new trial. For the latter problem, which is our main interest in this paper, it is important that there be multiple validations, involving overlapping populations, treatments, and outcomes, and that the model accurately predicts the results of all of the trials without using the results of any of them.

In this paper we have used the Archimedes model to illustrate these types of validations and the types of applications to which such a model can be put. However, it is important to note that over the past few years some other physiology-based models also have succeeded in predicting the results of some trials. For example, a physiology-based model of HIV resistance predicted the actual resistance rates seen in two independent trials not used to develop the model (Braithwaite et al., 2006). Similarly, physiology-based models for sepsis have been able to prospectively predict outcomes and cytokine patterns (in animals) after acute injury by applying large systems of differential equations that relate the insult to the cytokine production (Clermont et al., 2004a; Reynolds et al., 2006; Vodovotz et al., 2004).

In conclusion, the strengths and limitations of clinical trials are well known. Physiology-based models have substantial promise to, and a growing track record of, addressing many of these limitations. If carefully built and rigorously validated they can be used to enhance and extend the knowledge gained from trials.

EMERGING GENOMIC INFORMATION

Teri A. Manolio, M.D., Ph.D.
U.S. Department of Health and Human Services
National Institutes of Health
National Human Genome Research Institute

The recent advent of high-density, cost-effective, genomewide genotyping technologies as led to a virtual explosion of information on genetic variants related to common, complex diseases (Pearson and Manolio, 2008). In just the past 3 years, over 100 genetic variants associated with nearly 40 complex diseases and traits have been reliably identified and replicated using this revolutionary technology. Several of these findings have sufficient supporting evidence for functional significance or biologic plausibility, and many are sufficiently common that they provide real potential for translation into diagnostic, preventive, or therapeutic interventions. In this new era of genomic discovery, one of the most pressing questions for clinical effectiveness research is thus: What is needed to facilitate the reliable and timely introduction of emerging genetic information into research and clinical databases?

Genomewide Association Studies

The identification and mapping of the most common form of genetic variation, the single nucleotide polymorphism (SNP), has permitted the development of cost-effective genotyping platforms that utilize the patterns of association, or co-inheritance, among SNPs to assay the majority of common variants in the human population (Frazer et al., 2007; A haplotype map of the human genome, 2005; The International HapMap Project, 2003). Upward of 80–90 percent of common variants (those present at an allele frequency of 5 percent or more) can now be assayed by typing 500,000–1,000,000 carefully selected SNPs (Manolio et al., 2007). This allows a systematic approach to association testing that frees genomic investigation from dependence on what is as yet an imperfect understanding of genomic function, or on strongly supported prior hypotheses (Chanock et al., 2007; Frazer et al., 2007).

Success to Date of Genomewide Association Studies

The genomewide association (GWA) approach has been enormously successful in identifying genetic variants related to complex diseases, or diseases likely influenced by multiple genes and environmental factors. The first notable success of this method came in March 2005, with the identification of a variant in the gene for complement factor H (*CFH*) associated with age-related macular degeneration (Klein et al., 2005). This strong and highly significant relationship was simultaneously reported using two other study designs, and subsequently replicated many times (Edwards et al., 2005; Haines et al., 2005; Magnusson et al., 2006; Sepp et al., 2006; Zareparsi et al., 2005). Two additional GWA studies were published within that year, of Parkinson's disease and obesity (Herbert et al., 2006; Maraganore et al., 2005), but efforts at replicating these findings have been inconsistent (Hall et al., 2006; Lyon et al., 2007; Myers, 2006). Later in 2006, strong, robust associations with electrocardiographic QT interval prolongation (Arking et al., 2006), neovascular macular degeneration (Dewan et al., 2006), and inflammatory bowel disease (Duerr et al., 2006) were identified and have since been the subjects of a substantial body of follow-up research to determine gene function and population impact.

This pace of genomic discovery increased dramatically in 2007, following the increased availability of high-density genotyping platforms and experience in interpreting the results. Simultaneous publication of coordinated efforts in prostate cancer (Gudmundsson et al., 2007; Yeager et al., 2007), diabetes (Saxena et al., 2007; Scott et al., 2007; Zeggini et al., 2007), and breast cancer (Easton et al., 2007; Hunter et al., 2007; Stacey et al., 2007) demonstrated the power and value of collaborative projects involving multiple investigative efforts, often involving tens of thousands of study subjects. These were soon followed by publication of the landmark Wellcome Trust Case Control Consortium of 2,000 cases each of 7 common diseases and 3,000 shared controls (Wellcome Trust Case Control Consortium, 2007). Rapid progress has continued into 2008 with investigation of a wide variety of diseases and traits, though not all have produced definitive results (Table 3-2). Indeed, as Hunter and Kraft have noted, "There have been few, if any, similar bursts of discovery in the history of medical research" (Hunter and Kraft, 2007).

Recombination Rate

Unique aspects of the GWA methodology that have made these discoveries possible include its potential for examining inherited genetic variability at an unprecedented level of resolution. GWA studies allow the investigator to narrow an association region to a 5–10 kilobase length of DNA, in contrast to the 5–10 megabases usually detected in familial linkage studies. Because GWA regions typically contain only a few genes, rather than the dozens or hundreds implicated in linkage regions, potentially causative variants can be examined much more rapidly and in greater depth. As noted above, systematic interrogation of the entire genome frees the investigator from reliance on inaccurate prior hypotheses based on incomplete understanding of genome structure and function. The critical importance of this is illustrated by the fact that many of the associations identified to date, such as complement factor H in macular degeneration (Klein et al., 2005) and *TCF7L2* in Type 2 diabetes (Grant et al., 2006; Sladek et al., 2007) have not been with genes previously suspected of being related to the disease. Some, such as the strong associations of prostate cancer with SNPs in the 8q24 region (Scott et al., 2007), and Crohn's disease with the 5p13 region (Genome-wide association study of 14,000 cases of seven common diseases and 3,000 shared controls, 2007), have been in genomic regions containing no known genes at all. And because current genotyping assays capture the vast majority of human variation genomewide, rather than being focused on particular regions or pathways, once a GWA scan is completed it can be applied to any condition or trait measured in that same individual and consistent with his or her informed consent.

The potential for harnessing these data to examine additional traits has been amply demonstrated in GWA studies of anthropometric traits (such as obesity and height) and laboratory measures (such as serum urate and lipoproteins) performed in cohorts with a primary focus on diabetes

TABLE 3-2 Diseases and Traits Studied Using Genomewide Association Testing Assaying 100,000 Variants or More, March 2005–March 2008

Eye Diseases	**Neuropsychiatric Conditions**
• Macular Degeneration	• Parkinson's Disease
• Exfoliation Glaucoma	• Amyotrophic Lateral Sclerosis
• Macular Degeneration	• Multiple Sclerosis
• Exfoliation Glaucoma	• Progressive Supranuclear Palsy
	• MS Interferon Response
Cancer	• Alzheimer's Disease
• Lung Cancer	• Cognitive Ability
• Prostate Cancer	• Memory
• Breast Cancer	• Restless Legs Syndrome
• Colorectal Cancer	• Nicotine Dependence
	• Neuroticism
Gastrointestinal Diseases	• Schizophrenia
• Crohn's Disease	• Bipolar Disorder
• Celiac Disease	
• Gallstones	**Diabetes and Body Size**
• Irritable Bowel Syndrome	• Type 1 Diabetes
	• Type 2 Diabetes
Cardiovascular Conditions	• Diabetic Nephropathy
• QT Prolongation	• End-Stage Renal Disease
• Coronary Disease	• Obesity, BMI
• Stroke	• Height
• Hypertension	
• Atrial Fibrillation/Flutter	**Other Traits**
• Coronary Spasm	• F-Cell Distribution
• Lipids and Lipoproteins	• Fetal Hemoglobin Levels
	• 18 Groups of Traits in Framingham
Autoimmune and Infectious Disorders	Heart Study
• Rheumatoid Arthritis	• Pigmentation
• Childhood Asthma	• Uric Acid Levels
• Systemic Lupus Erythematosus	
• HIV Viral Setpoint	

NOTE: Adapted from Manolio et al., 2007.

or hypertension (Frayling et al., 2007; Wallace et al., 2008; Weedon et al., 2007; Willer et al., 2008). In addition, application of GWA genotyping to long-standing, extensively characterized cohorts such as the Framingham Heart Study and Women's Health Study (Cupples et al., 2007; Ridker et al., 2008) opens the door to investigation of the genetics of every disease and trait measured in these extensive studies and consistent with participants' informed consent, adding substantially to their research value both now and for the future.

Challenges of GWA Studies

Against the context of this remarkable flow of findings, however, lies a fundamental challenge of GWA studies: With hundreds of thousands of comparisons performed per study, the potential for spurious associations is unprecedented (Hunter and Kraft, 2007). This was widely recognized as a major shortcoming of candidate gene association studies, in which small sample sizes, publication bias, and the play of chance led to a rash of irreproducible results early on (Colhoun et al., 2003; Ioannidis et al., 2001). The problem was illustrated by Hirschhorn et al. in a seminal paper in 2002, who demonstrated that of 600 genetic associations reviewed, only 6 could be reliably reproduced (Hirschhorn et al., 2002). A variety of statistical approaches has been proposed for dealing with this problem in GWA studies, including the use of a standard Bonferroni correction, by dividing the conventional p-value (typically 0.05) by the number of tests performed (often 10^6 or more) (Yang et al., 2005). Other approaches include calculation of the false discovery rate or the false-positive report probability to estimate the proportion of significant associations that are actually false positives (Pearson and Manolio, 2008). But the approach most widely accepted is replication of findings (Todd, 2006), often in a staged design expanding from an initial set of 500 or 1,000 cases and similar number of matched controls to studies involving as many as 40,000 or 50,000 participants (Chanock et al., 2007; Hoover, 2007). These large numbers are necessitated by the very stringent p-values demanded by the hundreds of thousands of comparisons performed, and by the relatively modest effect sizes of the variants detected, typically carrying odds ratios of 1.5 or less (Pearson and Manolio, 2008). Such numbers have generally been achieved by combining many smaller studies (Easton et al., 2007; Frayling, 2007), but the potential for conducting this research in large healthcare systems involving hundreds of thousands or millions of participants should not be overlooked.

Use of GWA Information in Research and Clinical Databases

One way of using this emerging genomic technology in research and clinical databases is to perform GWA genotyping in patients with comprehensive (and typically, electronic) medical records and suitable consent to investigate a wide variety of past and current diagnoses or traits. Record linkage may also permit subsequent follow-up for development and progression of new clinical diagnoses or characteristics. Such studies are designed primarily for genomic discovery, to identify additional variants, genes, or regions associated with disease, which then require extensive additional investigation to identify causal variants, biologic mechanisms, and potential interventions. This approach is being used in large-scale biorepositories such as those organized by Kaiser Permanente (Research, 2008) and the Children's Hospital of Philadelphia in the United States (Philadelphia, 2008), deCODE Genetics in Iceland (Gulcher and Stefansson, 1998), and the UK Biobank in Britain (Palmer, 2007). GWA genotyping is also being applied to a more limited degree (that is, only to subsets of participants selected for presence or absence of disease in case control studies) in a number of biorepositories with electronic health records (EHRs), such as those participating in the National Human Genome Research Institute's eMERGE network (The eMERGE Network, 2008). Substantial efforts will be needed to examine the reliability and standardization of phenotypic measures derived from EHRs for genomic research, as well as the adequacy of participants' consent for the extensive investigation and widespread data sharing common in these studies.

A simpler and more immediate way of using emerging genomic information in research and clinical databases is to test only the variants that have been strongly implicated in disease causation or progression from GWA and other genomic discovery studies. This is particularly suited to clinical settings without the extensive research infrastructures needed for gene discovery (such as standardized phenotype and exposure measures, flexible informatics systems, biospecimen repositories, and consent for broad research uses), where real-world implications of these discoveries are best assessed. Limited genotyping for specific variants of interest in specific conditions can often be conducted more readily than GWA genotyping, assuming consent is adequate and phenotypic measures are reliable, allowing evaluation of the clinical and public health impact of these variants on a very large scale.

Genomic Information Suitable for Clinical Effectiveness Research

Assays of genetic variants related to two traits—Type 2 diabetes risk and warfarin dosing requirements—have sufficient scientific foundation and clinical availability to serve as prototypes for applying genomic information emerging from GWA studies to clinical effectiveness research. In a longer paper we also might have considered *CFH* and age-related macular degeneration (Klein et al., 2005), *IL23R* and inflammatory bowel disease (Duerr et al., 2006), or chromosome 8q24 variants and prostate cancer (Gudmundsson et al., 2007; Yeager et al., 2007), all of which would also lend themselves well to investigating questions of clinical effectiveness.

Type 2 Diabetes and TCF7L2

GWA studies have identified a number of variants associated with risk of diabetes to a modest degree, but the one first implicated by this approach, *TCF7L2*, clearly carries the greatest increased risk (Weedon,

2007). *TCF7L2* is a transcription factor that is part of the Wnt signaling pathway, a pathway critical for cell proliferation, motility, and development, particularly of the pancreas (Weedon, 2007). It is an excellent example of the power of the hypothesis-free approach exemplified by GWA studies, since this gene was not previously suspected of playing any role in diabetes. The variant was initially identified in a linkage study of diabetes in Icelanders by deCODE Genetics, Inc., and was shown to be present in 36 percent of patients with diabetes but only 28 percent of unaffected individuals (Grant et al., 2006). An estimated 38 percent of the Icelandic population was heterozygous for the risk allele, and 7 percent were homozygous. Each copy of the risk allele increased the odds of diabetes 1.56-fold with a p-value of 10^{-18} when the Icelandic study was combined with similar studies from Denmark and the United States (Grant et al., 2006).

When this finding was first published in January 2006, it evoked surprise and a certain degree of perplexity, since there was no *a priori* biologic information supporting such an association. The data presented, however, were quite robust and convincing, and the finding was subsequently replicated in a GWA study of French cases and controls in February 2007 (Sladek et al., 2007). Three additional GWA studies in British and Scandinavian participants published in April 2007 all found *TCF7L2* to be their strongest association signal (Saxena et al., 2007; Scott et al., 2007; Zeggini et al., 2007). These and subsequent studies have suggested a slightly lower odds ratio, closer to 1.4, but the association has been replicated in every population in which it has been examined (Frayling, 2007; Weedon, 2007).

Clinical testing for *TCF7L2* variants is currently offered by DNA Direct (DNA Direct, 2008) and deCODE Diagnostics (Genetics, 2008), the corporate home of the team that published the original paper (Grant et al., 2006). deCODE Diagnostics also offers DNA-based tests for assessing risk of atrial fibrillation, myocardial infarction, glaucoma, and prostate cancer, all conditions for which deCODE Genetics published the first or one of the first GWA studies (Gudbjartsson et al., 2007; Gudmundsson et al., 2007; Helgadottir et al., 2007; Thorleifsson et al., 2007). Information about *TCF7L2* testing (provided in a 4-gene panel referred to as deCODE T2™) is provided for physicians and patients on the company's website and describes the research conducted at deCODE and elsewhere demonstrating the *TCF7L2*–diabetes association (Genetics, 2008). Data from the NIH-sponsored clinical trial of diabetes prevention, the Diabetes Prevention Program (DPP), are cited showing that prediabetics homozygous for the risk allele were at 1.8-fold increased risk of developing diabetes in the next 4 years compared to heterozygotes or those without a risk allele (Florez et al., 2006). Evidence from the DPP on the effectiveness of weight loss and metformin treatment in reducing the risk of diabetes is also summarized, demonstrating the availability of clinical-trial proven interventions to reduce diabetes incidence in persons at risk for the disease. The website notes that deCODE offers a Clinical Laboratory Improvement Amendments (CLIA)-certified testing facility, that the test is not FDA-approved, and that information from the test may "offer a new means to help physicians decide which prediabetic patients they wish to treat more aggressively either through lifestyle modification or drug treatment." It also includes an important caveat: "Information gained from a genetic test does not itself prevent the development of disease, but can be used in formulating better preventive strategies. A positive genetic test result can emphasize the increased importance of using available and appropriate means in that regard" (deCODE, 2008).

Marketing or application of diagnostic genetic testing in this way has raised some anxieties, primarily due to the lack of evidence that genetic testing improves outcome or adds significantly to readily available clinical information (Haga et al., 2003; Janssens et al., 2006). Such evidence should be derivable, however, by linking genotypic data on these variants to phenotypic characteristics (such as presence of diagnosed diabetes or intermediate traits) and environmental exposures (such as lifestyle factors or medication use) in real-world clinical databases or ongoing research studies. If possible, it would be best to demonstrate that patients and/or their clinicians understood and retained the information and implemented appropriate interventions if improved outcomes are to be correctly attributed to the testing (Feero et al., 2008; Hunter et al., 2008).

Warfarin

Warfarin is a commonly used anticoagulant for prevention of pulmonary embolism in venous thromboembolic disease and of stroke in atrial fibrillation. Dosage must be maintained within a narrow range specific to each patient to prevent over-anticoagulation, and subsequent hemorrhage, or inadequate anticoagulation, and subsequent thrombosis. Dose requirements vary widely between individuals and are influenced by age, sex, body size, diet, medication use, and presence of other medical conditions (Kimmel, 2008). Variants in the cytochrome P450 system, specifically the *2 and *3 alleles of *CYP2C9*, have been shown to be associated with significantly lower dose requirements (Higashi et al., 2002). More recently, variants in the gene encoding vitamin K epoxide reductase complex 1 (*VKORC1*) have been shown to have similar effects (Figure 3-13 [Rieder et al., 2005]). A number of dosing algorithms have been proposed to reduce time to achieve therapeutic levels and avoid over-anticoagulation, incorporating a variety of clinical and genetic information (Kimmel, 2008).

Like *TCF7L2* and diabetes, the effectiveness of including pharmaco-

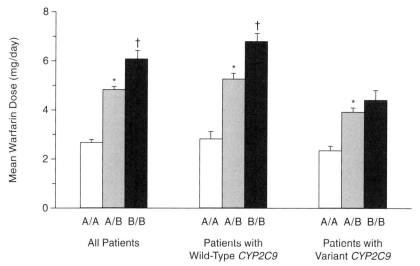

FIGURE 3-13 Patients were genotyped and assigned a *VKORC1* haplotype combination (A/A, A/B, or B/B). The patients were further classified according to *CYP2C9* genotype (the wild type or either the *2 or *3 variant). The total numbers of patients having a group A combination, a group B combination, or both were 182 (all patients), 124 (wild-type *CYP2C9*), and 58 (variant *CYP2C9*). The asterisks denote $P < 0.05$ for the comparison with combination A/A and the daggers $P < 0.05$ for the comparison with combination A/B. The T bars represent standard errors. SOURCE: Rieder, M. J., A. P. Reiner, B. F. Gage, D. A. Nickerson, C. S. Eby, H. L. McLeod, D. K. Blough, K. E. Thummel, D. L. Veenstra, and A. E. Rettie. 2005. Effect of vkorc1 haplotypes on transcriptional regulation and warfarin dose. *New England Journal of Medicine* 352(22):2285-2293. Copyright © 2005 Massachusetts Medical Society. All rights reserved.

genetic information in warfarin-dosing algorithms has yet to be demonstrated, despite clear evidence of dose dependence on a number of variants (Figure 3-14) (Anderson et al., 2007; Shurin and Nabel, 2008). Fortunately, a large, NIH-sponsored, randomized trial of genotype-guided warfarin therapy, designed to provide definitive answers to questions of clinical effectiveness, is about to get underway (Shurin and Nabel, 2008).

Incorporating Genomic Information into Clinical Effectiveness Research

With the examples of *TCF7L2* and warfarin-dosing-related variants in hand, we can return to our original question of what is needed to facilitate the reliable and timely introduction of emerging genomic information into

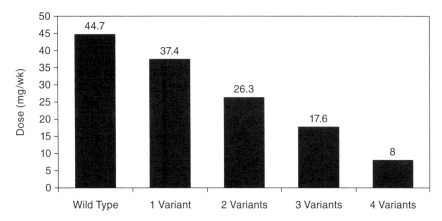

FIGURE 3-14 Average stable maintenance warfarin doses (mg/wk) by number of variant alleles (reproduced with permission from [Anderson et al., 2007]). Numbers of patients in each group: wild type (no variants), 56 (30%); 1 variant, 75 (43%); 2 variants, 36 (21%); 3 variants, 7 (4%); and 4 variants, 1 (0.6%). SEM is 2.0 for wild type and 1.4 for 1-, 2-, and 3-variant groups. Dose differences across groups are highly significant (P << 0.001).
SOURCE: Anderson, J. L., B. D. Horne, S. M. Stevens, A. S. Grove, S. Barton, Z. P. Nicholas, S. F. Kahn, H. T. May, K. M. Samuelson, J. B. Muhlestein, J. F. Carlquist; Couma-Gen Investigators. Randomized trial of genotype-guided versus standard war-farin dosing in patients initiating oral anticoagulation. *Circulation* 2007; 116:2563-2570.

research and clinical databases. Needs can be identified in several areas, including the information needed for rational clinical decision making likely to affect outcomes; the laboratory and clinical infrastructure needed to utilize this information in clinical practice; and the policy and educational infrastructures needed to facilitate this research.

Epidemiologic Information Needed

Much of the basic information needed for informed decision making about newly identified genetic variants relates to fundamental epidemiologic questions such as prevalence, risk, and potential for risk reduction. Genetic variants such as those in *TCF7L2*, *CYP2C9*, and *VKORC1* are essentially risk factors for complex diseases, similar in many ways to nongenetic risk factors such as obesity, smoking, or hypertension. Before recommending screening of *TCF7L2* variants (or any risk factor) in persons at risk for diabetes to increase the intensity of efforts to prevent diabetes, for example, or of *CYP2C9* or *VKORC1* variants to guide warfarin dosing, several pieces of information would be useful (Box 3-1). The prevalence of the variant is an important factor—testing for common variants is likely to be more useful and cost-effective than testing for rare ones. It may still be important to measure rare variants if their effects are devastating and essentially avoidable (such as *TPMT* variants in 6-mercaptopurine dosing [Wang and Weinshilboum, 2006] or phenylalanine hydroxylase deficiency in phenylketonuria [Scriver, 2007]), but even there information on prevalence is useful in estimating the costs of screening or the magnitude of the population likely to need intervention, if interventions are available.

Magnitude of increased risk associated with the variant is also important—variants of large effect would likely have more impact than those of small effect. Differences in the presence or magnitude of associated risk across different demographic groups, such as those defined by age, sex, or race/ethnicity, or in persons with particular medical conditions, lifestyle factors, or medications, would be useful in targeting testing or interpreting results. Independence of the association from other known risk factors, such as body mass, family history, or age, also would be important—it would seem unwise at present to substitute a genetic test for other information that is readily available clinically. Association of the variant with earlier onset or more severe course, or with response to treatment, might suggest targeted interventions or time-sensitive ones, or provide clues to pathogenesis. Evidence that knowledge of the variant would improve patients' adherence to effective interventions also would be useful.

Much of this epidemiologic information about genetic variants identified as potentially causally associated with complex diseases can be readily obtained by assaying them in well-characterized population studies.

BOX 3-1
Epidemiologic Information Needed to Assess the Usefulness of Genetic Variants in Clinical Practice

- Prevalence
- Magnitude of increased risk associated with variant
- Consistency of increased risk across multiple groups defined by age, sex, race/ethnicity, exposures
- Independence of associated risk from other known risk factors
- Association of variant with earlier onset or more severe disease course
- Association of variant with response to treatment (gene–environment interaction)

Genomewide genotyping in cohorts such as the Framingham Heart Study or the Women's Health Study (Cupples et al., 2007; Ridker et al., 2008), will provide this type of information, as will typing of specific variants in large numbers of extensively phenotyped participants in other cross-sectional studies, prospective cohorts, and clinical trials. Such efforts have been quite valuable in understanding the epidemiology of diabetes risk variants as studied in the Diabetes Prevention Program (Florez et al., 2006, 2007), particularly when the resulting prevalence and association data are made widely available. The National Human Genome Research Institute (NHGRI) is initiating a program to expand genotyping of putative causal variants in large-scale population studies and disseminate the results, as permitted by participants' informed consent, for application in research and clinical settings (Services, 2007).

Genetic Information Needed

Detailed information about the genomic region proposed for testing is also needed (Box 3-2). The *TCF7L2* gene, for example, is large and complex, with 17 exons and 4 alternate splice sites yielding multiple isoforms (John Hopkins University, 2008). The markers first identified as associated with diabetes lay in the third intron of the gene, in a well-defined linkage disequilibrium (LD) block spanning 92 kb (Figure 3-15 [Grant et al., 2006]). Conceivably, any of the variants in this block, which encompasses all of exon 4 and parts of introns 3 and 4, could be responsible for the observed association, since they would all tend to be inherited together. This would include variants that were not assayed on the original genotyping platform or, possibly, not even yet known to exist. Substantial investigative effort was needed to narrow this down; in this instance, the deCODE investigators identified another SNP, rs7903146, that carried a higher relative risk at a

---

BOX 3-2
Genetic Information Needed to Select Genetic Variants for Use in Clinical Effectiveness Research

- Location and frequency of variants in and near association region
- Allelic forms including insertions, deletions, and duplications, as well as single nucleotide polymorphisms
- Linkage-disequilibrium relationships among these variants
- Type of variants: coding, promoter, splice site
- Ease of typing and reliability of assay for each variant

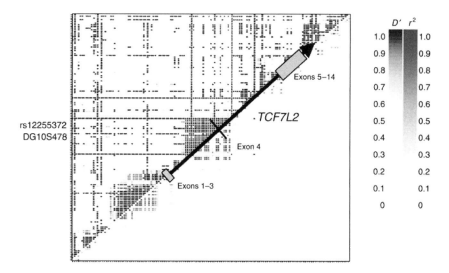

FIGURE 3-15 Region of interest in *TCF7L2* and associated linkage disequilibrium (LD) pattern. LD between pairs of SNPs is shown by standard D′ (upper left) or r^2 measures (lower right); the 216-kb gene spans several LD blocks as shown by the black arrow, indicating the direction of transcription and position of exons. Relative location of two of the most strongly associated markers, rs12255372 and DG10S478, are also shown.
SOURCE: Reprinted by permission from Macmillan Publishers, Ltd. *Nature Genetics* 38(3):320-323. Copyright © 2006.

much stronger significance level (Grant et al., 2006). It is this variant that is reported from deCODE T2™. One might want to demonstrate, however, that assaying this variant is sufficient to measure all of the relevant variation in the region, as LD blocks may contain multiple independent signals (Haiman et al., 2007).

Similarly for *CYP2C9* and *VKORC1*, it would be important to determine exactly which variants to test from the frequency and association patterns of SNPs in the genetic region surrounding the association signal. These patterns may not be known, but they may be possible to infer from available LD patterns in well-characterized samples such as those included in the HapMap (A haplotype map of the human genome, 2005). The relationship of LD patterns in these defined populations, however, to those in the clinical populations to be tested may be unclear, and this should be recognized as a limitation of proposed testing strategies.

Information on rarer SNPs and structural variants such as insertions, deletions, and duplications not captured through the HapMap also is needed, as these may be causing an underlying association signal but may not be identified by existing genotyping platforms (Pearson and Manolio, 2008). Sequencing of association regions in hundreds or thousands of people may be needed to identify these rarer variants, and such efforts are ongoing on a small scale in follow-up to GWA findings. In-depth sequencing of the entire human genome is the best way to develop a comprehensive catalog of rarer variants, and an international effort to do just this has recently gotten underway (Genomes, 2008). Efforts to identify functional variants and their phenotypic effects also are continuing with projects such as ENCODE and the Knockout Mouse Project (Austin et al., 2004; Birney et al., 2007) which should help to extend and refine testing and interpretation of genomic regions associated with complex diseases and traits. Approaches are needed for updating clinical testing strategies and intervention approaches with this emerging information.

Laboratory and Clinical Infrastructure

Incorporation of genomic information into clinical effectiveness research also requires broad capacity to conduct testing and interpret the results (Box 3-3). First, we would need a laboratory infrastructure that could support such research, including a test that is valid, readily available, affordable, and (preferably) FDA-certified, and that is conducted under the auspices of a CLIA-certified laboratory. It would be important to have available a test for whatever genetic variant(s) one is interested in. Such a test should be eligible, or preferably approved, for reimbursement by insurers, though this raises the conundrum that even provisional approval requires a sufficient evidence base to support use of the test. It also would need to meet estab-

---

BOX 3-3
Laboratory and Clinical Infrastructure Needed to Conduct Clinical Effectiveness Research on Genetic Variants

- Valid FDA-approved test
- Insurer-approved reimbursement
- CLIA-certified laboratory
- Available/affordable testing
- Electronic health records
- Confidentiality/privacy protections
- Large-scale databases for sharing of research data with qualified investigators

lished guidelines for analytic validity, clinical validity, clinical utility, and public health utility (Grosse and Khoury, 2006; National Human Genome Research Institute, 2008b).

Flexible, comprehensive, accessible, user-friendly EHRs and personal health records (PHRs) also would be important for receiving and providing the results of genetic testing and related phenotypic or other measures. Such systems would need adequate privacy protections, as does all protected health information (U.S. Department of Health and Human Services, 1996) and ideally should provide point of care performance feedback so that clinicians or patients who receive results of genetic testing will know what actions they should then take. Automated prompts and patient management tools recommending genetic testing for patients in whom it has been demonstrated to improve outcomes, particularly in response to changing clinical parameters also recorded in the EHR, would also be useful. Testing might be recommended, for example, in persons who cross a certain threshold of increased risk for diabetes based on obesity or fasting glucose, or those who need to initiate warfarin therapy. To facilitate research as well as practice, a secure network of interoperable EHR and PHR systems (Murphy et al., 2006; Murray et al., 2003) would make possible rapid, large-scale, multicenter clinical studies to assess the effectiveness of testing for specific genetic variants and the interventions that follow. Additional standardized, structured nomenclatures for genomic applications in such systems also may be needed.

Accessible but secure large-scale databases to receive, archive, and distribute results of studies of genotype–phenotype associations are needed, such as the database of Genotype and Phenotype (dbGaP) (Mailman et al., 2007). Developed and maintained by the National Center for Biotechnology Information of the NIH, dbGaP includes genotype and phenotype data from genomewide association studies, medical sequencing, and molecular diagnostic assays, as well as phenotypic and clinical characteristics and environmental and lifestyle exposures. dbGaP provides access to data at two levels—open and controlled—allowing for both the broad release of summary data on allele frequencies and associations while also restricting access and ensuring investigator accountability for sensitive datasets involving individual-level genotype and phenotype data. By NIH policy, data in dbGaP are assumed to be pre-competitive and are expected to remain unencumbered by premature intellectual property claims (U.S. Department of Health and Human Services, 2007). On the open access public site, dbGaP supports searches for studies, protocols, and questionnaires. Visitors to dbGaP can view phenotype summary data, genotype summary data, and pre-computed or published genetic associations. As such it provides a powerful tool for identifying emerging genomic information that may potentially be applied to clinical effectiveness research, but as yet the association information is not readily searchable and may be difficult to extract and distill. Published genomewide association studies also are catalogued by the National Human Genome Research Institute (2008a) and the Centers for Disease Control and Prevention (Centers for Disease Control and Prevention, 2008). Such catalogues provide information on genetic associations that may be closer to practical application than those in dbGaP, but as noted above, much additional investigation is needed following an initial genomewide association report before one can contemplate applying them to clinical research.

Policy and Educational Infrastructure

The need to ensure confidentiality and privacy is vitally important to databases containing individual-level genotype or phenotype information, whether they be research databases such as dbGaP or clinical databases derived from EHRs used in clinical care. Major, justified, and unresolved concerns about the potential for persons with genetic variants putting them at increased disease risk becoming the object of discrimination by employers or insurers must be addressed. Clinical effectiveness research on genomic information will be difficult, if not impossible, to conduct on a large scale without the formal legal protection against discrimination provided by the Genetic Information Non-Discrimination Act (GINA). The Act would protect individuals against discrimination based on their genetic information in health insurance and employment. Enactment would prohibit insurers from denying health insurance coverage or charging higher premiums or employers from using genetic information in hiring or firing decisions. These protections are intended to encourage Americans to take advantage of genetic testing as part of their medical care and to participate in genetic research. Originally introduced over a decade ago, genetic non-discrimination legislation was passed unanimously by the Senate in both the 108th and 109th Congresses, but, until this year had never been passed by the House. The Genetic Nondiscrimination Act of 2007 was passed in the House by a vote of 420-3, and has the support of the current administration, but as of this writing has yet to be voted on in the Senate. This kind of policy infrastructure is absolutely crucial not only to clinical effectiveness research but also to any genomic research and its incorporation in clinical care.

Additional needs include consensus on reporting of variants or abnormalities to patients, consent requirements for research, approaches to counseling, and education of clinicians and patients (Box 3-4). Debate continues on whether, when, and how results of genetic tests, especially for common, complex diseases for which genetic variants are not deterministic, should be reported to patients, particularly in research settings (Bookman et al., 2006). This is a legacy in part of the era of Mendelian genetics when

---

BOX 3-4
Policy and Educational Infrastructure

- Genetic Information Non-Discrimination Act (GINA)
- Consensus or decisions on what should be reported to patients
- Adequate consent and consistent IRB approach
- Flexible approach to counseling that does not require one-on-one sessions with certified genetic counselor
- Education of clinicians
- Education of patients and family members

---

identification of at risk variants such as those for Huntington's disease carried grave implications, often with little in the way of effective intervention (Manolio, 2006). Many research studies have taken the approach of informing patients in the consent form that under no circumstances will any results of genetic testing be provided to them, their physicians, or anyone outside the research setting, but this also precludes informing patients of the presence of potentially modifiable genetic risk that this research is specifically intended to identify (Bookman et al., 2006).

Research to develop valid, feasible approaches to informing patients of the modest increased risk conferred by many variants associated with complex diseases, and the avenues open to them for reducing that risk, is needed if this work is to be conducted in a way that maximizes benefits and minimizes risks to research participants. To that end, consistent and agreed-upon consent policies and procedures also are needed, as well as consistent policies by Institutional Review Boards (IRBs), particularly for multicenter research and practice. Flexible approaches to genetic counseling also are needed, including approaches for providing adequate counseling, where appropriate, through means other than one-on-one counseling with a certified genetic counselor. There are simply not enough certified genetic counselors available, nor is that level of counseling necessary for variants of modest effect, to provide it for every genetic test performed in the course of clinical care or effectiveness research. Less cumbersome alternatives that still bring qualified expertise to the discussion are needed. Finally, a better educational infrastructure is needed to improve "genomic literacy" for clinicians, research participants, and patients. Importantly, education should extend to family members who may be in a decision-making or advisory role and who may well be personally affected by genetic information provided to a blood relative with whom they share many of the same genetic variants. Rapid and reliable systems also are needed for updating clinicians and the public on emerging genomic information, without the hyperbole that can sometimes accompany initial media reports.

As genomic information evolves and clinical effectiveness research progresses, the lines between research and patient care will blur and the two purposes may well merge. A number of other issues will need to be addressed, such as whose responsibility it will be to contact patients who have been genotyped for markers of unknown or questionable significance, in either the research or clinical setting, once actionable information on them becomes available. Whose responsibility will it be to store and maintain the data long term? What if a clinician acts on a marker and later the association is shown to be of lesser importance or have different implications than initially thought? Will clinicians be criticized or held accountable for inaction on risk variants of questionable clinical but very strong statistical significance? The agenda for clinical effectiveness research on emerging genomic information is clearly substantial and will likely continue for some time after initial identification of a clinically important variant.

Conclusion

Advances in genotyping technology coupled with expanding knowledge of genome structure and function have fueled a virtual explosion of genomic information on common, complex diseases. New insights into disease mechanisms, and new avenues to diagnosis, prevention, and treatment, are opening more rapidly than we can keep pace with them, but most remain many steps away from actual clinical application. Incorporation of this information into research and clinical databases, and ultimately into effective clinical practice, will require substantial additional epidemiologic and genetic information. It also will require a substantial infrastructure, including a valid, certified, reimbursable, available test; secure, interoperable, and transportable electronic medical records; genetic information, non-discrimination legislation; guidelines for reporting results to patients; guidelines for obtaining consent and institutional review; practical approaches to counseling; and genomically literate clinicians and patients. Although this is a tall order, it is one we must fill if we are to capitalize on the enormous investment, and the enormous promise, of genomic research in common, complex diseases.

REFERENCES

Anderson, J. L., B. D. Horne, S. M. Stevens, A. S. Grove, S. Barton, Z. P. Nicholas, S. F. Kahn, H. T. May, K. M. Samuelson, J. B. Muhlestein, and J. F. Carlquist. 2007. Randomized trial of genotype-guided versus standard warfarin dosing in patients initiating oral anticoagulation. *Circulation* 116(22):2563-2570.

Angrist, J. D. 1996. Identification of casual effects using instrumental variables *Journal of the American Statistical Association* (91):444-455.

Arking, D. E., A. Pfeufer, W. Post, W. H. Kao, C. Newton-Cheh, M. Ikeda, K. West, C. Kashuk, M. Akyol, S. Perz, S. Jalilzadeh, T. Illig, C. Gieger, C. Y. Guo, M. G. Larson, H. E. Wichmann, E. Marban, C. J. O'Donnell, J. N. Hirschhorn, S. Kaab, P. M. Spooner, T. Meitinger, and A. Chakravarti. 2006. A common genetic variant in the NOS1 regulator NOS1AP modulates cardiac repolarization. *Nature Genetics* 38(6):644-651.

Armitage, J., R. Souhami, L. Friedman, L. Hilbrich, J. Holland, L. H. Muhlbaier, J. Shannon, and A. Van Nie. 2008. The impact of privacy and confidentiality laws on the conduct of clinical trials. *Clinical Trials* 5(1):70-74.

Austin, C. P., J. F. Battey, A. Bradley, M. Bucan, M. Capecchi, F. S. Collins, W. F. Dove, G. Duyk, S. Dymecki, J. T. Eppig, F. B. Grieder, N. Heintz, G. Hicks, T. R. Insel, A. Joyner, B. H. Koller, K. C. Lloyd, T. Magnuson, M. W. Moore, A. Nagy, J. D. Pollock, A. D. Roses, A. T. Sands, B. Seed, W. C. Skarnes, J. Snoddy, P. Soriano, D. J. Stewart, F. Stewart, B. Stillman, H. Varmus, L. Varticovski, I. M. Verma, T. F. Vogt, H. von Melchner, J. Witkowski, R. P. Woychik, W. Wurst, G. D. Yancopoulos, S. G. Young, and B. Zambrowicz. 2004. The knockout mouse project. *Nature Genetics* 36(9):921-924.

Baigent, C., F. E. Harrell, M. Buyse, J. R. Emberson, and D. G. Altman. 2008. Ensuring trial validity by data quality assurance and diversification of monitoring methods. *Clinical Trials* 5(1):49-55.

Benjamin, D. K., Jr., P. B. Smith, M. D. Murphy, R. Roberts, L. Mathis, D. Avant, R. M. Califf, and J. S. Li. 2006. Peer-reviewed publication of clinical trials completed for pediatric exclusivity. *Journal of the American Medical Association* 296(10):1266-1273.

Berry, D. A. 1996. *Statistics: A Bayesian Perspective*. Belmont, CA: Duxbury Press.

———. 2006. Bayesian clinical studies. *Nature Reviews and Drug Discovery* (5):27-36.

Berry, D. A., K. A. Cronin, S. K. Plevritis, D. G. Fryback, L. Clarke, M. Zelen, J. S. Mandelblatt, A. Y. Yakovlev, J. D. Habbema, and E. J. Feuer. 2005. Effect of screening and adjuvant therapy on mortality from breast cancer. *New England Journal of Medicine* 353(17):1784-1792.

Berry, D. A., L. Inoue, Y. Shen, J. Venier, D. Cohen, M. Bondy, R. Theriault, and M. F. Munsell. 2006. Modeling the impact of treatment and screening on U.S. breast cancer mortality: A Bayesian approach. *Journal of the National Cancer Institute Monographs* (36):30-36.

Birney, E., J. A. Stamatoyannopoulos, A. Dutta, R. Guigo, T. R. Gingeras, E. H. Margulies, Z. Weng, M. Snyder, E. T. Dermitzakis, R. E. Thurman, M. S. Kuehn, C. M. Taylor, S. Neph, C. M. Koch, S. Asthana, A. Malhotra, I. Adzhubei, J. A. Greenbaum, R. M. Andrews, P. Flicek, P. J. Boyle, H. Cao, N. P. Carter, G. K. Clelland, S. Davis, N. Day, P. Dhami, S. C. Dillon, M. O. Dorschner, H. Fiegler, P. G. Giresi, J. Goldy, M. Hawrylycz, A. Haydock, R. Humbert, K. D. James, B. E. Johnson, E. M. Johnson, T. T. Frum, E. R. Rosenzweig, N. Karnani, K. Lee, G. C. Lefebvre, P. A. Navas, F. Neri, S. C. Parker, P. J. Sabo, R. Sandstrom, A. Shafer, D. Vetrie, M. Weaver, S. Wilcox, M. Yu, F. S. Collins, J. Dekker, J. D. Lieb, T. D. Tullius, G. E. Crawford, S. Sunyaev, W. S. Noble, I. Dunham, F. Denoeud, A. Reymond, P. Kapranov, J. Rozowsky, D. Zheng, R. Castelo, A. Frankish, J. Harrow, S. Ghosh, A. Sandelin, I. L. Hofacker, R. Baertsch, D. Keefe, S. Dike, J. Cheng, H. A. Hirsch, E. A. Sekinger, J. Lagarde, J. F. Abril, A. Shahab, C. Flamm, C. Fried, J. Hackermuller, J. Hertel, M. Lindemeyer, K. Missal, A. Tanzer, S. Washietl, J. Korbel, O. Emanuelsson, J. S. Pedersen, N. Holroyd, R. Taylor, D. Swarbreck, N. Matthews, M. C. Dickson, D. J. Thomas, M. T. Weirauch, J. Gilbert, J. Drenkow, I. Bell, X. Zhao, K. G. Srinivasan, W. K. Sung, H. S. Ooi, K. P. Chiu, S. Foissac, T. Alioto, M. Brent, L. Pachter, M. L. Tress, A. Valencia, S. W. Choo, C. Y. Choo, C. Ucla, C. Manzano, C. Wyss, E. Cheung, T. G. Clark, J. B. Brown, M. Ganesh, S. Patel, H. Tammana, J. Chrast, C. N.

Henrichsen, C. Kai, J. Kawai, U. Nagalakshmi, J. Wu, Z. Lian, J. Lian, P. Newburger, X. Zhang, P. Bickel, J. S. Mattick, P. Carninci, Y. Hayashizaki, S. Weissman, T. Hubbard, R. M. Myers, J. Rogers, P. F. Stadler, T. M. Lowe, C. L. Wei, Y. Ruan, K. Struhl, M. Gerstein, S. E. Antonarakis, Y. Fu, E. D. Green, U. Karaoz, A. Siepel, J. Taylor, L. A. Liefer, K. A. Wetterstrand, P. J. Good, E. A. Feingold, M. S. Guyer, G. M. Cooper, G. Asimenos, C. N. Dewey, M. Hou, S. Nikolaev, J. I. Montoya-Burgos, A. Loytynoja, S. Whelan, F. Pardi, T. Massingham, H. Huang, N. R. Zhang, I. Holmes, J. C. Mullikin, A. Ureta-Vidal, B. Paten, M. Seringhaus, D. Church, K. Rosenbloom, W. J. Kent, E. A. Stone, S. Batzoglou, N. Goldman, R. C. Hardison, D. Haussler, W. Miller, A. Sidow, N. D. Trinklein, Z. D. Zhang, L. Barrera, R. Stuart, D. C. King, A. Ameur, S. Enroth, M. C. Bieda, J. Kim, A. A. Bhinge, N. Jiang, J. Liu, F. Yao, V. B. Vega, C. W. Lee, P. Ng, A. Yang, Z. Moqtaderi, Z. Zhu, X. Xu, S. Squazzo, M. J. Oberley, D. Inman, M. A. Singer, T. A. Richmond, K. J. Munn, A. Rada-Iglesias, O. Wallerman, J. Komorowski, J. C. Fowler, P. Couttet, A. W. Bruce, O. M. Dovey, P. D. Ellis, C. F. Langford, D. A. Nix, G. Euskirchen, S. Hartman, A. E. Urban, P. Kraus, S. Van Calcar, N. Heintzman, T. H. Kim, K. Wang, C. Qu, G. Hon, R. Luna, C. K. Glass, M. G. Rosenfeld, S. F. Aldred, S. J. Cooper, A. Halees, J. M. Lin, H. P. Shulha, M. Xu, J. N. Haidar, Y. Yu, V. R. Iyer, R. D. Green, C. Wadelius, P. J. Farnham, B. Ren, R. A. Harte, A. S. Hinrichs, H. Trumbower, H. Clawson, J. Hillman-Jackson, A. S. Zweig, K. Smith, A. Thakkapallayil, G. Barber, R. M. Kuhn, D. Karolchik, L. Armengol, C. P. Bird, P. I. de Bakker, A. D. Kern, N. Lopez-Bigas, J. D. Martin, B. E. Stranger, A. Woodroffe, E. Davydov, A. Dimas, E. Eyras, I. B. Hallgrimsdottir, J. Huppert, M. C. Zody, G. R. Abecasis, X. Estivill, G. G. Bouffard, X. Guan, N. F. Hansen, J. R. Idol, V. V. Maduro, B. Maskeri, J. C. McDowell, M. Park, P. J. Thomas, A. C. Young, R. W. Blakesley, D. M. Muzny, E. Sodergren, D. A. Wheeler, K. C. Worley, H. Jiang, G. M. Weinstock, R. A. Gibbs, T. Graves, R. Fulton, E. R. Mardis, R. K. Wilson, M. Clamp, J. Cuff, S. Gnerre, D. B. Jaffe, J. L. Chang, K. Lindblad-Toh, E. S. Lander, M. Koriabine, M. Nefedov, K. Osoegawa, Y. Yoshinaga, B. Zhu, and P. J. de Jong. 2007. Identification and analysis of functional elements in 1% of the human genome by the encode pilot project. *Nature* 447(7146):799-816.

Bookman, E. B., A. A. Langehorne, J. H. Eckfeldt, K. C. Glass, G. P. Jarvik, M. Klag, G. Koski, A. Motulsky, B. Wilfond, T. A. Manolio, R. R. Fabsitz, and R. V. Luepker. 2006. Reporting genetic results in research studies: Summary and recommendations of an NHLBI working group. *American Journal of Medical Genetics Part A* 140(10):1033-1040.

Braithwaite, R. S., S. Shechter, M. S. Roberts, A. Schaefer, D. R. Bangsberg, P. R. Harrigan, and A. C. Justice. 2006. Explaining variability in the relationship between antiretroviral adherence and HIV mutation accumulation. *Journal of Antimicrobial Chemotherapy* 58(5):1036-1043.

Braithwaite, R. S., M. S. Roberts, C. C. Chang, M. B. Goetz, C. L. Gibert, M. C. Rodriguez-Barradas, S. Shechter, A. Schaefer, K. Nucifora, R. Koppenhaver, and A. C. Justice. 2008. Influence of alternative thresholds for initiating HIV treatment on quality-adjusted life expectancy: A decision model. *Annals of Internal Medicine* 148(3):178-185.

Brookhart, M. A. 2007. Evaluating the validity of an instrumental variable study of nueroleptics: Can between-physician differences in prescribing patterns be used to estimate treatment effects? *Medical Care* 45(10):116-122.

Brookhart, M. A., S. Schneeweiss, K. J. Rothman, R. J. Glynn, J. Avorn, and T. Sturmer. 2006. Variable selection for propensity score models. *American Journal of Epidemiology* 163(12):1149-1156.

Brookhart, M. A., J. A. Rassen, P. S. Wang, C. Dormuth, H. Mogun, and S. Schneeweiss. 2007. Evaluating the validity of an instrumental variable study of neuroleptics: Can between-physician differences in prescribing patterns be used to estimate treatment effects? *Medical Care* 45(10 Suppl 2):S116-S122.

Califf, R. M., and R. A. Rosati. 1981. The doctor and the computer. *Western Journal of Medicine* 135(4):321-323.

Califf, R. M., E. D. Peterson, R. J. Gibbons, A. Garson, Jr., R. G. Brindis, G. A. Beller, and S. C. Smith, Jr. 2002. Integrating quality into the cycle of therapeutic development. *Journal of the American College of Cardiology* 40(11):1895-1901.

Califf, R. M., R. A. Harrington, L. K. Madre, E. D. Peterson, D. Roth, and K. A. Schulman. 2007. Curbing the cardiovascular disease epidemic: Aligning industry, government, payers, and academics. *Health Affairs (Millwood)* 26(1):62-74.

Centers for Disease Control and Prevention. 2008. *HuGE Literature Finder*. http://www.hugenavigator.net/ (accessed July 9, 2008).

Chanock, S. J., T. Manolio, M. Boehnke, E. Boerwinkle, D. J. Hunter, G. Thomas, J. N. Hirschhorn, G. Abecasis, D. Altshuler, J. E. Bailey-Wilson, L. D. Brooks, L. R. Cardon, M. Daly, P. Donnelly, J. F. Fraumeni, Jr., N. B. Freimer, D. S. Gerhard, C. Gunter, A. E. Guttmacher, M. S. Guyer, E. L. Harris, J. Hoh, R. Hoover, C. A. Kong, K. R. Merikangas, C. C. Morton, L. J. Palmer, E. G. Phimister, J. P. Rice, J. Roberts, C. Rotimi, M. A. Tucker, K. J. Vogan, S. Wacholder, E. M. Wijsman, D. M. Winn, and F. S. Collins. 2007. Replicating genotype-phenotype associations. *Nature* 447(7145):655-660.

Children's Hospital of Philadelphia. 2008. *Center for Applied Genomics*. http://www.chop.edu/consumer/jsp/division/generic.jsp?id=84930 (accessed July 9, 2008).

Clermont, G., J. Bartels, R. Kumar, G. Constantine, Y. Vodovotz, and C. Chow. 2004a. In silico design of clinical trials: A method coming of age. *Critical Care Medicine* 32(10):2061-2070.

Clermont, G., V. Kaplan, R. Moreno, J. L. Vincent, W. T. Linde-Zwirble, B. V. Hout, and D. C. Angus. 2004b. Dynamic microsimulation to model multiple outcomes in cohorts of critically ill patients. *Intensive Care Medicine* 30(12):2237-2244.

Colhoun, H. M., P. M. McKeigue, and G. Davey Smith. 2003. Problems of reporting genetic associations with complex outcomes. *Lancet* 361(9360):865-872.

Cook, D., A. Moore-Cox, D. Xavier, F. Lauzier, and I. Roberts. 2008. Randomized trials in vulnerable populations. *Clinical Trials* 5(1):61-69.

Cupples, L. A., H. T. Arruda, E. J. Benjamin, R. B. D'Agostino, Sr., S. Demissie, A. L. DeStefano, J. Dupuis, K. M. Falls, C. S. Fox, D. J. Gottlieb, D. R. Govindaraju, C. Y. Guo, N. L. Heard-Costa, S. J. Hwang, S. Kathiresan, D. P. Kiel, J. M. Laramie, M. G. Larson, D. Levy, C. Y. Liu, K. L. Lunetta, M. D. Mailman, A. K. Manning, J. B. Meigs, J. M. Murabito, C. Newton-Cheh, G. T. O'Connor, C. J. O'Donnell, M. Pandey, S. Seshadri, R. S. Vasan, Z. Y. Wang, J. B. Wilk, P. A. Wolf, Q. Yang, and L. D. Atwood. 2007. The Framingham Heart Study 100k SNP genome-wide association study resource: Overview of 17 phenotype working group reports. *BMC Medical Genetics* 8(Supl 1):S1.

Davis, J. R. 1999. *Assuring data quality and validiy in clinical trials for regulatory descision making*. Washington, D.C.

Day, J., J. Rubin, Y. Vodovotz, C. C. Chow, A. Reynolds, and G. Clermont. 2006. A reduced mathematical model of the acute inflammatory response II. Capturing scenarios of repeated endotoxin administration. *Journal of Theoretical Biology* 242(1):237-256.

deCODE. 2008. *deCODE Diagnostics*. http://www.decodediagnostics.com (accessed June 21, 2010).

DeMets, D. L., and R. M. Califf. 2002a. Lessons learned from recent cardiovascular clinical trials: Part I. *Circulation* 106(6):746-751.

———. 2002b. Lessons learned from recent cardiovascular clinical trials: Part II. *Circulation* 106(7):880-886.

Department of Health and Human Services. 2007. *Epidemiologic Investigation of Putative Causal Genetic Variants—Study Investigators (u01)*. http://grants.nih.gov/grants/guide/rfa-files/RFA-HG-07-014.html (accessed July 9, 2008).

Dewan, A., M. Liu, S. Hartman, S. S. Zhang, D. T. Liu, C. Zhao, P. O. Tam, W. M. Chan, D. S. Lam, M. Snyder, C. Barnstable, C. P. Pang, and J. Hoh. 2006. HTRA1 promoter polymorphism in wet age-related macular degeneration. *Science* 314(5801):989-992.

Dilts, D. M., A. Sandler, S. Cheng, J. Crites, L. Ferranti, A. Wu, R. Gray, J. Macdonald, D. Marinucci, and R. Comis. 2008. Development of clinical trials in a cooperative group setting: The Eastern Cooperative Oncology Group. *Clinical Cancer Research* 14(11):3427-3433.

DNA Direct. 2008. *Decode T2™—Diabetes Risk Marker*. http://www.dnadirect.com/ patients/tests/decode_diabetes/decode_t2.jsp (accessed July 9, 2008).

Duerr, R. H., K. D. Taylor, S. R. Brant, J. D. Rioux, M. S. Silverberg, M. J. Daly, A. H. Steinhart, C. Abraham, M. Regueiro, A. Griffiths, T. Dassopoulos, A. Bitton, H. Yang, S. Targan, L. W. Datta, E. O. Kistner, L. P. Schumm, A. T. Lee, P. K. Gregersen, M. M. Barmada, J. I. Rotter, D. L. Nicolae, and J. H. Cho. 2006. A genome-wide association study identifies IL23R as an inflammatory bowel disease gene. *Science* 314(5804):1461-1463.

Duley, L., K. Antman, J. Arena, A. Avezum, M. Blumenthal, J. Bosch, S. Chrolavicius, T. Li, S. Ounpuu, A. C. Perez, P. Sleight, R. Svard, R. Temple, Y. Tsouderous, C. Yunis, and S. Yusuf. 2008. Specific barriers to the conduct of randomized trials. *Clinical Trials* 5(1):40-48.

Easton, D. F., K. A. Pooley, A. M. Dunning, P. D. Pharoah, D. Thompson, D. G. Ballinger, J. P. Struewing, J. Morrison, H. Field, R. Luben, N. Wareham, S. Ahmed, C. S. Healey, R. Bowman, K. B. Meyer, C. A. Haiman, L. K. Kolonel, B. E. Henderson, L. Le Marchand, P. Brennan, S. Sangrajrang, V. Gaborieau, F. Odefrey, C. Y. Shen, P. E. Wu, H. C. Wang, D. Eccles, D. G. Evans, J. Peto, O. Fletcher, N. Johnson, S. Seal, M. R. Stratton, N. Rahman, G. Chenevix-Trench, S. E. Bojesen, B. G. Nordestgaard, C. K. Axelsson, M. Garcia-Closas, L. Brinton, S. Chanock, J. Lissowska, B. Peplonska, H. Nevanlinna, R. Fagerholm, H. Eerola, D. Kang, K. Y. Yoo, D. Y. Noh, S. H. Ahn, D. J. Hunter, S. E. Hankinson, D. G. Cox, P. Hall, S. Wedren, J. Liu, Y. L. Low, N. Bogdanova, P. Schurmann, T. Dork, R. A. Tollenaar, C. E. Jacobi, P. Devilee, J. G. Klijn, A. J. Sigurdson, M. M. Doody, B. H. Alexander, J. Zhang, A. Cox, I. W. Brock, G. MacPherson, M. W. Reed, F. J. Couch, E. L. Goode, J. E. Olson, H. Meijers-Heijboer, A. van den Ouweland, A. Uitterlinden, F. Rivadeneira, R. L. Milne, G. Ribas, A. Gonzalez-Neira, J. Benitez, J. L. Hopper, M. McCredie, M. Southey, G. G. Giles, C. Schroen, C. Justenhoven, H. Brauch, U. Hamann, Y. D. Ko, A. B. Spurdle, J. Beesley, X. Chen, A. Mannermaa, V. M. Kosma, V. Kataja, J. Hartikainen, N. E. Day, D. R. Cox, and B. A. Ponder. 2007. Genome-wide association study identifies novel breast cancer susceptibility loci. *Nature* 447(7148):1087-1093.

Eddy, D. M., and L. Schlessinger. 2003a. Archimedes: A trial-validated model of diabetes. *Diabetes Care* 26(11):3093-3101.

———. 2003b. Validation of the Archimedes diabetes model. *Diabetes Care* 26(11):3102-3110.

Edwards, A. O., R. Ritter, 3rd, K. J. Abel, A. Manning, C. Panhuysen, and L. A. Farrer. 2005. Complement factor H polymorphism and age-related macular degeneration. *Science* 308(5720):421-424.

Eisenstein, E. L., R. Collins, B. S. Cracknell, O. Podesta, E. D. Reid, P. Sandercock, Y. Shakhov, M. L. Terrin, M. A. Sellers, R. M. Califf, C. B. Granger, and R. Diaz. 2008. Sensible approaches for reducing clinical trial costs. *Clinical Trials* 5(1):75-84.

The eMERGE Network. 2008. *Electronics Medical Records and Genomics*. http://www.gwas. net (accessed July 9, 2008).

Feero, W. G., A. E. Guttmacher, and F. S. Collins. 2008. The genome gets personal—almost. *Journal of the American Medical Association* 299(11):1351-1352.

Ferguson, T. B., Jr., S. W. Dziuban, Jr., F. H. Edwards, M. C. Eiken, A. L. Shroyer, P. C. Pairolero, R. P. Anderson, and F. L. Grover. 2000. The STS national database: Current changes and challenges for the new millennium. Committee to Establish a National Database in Cardiothoracic Surgery, The Society of Thoracic Surgeons. *Annals of Thoracic Surgery* 69(3):680-691.

Florez, J. C., K. A. Jablonski, N. Bayley, T. I. Pollin, P. I. de Bakker, A. R. Shuldiner, W. C. Knowler, D. M. Nathan, and D. Altshuler. 2006. Tcf7l2 polymorphisms and progression to diabetes in the diabetes prevention program. *New England Journal of Medicine* 355(3):241-250.

Florez, J. C., K. A. Jablonski, M. W. Sun, N. Bayley, S. E. Kahn, H. Shamoon, R. F. Hamman, W. C. Knowler, D. M. Nathan, and D. Altshuler. 2007. Effects of the type 2 diabetes-associated PPARG P12A polymorphism on progression to diabetes and response to troglitazone. *Journal of Clinical Endocrinology & Metabolism* 92(4):1502-1509.

Frayling, T. M. 2007. Genome-wide association studies provide new insights into type 2 diabetes aetiology. *Nature Reviews Genetics* 8(9):657-662.

Frayling, T. M., N. J. Timpson, M. N. Weedon, E. Zeggini, R. M. Freathy, C. M. Lindgren, J. R. Perry, K. S. Elliott, H. Lango, N. W. Rayner, B. Shields, L. W. Harries, J. C. Barrett, S. Ellard, C. J. Groves, B. Knight, A. M. Patch, A. R. Ness, S. Ebrahim, D. A. Lawlor, S. M. Ring, Y. Ben-Shlomo, M. R. Jarvelin, U. Sovio, A. J. Bennett, D. Melzer, L. Ferrucci, R. J. Loos, I. Barroso, N. J. Wareham, F. Karpe, K. R. Owen, L. R. Cardon, M. Walker, G. A. Hitman, C. N. Palmer, A. S. Doney, A. D. Morris, G. D. Smith, A. T. Hattersley, and M. I. McCarthy. 2007. A common variant in the FTO gene is associated with body mass index and predisposes to childhood and adult obesity. *Science* 316(5826):889-894.

Frazer, K. A., D. G. Ballinger, D. R. Cox, D. A. Hinds, L. L. Stuve, R. A. Gibbs, J. W. Belmont, A. Boudreau, P. Hardenbol, S. M. Leal, S. Pasternak, D. A. Wheeler, T. D. Willis, F. Yu, H. Yang, C. Zeng, Y. Gao, H. Hu, W. Hu, C. Li, W. Lin, S. Liu, H. Pan, X. Tang, J. Wang, W. Wang, J. Yu, B. Zhang, Q. Zhang, H. Zhao, J. Zhou, S. B. Gabriel, R. Barry, B. Blumenstiel, A. Camargo, M. Defelice, M. Faggart, M. Goyette, S. Gupta, J. Moore, H. Nguyen, R. C. Onofrio, M. Parkin, J. Roy, E. Stahl, E. Winchester, L. Ziaugra, D. Altshuler, Y. Shen, Z. Yao, W. Huang, X. Chu, Y. He, L. Jin, Y. Liu, W. Sun, H. Wang, Y. Wang, X. Xiong, L. Xu, M. M. Waye, S. K. Tsui, H. Xue, J. T. Wong, L. M. Galver, J. B. Fan, K. Gunderson, S. S. Murray, A. R. Oliphant, M. S. Chee, A. Montpetit, F. Chagnon, V. Ferretti, M. Leboeuf, J. F. Olivier, M. S. Phillips, S. Roumy, C. Sallee, A. Verner, T. J. Hudson, P. Y. Kwok, D. Cai, D. C. Koboldt, R. D. Miller, L. Pawlikowska, P. Taillon-Miller, M. Xiao, L. C. Tsui, W. Mak, Y. Q. Song, P. K. Tam, Y. Nakamura, T. Kawaguchi, T. Kitamoto, T. Morizono, A. Nagashima, Y. Ohnishi, A. Sekine, T. Tanaka, T. Tsunoda, P. Deloukas, C. P. Bird, M. Delgado, E. T. Dermitzakis, R. Gwilliam, S. Hunt, J. Morrison, D. Powell, B. E. Stranger, P. Whittaker, D. R. Bentley, M. J. Daly, P. I. de Bakker, J. Barrett, Y. R. Chretien, J. Maller, S. McCarroll, N. Patterson, I. Pe'er, A. Price, S. Purcell, D. J. Richter, P. Sabeti, R. Saxena, S. F. Schaffner, P. C. Sham, P. Varilly, L. D. Stein, L. Krishnan, A. V. Smith, M. K. Tello-Ruiz, G. A. Thorisson, A. Chakravarti, P. E. Chen, D. J. Cutler, C. S. Kashuk, S. Lin, G. R. Abecasis, W. Guan, Y. Li, H. M. Munro, Z. S. Qin, D. J. Thomas, G. McVean, A. Auton, L. Bottolo, N. Cardin, S. Eyheramendy, C. Freeman, J. Marchini, S. Myers, C. Spencer, M. Stephens, P. Donnelly, L. R. Cardon, G. Clarke, D. M. Evans, A. P. Morris, B. S. Weir, J. C. Mullikin, S. T. Sherry, M. Feolo, A. Skol, H. Zhang, I. Matsuda, Y. Fukushima, D. R. Macer, E. Suda, C. N. Rotimi, C. A. Adebamowo, I. Ajayi, T. Aniagwu, P. A. Marshall, C. Nkwodimmah, C. D. Royal, M. F. Leppert, M. Dixon, A. Peiffer, R. Qiu, A. Kent, K. Kato, N. Niikawa, I. F. Adewole, B. M. Knoppers, M. W. Foster, E. W. Clayton, J. Watkin, D. Muzny, L. Nazareth, E. Sodergren, G. M. Weinstock, I. Yakub, B. W. Birren, R. K. Wilson, L. L. Fulton, J. Rogers, J. Burton, N. P. Carter, C. M. Clee, M. Griffiths, M. C. Jones, K. McLay, R. W. Plumb, M. T. Ross,

S. K. Sims, D. L. Willey, Z. Chen, H. Han, L. Kang, M. Godbout, J. C. Wallenburg, P. L'Archeveque, G. Bellemare, K. Saeki, D. An, H. Fu, Q. Li, Z. Wang, R. Wang, A. L. Holden, L. D. Brooks, J. E. McEwen, M. S. Guyer, V. O. Wang, J. L. Peterson, M. Shi, J. Spiegel, L. M. Sung, L. F. Zacharia, F. S. Collins, K. Kennedy, R. Jamieson, and J. Stewart. 2007. A second generation human haplotype map of over 3.1 million SNPS. *Nature* 449(7164):851-861.

Genomes. 2008. *A Deep Catalog of Human Genetic Variation.* http://www.1000genomes.org/ (accessed July 9, 2008).

Giles, F. J., H. M. Kantarjian, J. E. Cortes, G. Garcia-Manero, S. Verstovsek, S. Faderl, D. A. Thomas, A. Ferrajoli, S. O'Brien, J. K. Wathen, L. C. Xiao, D. A. Berry, and E. H. Estey. 2003. Adaptive randomized study of idarubicin and cytarabine versus troxacitabine and cytarabine versus troxacitabine and idarubicin in untreated patients 50 years or older with adverse karyotype acute myeloid leukemia. *Journal of Clinical Oncology* 21(9):1722-1727.

Granger, C. B., V. Vogel, S. R. Cummings, P. Held, F. Fiedorek, M. Lawrence, B. Neal, H. Reidies, L. Santarelli, R. Schroyer, N. L. Stockbridge, and Z. Feng. 2008. Do we need to adjudicate major clinical events? *Clinical Trials* 5(1):56-60.

Grant, S. F., G. Thorleifsson, I. Reynisdottir, R. Benediktsson, A. Manolescu, J. Sainz, A. Helgason, H. Stefansson, V. Emilsson, A. Helgadottir, U. Styrkarsdottir, K. P. Magnusson, G. B. Walters, E. Palsdottir, T. Jonsdottir, T. Gudmundsdottir, A. Gylfason, J. Saemundsdottir, R. L. Wilensky, M. P. Reilly, D. J. Rader, Y. Bagger, C. Christiansen, V. Gudnason, G. Sigurdsson, U. Thorsteinsdottir, J. R. Gulcher, A. Kong, and K. Stefansson. 2006. Variant of transcription factor 7-like 2 (TCF7L2) gene confers risk of type 2 diabetes. *Nature Genetics* 38(3):320-323.

Grosse, S. D., and M. J. Khoury. 2006. What is the clinical utility of genetic testing? *Journal of Medical Genetics* 8(7):448-450.

Gudbjartsson, D. F., D. O. Arnar, A. Helgadottir, S. Gretarsdottir, H. Holm, A. Sigurdsson, A. Jonasdottir, A. Baker, G. Thorleifsson, K. Kristjansson, A. Palsson, T. Blondal, P. Sulem, V. M. Backman, G. A. Hardarson, E. Palsdottir, A. Helgason, R. Sigurjonsdottir, J. T. Sverrisson, K. Kostulas, M. C. Ng, L. Baum, W. Y. So, K. S. Wong, J. C. Chan, K. L. Furie, S. M. Greenberg, M. Sale, P. Kelly, C. A. MacRae, E. E. Smith, J. Rosand, J. Hillert, R. C. Ma, P. T. Ellinor, G. Thorgeirsson, J. R. Gulcher, A. Kong, U. Thorsteinsdottir, and K. Stefansson. 2007. Variants conferring risk of atrial fibrillation on chromosome 4Q25. *Nature* 448(7151):353-357.

Gudmundsson, J., P. Sulem, A. Manolescu, L. T. Amundadottir, D. Gudbjartsson, A. Helgason, T. Rafnar, J. T. Bergthorsson, B. A. Agnarsson, A. Baker, A. Sigurdsson, K. R. Benediktsdottir, M. Jakobsdottir, J. Xu, T. Blondal, J. Kostic, J. Sun, S. Ghosh, S. N. Stacey, M. Mouy, J. Saemundsdottir, V. M. Backman, K. Kristjansson, A. Tres, A. W. Partin, M. T. Albers-Akkers, J. Godino-Ivan Marcos, P. C. Walsh, D. W. Swinkels, S. Navarrete, S. D. Isaacs, K. K. Aben, T. Graif, J. Cashy, M. Ruiz-Echarri, K. E. Wiley, B. K. Suarez, J. A. Witjes, M. Frigge, C. Ober, E. Jonsson, G. V. Einarsson, J. I. Mayordomo, L. A. Kiemeney, W. B. Isaacs, W. J. Catalona, R. B. Barkardottir, J. R. Gulcher, U. Thorsteinsdottir, A. Kong, and K. Stefansson. 2007. Genome-wide association study identifies a second prostate cancer susceptibility variant at 8Q24. *Nature Genetics* 39(5):631-637.

Gulcher, J., and K. Stefansson. 1998. Population genomics: Laying the groundwork for genetic disease modeling and targeting. *Clinical Chemistry and Laboratory Medicine* 36(8):523-527.

Haga, S. B., M. J. Khoury, and W. Burke. 2003. Genomic profiling to promote a healthy lifestyle: Not ready for prime time. *Nature Genetics* 34(4):347-350.

Haiman, C. A., N. Patterson, M. L. Freedman, S. R. Myers, M. C. Pike, A. Waliszewska, J. Neubauer, A. Tandon, C. Schirmer, G. J. McDonald, S. C. Greenway, D. O. Stram, L. Le Marchand, L. N. Kolonel, M. Frasco, D. Wong, L. C. Pooler, K. Ardlie, I. Oakley-Girvan, A. S. Whittemore, K. A. Cooney, E. M. John, S. A. Ingles, D. Altshuler, B. E. Henderson, and D. Reich. 2007. Multiple regions within 8Q24 independently affect risk for prostate cancer. *Nature Genetics* 39(5):638-644.

Haines, J. L., M. A. Hauser, S. Schmidt, W. K. Scott, L. M. Olson, P. Gallins, K. L. Spencer, S. Y. Kwan, M. Noureddine, J. R. Gilbert, N. Schnetz-Boutaud, A. Agarwal, E. A. Postel, and M. A. Pericak-Vance. 2005. Complement factor H variant increases the risk of age-related macular degeneration. *Science* 308(5720):419-421.

Hall, D. H., T. Rahman, P. J. Avery, and B. Keavney. 2006. INSIG-2 promoter polymorphism and obesity related phenotypes: Association study in 1428 members of 248 families. *BMC Medical Genetics* 7:83.

Heikes, K. E., D. M. Eddy, B. Arondekar, and L. Schlessinger. 2007. Diabetes risk calculator: A simple tool for detecting undiagnosed diabetes and prediabetes. *Diabetes Care* 31(5):1040-1045.

Helgadottir, A., G. Thorleifsson, A. Manolescu, S. Gretarsdottir, T. Blondal, A. Jonasdottir, A. Sigurdsson, A. Baker, A. Palsson, G. Masson, D. F. Gudbjartsson, K. P. Magnusson, K. Andersen, A. I. Levey, V. M. Backman, S. Matthiasdottir, T. Jonsdottir, S. Palsson, H. Einarsdottir, S. Gunnarsdottir, A. Gylfason, V. Vaccarino, W. C. Hooper, M. P. Reilly, C. B. Granger, H. Austin, D. J. Rader, S. H. Shah, A. A. Quyyumi, J. R. Gulcher, G. Thorgeirsson, U. Thorsteinsdottir, A. Kong, and K. Stefansson. 2007. A common variant on chromosome 9P21 affects the risk of myocardial infarction. *Science* 316(5830):1491-1493.

Herbert, A., N. P. Gerry, M. B. McQueen, I. M. Heid, A. Pfeufer, T. Illig, H. E. Wichmann, T. Meitinger, D. Hunter, F. B. Hu, G. Colditz, A. Hinney, J. Hebebrand, K. Koberwitz, X. Zhu, C. Cooper, K. Ardlie, H. Lyon, J. N. Hirschhorn, N. M. Laird, M. E. Lenburg, C. Lange, and M. F. Christman. 2006. A common genetic variant is associated with adult and childhood obesity. *Science* 312(5771):279-283.

Higashi, M. K., D. L. Veenstra, L. M. Kondo, A. K. Wittkowsky, S. L. Srinouanprachanh, F. M. Farin, and A. E. Rettie. 2002. Association between CYP2C9 genetic variants and anticoagulation-related outcomes during warfarin therapy. *Journal of the American Medical Association* 287(13):1690-1698.

Hirschhorn, J. N., K. Lohmueller, E. Byrne, and K. Hirschhorn. 2002. A comprehensive review of genetic association studies. *Journal of Medical Genetics* 4(2):45-61.

Hlatky, M. A., R. M. Califf, F. E. Harrell, Jr., K. L. Lee, D. B. Mark, and D. B. Pryor. 1988. Comparison of predictions based on observational data with the results of randomized controlled clinical trials of coronary artery bypass surgery. *Journal of the American College of Cardiology* 11(2):237-245.

Hoover, R. N. 2007. The evolution of epidemiologic research: From cottage industry to "big" science. *Epidemiology* 18(1):13-17.

Hunter, D. J., and P. Kraft. 2007. Drinking from the fire hose—statistical issues in genomewide association studies. *New England Journal of Medicine* 357(5):436-439.

Hunter, D. J., P. Kraft, K. B. Jacobs, D. G. Cox, M. Yeager, S. E. Hankinson, S. Wacholder, Z. Wang, R. Welch, A. Hutchinson, J. Wang, K. Yu, N. Chatterjee, N. Orr, W. C. Willett, G. A. Colditz, R. G. Ziegler, C. D. Berg, S. S. Buys, C. A. McCarty, H. S. Feigelson, E. E. Calle, M. J. Thun, R. B. Hayes, M. Tucker, D. S. Gerhard, J. F. Fraumeni, Jr., R. N. Hoover, G. Thomas, and S. J. Chanock. 2007. A genome-wide association study identifies alleles in FGFR2 associated with risk of sporadic postmenopausal breast cancer. *Nature Genetics* 39(7):870-874.

Hunter, D. J., M. J. Khoury, and J. M. Drazen. 2008. Letting the genome out of the bottle—will we get our wish? *New England Journal of Medicine* 358(2):105-107.

The International HapMap Consortium. 2003. The International HapMap Project. *Nature* 426(6968):789-796.

———. 2005. *Nature* 437(7063):1299-1320.

Ioannidis, J. P., E. E. Ntzani, T. A. Trikalinos, and D. G. Contopoulos-Ioannidis. 2001. Replication validity of genetic association studies. *Nature Genetics* 29(3):306-309.

IOM (Institute of Medicine). 2001. *Crossing the Quality Chasm: A New Health System for the 21st Century.* Washington, DC: National Academy Press.

Janssens, A. C., M. Gwinn, R. Valdez, K. M. Narayan, and M. J. Khoury. 2006. Predictive genetic testing for type 2 diabetes. *British Medical Journal* 333(7567):509-510.

Johns Hopkins University. 2008. *Online Mendelian Inheritance in Man.* http://www.ncbi.nlm.nih.gov/omim/ (accessed July 9, 2008).

Kaiser Permanente Medical Plan of Northern California. 2008. *Research Program on Genes, Environment, and Health.* http://www.dor.kaiser.org/studies/rpgeh/ (accessed July 9, 2008).

Kimmel, S. E. 2008. Warfarin therapy: In need of improvement after all these years. *Expert Opinion on Pharmacotherapy* 9(5):677-686.

Klein, R. J., C. Zeiss, E. Y. Chew, J. Y. Tsai, R. S. Sackler, C. Haynes, A. K. Henning, J. P. SanGiovanni, S. M. Mane, S. T. Mayne, M. B. Bracken, F. L. Ferris, J. Ott, C. Barnstable, and J. Hoh. 2005. Complement factor H polymorphism in age-related macular degeneration. *Science* 308(5720):385-389.

Li, J. S., E. L. Eisenstein, H. G. Grabowski, E. D. Reid, B. Mangum, K. A. Schulman, J. V. Goldsmith, M. D. Murphy, R. M. Califf, and D. K. Benjamin, Jr. 2007. Economic return of clinical trials performed under the pediatric exclusivity program. *Journal of the American Medical Association* 297(5):480-488.

Lyon, H. N., V. Emilsson, A. Hinney, I. M. Heid, J. Lasky-Su, X. Zhu, G. Thorleifsson, S. Gunnarsdottir, G. B. Walters, U. Thorsteinsdottir, A. Kong, J. Gulcher, T. T. Nguyen, A. Scherag, A. Pfeufer, T. Meitinger, G. Bronner, W. Rief, M. E. Soto-Quiros, L. Avila, B. Klanderman, B. A. Raby, E. K. Silverman, S. T. Weiss, N. Laird, X. Ding, L. Groop, T. Tuomi, B. Isomaa, K. Bengtsson, J. L. Butler, R. S. Cooper, C. S. Fox, C. J. O'Donnell, C. Vollmert, J. C. Celedon, H. E. Wichmann, J. Hebebrand, K. Stefansson, C. Lange, and J. N. Hirschhorn. 2007. The association of a SNP upstream of INSIG2 with body mass index is reproduced in several but not all cohorts. *PLoS Genetics* 3(4):e61.

Magnusson, K. P., S. Duan, H. Sigurdsson, H. Petursson, Z. Yang, Y. Zhao, P. S. Bernstein, J. Ge, F. Jonasson, E. Stefansson, G. Helgadottir, N. A. Zabriskie, T. Jonsson, A. Bjornsson, T. Thorlacius, P. V. Jonsson, G. Thorleifsson, A. Kong, H. Stefansson, K. Zhang, K. Stefansson, and J. R. Gulcher. 2006. CFH Y402H confers similar risk of soft drusen and both forms of advanced AMD. *PLoS Medicine* 3(1):e5.

Mailman, M. D., M. Feolo, Y. Jin, M. Kimura, K. Tryka, R. Bagoutdinov, L. Hao, A. Kiang, J. Paschall, L. Phan, N. Popova, S. Pretel, L. Ziyabari, M. Lee, Y. Shao, Z. Y. Wang, K. Sirotkin, M. Ward, M. Kholodov, K. Zbicz, J. Beck, M. Kimelman, S. Shevelev, D. Preuss, E. Yaschenko, A. Graeff, J. Ostell, and S. T. Sherry. 2007. The NCBI dbGaP database of genotypes and phenotypes. *Nature Genetics* 39(10):1181-1186.

Manolio, T. A. 2006. Taking our obligations to research participants seriously: Disclosing individual results of genetic research. *American Journal of Bioethics* 6(6):32-34; author reply W10-W32.

Manolio, T. A., L. L. Rodriguez, L. Brooks, G. Abecasis, D. Ballinger, M. Daly, P. Donnelly, S. V. Faraone, K. Frazer, S. Gabriel, P. Gejman, A. Guttmacher, E. L. Harris, T. Insel, J. R. Kelsoe, E. Lander, N. McCowin, M. D. Mailman, E. Nabel, J. Ostell, E. Pugh, S. Sherry, P. F. Sullivan, J. F. Thompson, J. Warram, D. Wholley, P. M. Milos, and F. S. Collins. 2007. New models of collaboration in genome-wide association studies: The genetic association information network. *Nature Genetics* 39(9):1045-1051.

Maraganore, D. M., M. de Andrade, T. G. Lesnick, K. J. Strain, M. J. Farrer, W. A. Rocca, P. V. Pant, K. A. Frazer, D. R. Cox, and D. G. Ballinger. 2005. High-resolution whole-genome association study of Parkinson's disease. *American Journal of Human Genetics* 77(5):685-693.

Mazor, K. M., J. E. Sabin, D. Boudreau, M. J. Goodman, J. H. Gurwitz, L. J. Herrinton, M. A. Raebel, D. Roblin, D. H. Smith, V. Meterko, and R. Platt. 2007. Cluster randomized trials: Opportunities and barriers identified by leaders of eight health plans. *Medical Care* 45(10 Supl 2):S29-S37.

McClellan, M., B. J. McNeil, and J. P. Newhouse. 1994. Does more intensive treatment of acute myocardial infarction in the elderly reduce mortality? Analysis using instrumental variables. *Journal of the American Medical Association* 272(11):859-866.

Michener, J. L., S. Yaggy, M. Lyn, S. Warburton, M. Champagne, M. Black, M. Cuffe, R. Califf, C. Gilliss, R. S. Williams, and V. J. Dzau. 2008. Improving the health of the community: Duke's experience with community engagement. *Academic Medicine* 83(4):408-413.

Mount Hood Modeling Group. 2007. Computer modeling of diabetes and its complications: A report on the fourth Mount Hood challenge meeting. *Diabetes Care* 30(6):1638-1646.

MRC Streptomycin in Tuberculosis Studies Committee. 1948. Streptomycin treatment of pulmonary tuberculosis: A medical research council investigation. *British Medical Journal* 2(4582):769-782.

Murphy, S. N., M. E. Mendis, D. A. Berkowitz, I. Kohane, and H. C. Chueh. 2006. Integration of clinical and genetic data in the I2B2 architecture. *AMIA Annual Symposium Proceedings* 1040.

Murray, M. D., F. E. Smith, J. Fox, E. Y. Teal, J. G. Kesterson, T. A. Stiffler, R. J. Ambuehl, J. Wang, M. Dibble, D. O. Benge, L. J. Betley, W. M. Tierney, and C. J. McDonald. 2003. Structure, functions, and activities of a research support informatics section. *Journal of the American Medical Informatics Association* 10(4):389-398.

Myers, R. H. 2006. Considerations for genomewide association studies in Parkinson disease. *American Journal of Human Genetics* 78(6):1081-1082.

National Human Genome Research Institute. 2008a. *A Catalog of Published Genome-wide Association Studies.* http://www.genome.gov/GWAstudies/ (accessed July 9, 2008).

————. 2008b. *Promoting Safe and Effective Genetic Testing in the United States.* http://www.genome.gov/10001733 (accessed July 9, 2008).

Palmer, L. J. 2007. UK biobank: Bank on it. *Lancet* 369(9578):1980-1982.

Pearson, T. A., and T. A. Manolio. 2008. How to interpret a genome-wide association study. *Journal of the American Medical Association* 299(11):1335-1344.

Peto, R., R. Collins, and R. Gray. 1995. Large-scale randomized evidence: Large, simple trials and overviews of trials. *Journal of Clinical Epidemiology* 48(1):23-40.

Rassen, J. A., M. A. Brookhart, et al. 2009. Instrumental variables II: Instrumental variable application—in 25 variations, the physician prescribing preference generally was strong and reduced covariate imbalance. *Journal of Clinical Epidemiology* 62(12):1233-1241.

Reynolds, A., J. Rubin, G. Clermont, J. Day, Y. Vodovotz, and G. Bard Ermentrout. 2006. A reduced mathematical model of the acute inflammatory response: I. Derivation of model and analysis of anti-inflammation. *Journal of Theoretical Biology* 242(1):220-236.

Ridker, P. M., D. I. Chasman, R. Y. Zee, A. Parker, L. Rose, N. R. Cook, and J. E. Buring. 2008. Rationale, design, and methodology of the women's genome health study: A genome-wide association study of more than 25,000 initially healthy American women. *Clinical Chemistry* 54(2):249-255.

Rieder, M. J., A. P. Reiner, B. F. Gage, D. A. Nickerson, C. S. Eby, H. L. McLeod, D. K. Blough, K. E. Thummel, D. L. Veenstra, and A. E. Rettie. 2005. Effect of VKORC1 haplotypes on transcriptional regulation and warfarin dose. *New England Journal of Medicine* 352(22):2285-2293.

Saka, G., J. E. Kreke, A. J. Schaefer, C. C. Chang, M. S. Roberts, and D. C. Angus. 2007. Use of dynamic microsimulation to predict disease progression in patients with pneumonia-related sepsis. *Critical Care* 11(3):R65.

Saxena, R., B. F. Voight, V. Lyssenko, N. P. Burtt, P. I. de Bakker, H. Chen, J. J. Roix, S. Kathiresan, J. N. Hirschhorn, M. J. Daly, T. E. Hughes, L. Groop, D. Altshuler, P. Almgren, J. C. Florez, J. Meyer, K. Ardlie, K. Bengtsson Bostrom, B. Isomaa, G. Lettre, U. Lindblad, H. N. Lyon, O. Melander, C. Newton-Cheh, P. Nilsson, M. Orho-Melander, L. Rastam, E. K. Speliotes, M. R. Taskinen, T. Tuomi, C. Guiducci, A. Berglund, J. Carlson, L. Gianniny, R. Hackett, L. Hall, J. Holmkvist, E. Laurila, M. Sjogren, M. Sterner, A. Surti, M. Svensson, R. Tewhey, B. Blumenstiel, M. Parkin, M. Defelice, R. Barry, W. Brodeur, J. Camarata, N. Chia, M. Fava, J. Gibbons, B. Handsaker, C. Healy, K. Nguyen, C. Gates, C. Sougnez, D. Gage, M. Nizzari, S. B. Gabriel, G. W. Chirn, Q. Ma, H. Parikh, D. Richardson, D. Ricke, and S. Purcell. 2007. Genome-wide association analysis identifies loci for type 2 diabetes and triglyceride levels. *Science* 316(5829):1331-1336.

Schlessinger, L., and D. M. Eddy. 2002. Archimedes: A new model for simulating health care systems—the mathematical formulation. *Journal of Biomedical Information* 35(1): 37-50.

Schneeweiss, S. 2006. Sensitivity analysis and external adjustment for unmeasured confounders in epidemiologic database studies of therapeutics. *Pharmacoepidemiology and Drug Safety* 15(5):291-303.

Schneeweiss, S., R. J. Glynn, J. Avorn, and D. H. Solomon. 2005. A medicare database review found that physician preferences increasingly outweighed patient characteristics as determinants of first-time prescriptions for cox-2 inhibitors. *Journal of Clinical Epidemiology* 58(1):98-102.

Schneeweiss, S., D. H. Solomon, P. S. Wang, J. Rassen, and M. A. Brookhart. 2006. Simultaneous assessment of short-term gastrointestinal benefits and cardiovascular risks of selective cyclooxygenase 2 inhibitors and nonselective nonsteroidal antiinflammatory drugs: An instrumental variable analysis. *Arthritis and Rheumatism* 54(11):3390-3398.

Scott, L. J., K. L. Mohlke, L. L. Bonnycastle, C. J. Willer, Y. Li, W. L. Duren, M. R. Erdos, H. M. Stringham, P. S. Chines, A. U. Jackson, L. Prokunina-Olsson, C. J. Ding, A. J. Swift, N. Narisu, T. Hu, R. Pruim, R. Xiao, X. Y. Li, K. N. Conneely, N. L. Riebow, A. G. Sprau, M. Tong, P. P. White, K. N. Hetrick, M. W. Barnhart, C. W. Bark, J. L. Goldstein, L. Watkins, F. Xiang, J. Saramies, T. A. Buchanan, R. M. Watanabe, T. T. Valle, L. Kinnunen, G. R. Abecasis, E. W. Pugh, K. F. Doheny, R. N. Bergman, J. Tuomilehto, F. S. Collins, and M. Boehnke. 2007. A genome-wide association study of type 2 diabetes in Finns detects multiple susceptibility variants. *Science* 316(5829):1341-1345.

Scriver, C. R. 2007. The PAH gene, phenylketonuria, and a paradigm shift. *Human Mutation* 28(9):831-845.

Sepp, T., J. C. Khan, D. A. Thurlby, H. Shahid, D. G. Clayton, A. T. Moore, A. C. Bird, and J. R. Yates. 2006. Complement factor H variant Y402H is a major risk determinant for geographic atrophy and choroidal neovascularization in smokers and nonsmokers. *Investigative Ophthalmology Visual Science* 47(2):536-540.

Sherwin, R. S., R. M. Anderson, J. B. Buse, M. H. Chin, D. Eddy, J. Fradkin, T. G. Ganiats, H. N. Ginsberg, R. Kahn, R. Nwankwo, M. Rewers, L. Schlessinger, M. Stern, F. Vinicor, and B. Zinman. 2004. Prevention or delay of type 2 diabetes. *Diabetes Care* 27(Supl 1): S47-S54.

Shurin, S. B., and E. G. Nabel. 2008. Pharmacogenomics—ready for prime time? *New England Journal of Medicine* 358(10):1061-1063.

Sladek, R., G. Rocheleau, J. Rung, C. Dina, L. Shen, D. Serre, P. Boutin, D. Vincent, A. Belisle, S. Hadjadj, B. Balkau, B. Heude, G. Charpentier, T. J. Hudson, A. Montpetit, A. V. Pshezhetsky, M. Prentki, B. I. Posner, D. J. Balding, D. Meyre, C. Polychronakos, and P. Froguel. 2007. A genome-wide association study identifies novel risk loci for type 2 diabetes. *Nature* 445(7130):881-885.

Solomon, D. H., S. Schneeweiss, R. J. Glynn, R. Levin, and J. Avorn. 2003. Determinants of selective cyclooxygenase-2 inhibitor prescribing: Are patient or physician characteristics more important? *American Journal of Medicine* 115(9):715-720.

Spiegelhlater, D. A. K., Myles, J. 2004. *Bayesian Approaches to Clinical Trials and Health-care Evaluation.* Chichester, West Sussex, UK: John Wiley & Sons.

Stacey, S. N., A. Manolescu, P. Sulem, T. Rafnar, J. Gudmundsson, S. A. Gudjonsson, G. Masson, M. Jakobsdottir, S. Thorlacius, A. Helgason, K. K. Aben, L. J. Strobbe, M. T. Albers-Akkers, D. W. Swinkels, B. E. Henderson, L. N. Kolonel, L. Le Marchand, E. Millastre, R. Andres, J. Godino, M. D. Garcia-Prats, E. Polo, A. Tres, M. Mouy, J. Saemundsdottir, V. M. Backman, L. Gudmundsson, K. Kristjansson, J. T. Bergthorsson, J. Kostic, M. L. Frigge, F. Geller, D. Gudbjartsson, H. Sigurdsson, T. Jonsdottir, J. Hrafnkelsson, J. Johannsson, T. Sveinsson, G. Myrdal, H. N. Grimsson, T. Jonsson, S. von Holst, B. Werelius, S. Margolin, A. Lindblom, J. I. Mayordomo, C. A. Haiman, L. A. Kiemeney, O. T. Johannsson, J. R. Gulcher, U. Thorsteinsdottir, A. Kong, and K. Stefansson. 2007. Common variants on chromosomes 2q35 and 16q12 confer susceptibility to estrogen receptor-positive breast cancer. *Nature Genetics* 39(7):865-869.

Stangl, D. K. B., D.A. 2000. *Meta-analysis in Medicine and Health Policy.* New York: Marcel Dekker.

Stukel, T. A., E. S. Fisher, D. E. Wennberg, D. A. Alter, D. J. Gottlieb, and M. J. Vermeulen. 2007. Analysis of observational studies in the presence of treatment selection bias: Effects of invasive cardiac management on AMI survival using propensity score and instrumental variable methods. *Journal of the American Medical Association* 297(3):278-285.

Thorleifsson, G., K. P. Magnusson, P. Sulem, G. B. Walters, D. F. Gudbjartsson, H. Stefansson, T. Jonsson, A. Jonasdottir, G. Stefansdottir, G. Masson, G. A. Hardarson, H. Petursson, A. Arnarsson, M. Motallebipour, O. Wallerman, C. Wadelius, J. R. Gulcher, U. Thorsteinsdottir, A. Kong, F. Jonasson, and K. Stefansson. 2007. Common sequence variants in the LOXL1 gene confer susceptibility to exfoliation glaucoma. *Science* 317(5843):1397-1400.

Todd, J. A. 2006. Statistical false positive or true disease pathway? *Nature Genetics* 38(7): 731-733.

Tunis, S. R., D. B. Stryer, and C. M. Clancy. 2003. Practical clinical trials: Increasing the value of clinical research for decision making in clinical and health policy. *Journal of the American Medical Association* 290(12):1624-1632.

U.S. Department of Health and Human Services. 1996. *Health Insurance Portability and Accountability Act of 1996.* http://aspe.hhs.gov/admnsimp/pL104191.htm (accessed July 10, 2008).

———. 2007. *Policy for Sharing of Data Obtained in NIH Supported or Conducted Genomewide Association Studies (GWAS).* http://grants.nih.gov/grants/guide/notice-files/NOT-OD-07-088.html (accessed July 10, 2008).

Vodovotz, Y., G. Clermont, C. Chow, and G. An. 2004. Mathematical models of the acute inflammatory response. *Current Opinion in Critical Care* 10(5):383-390.

Wallace, C., S. J. Newhouse, P. Braund, F. Zhang, M. Tobin, M. Falchi, K. Ahmadi, R. J. Dobson, A. C. Marcano, C. Hajat, P. Burton, P. Deloukas, M. Brown, J. M. Connell, A. Dominiczak, G. M. Lathrop, J. Webster, M. Farrall, T. Spector, N. J. Samani, M. J. Caulfield, and P. B. Munroe. 2008. Genome-wide association study identifies genes for biomarkers of cardiovascular disease: Serum urate and dyslipidemia. *American Journal of Human Genetics* 82(1):139-149.

Wang, L., and R. Weinshilboum. 2006. Thiopurine s-methyltransferase pharmacogenetics: Insights, challenges and future directions. *Oncogene* 25(11):1629-1638.

Weedon, M. N. 2007. The importance of TCF7L2. *Diabetes Medicine* 24(10):1062-1066.

Weedon, M. N., G. Lettre, R. M. Freathy, C. M. Lindgren, B. F. Voight, J. R. Perry, K. S. Elliott, R. Hackett, C. Guiducci, B. Shields, E. Zeggini, H. Lango, V. Lyssenko, N. J. Timpson, N. P. Burtt, N. W. Rayner, R. Saxena, K. Ardlie, J. H. Tobias, A. R. Ness, S. M. Ring, C. N. Palmer, A. D. Morris, L. Peltonen, V. Salomaa, G. Davey Smith, L. C. Groop, A. T. Hattersley, M. I. McCarthy, J. N. Hirschhorn, and T. M. Frayling. 2007. A common variant of HMGA2 is associated with adult and childhood height in the general population. *Nature Genetics* 39(10):1245-1250.

Wellcome Trust Case Control Consortium. 2007. Genome-wide association study of 14,000 cases of seven common diseases and 3,000 shared controls. *Nature* 447(7145):661-678.

Willer, C. J., S. Sanna, A. U. Jackson, A. Scuteri, L. L. Bonnycastle, R. Clarke, S. C. Heath, N. J. Timpson, S. S. Najjar, H. M. Stringham, J. Strait, W. L. Duren, A. Maschio, F. Busonero, A. Mulas, G. Albai, A. J. Swift, M. A. Morken, N. Narisu, D. Bennett, S. Parish, H. Shen, P. Galan, P. Meneton, S. Hercberg, D. Zelenika, W. M. Chen, Y. Li, L. J. Scott, P. A. Scheet, J. Sundvall, R. M. Watanabe, R. Nagaraja, S. Ebrahim, D. A. Lawlor, Y. Ben-Shlomo, G. Davey-Smith, A. R. Shuldiner, R. Collins, R. N. Bergman, M. Uda, J. Tuomilehto, A. Cao, F. S. Collins, E. Lakatta, G. M. Lathrop, M. Boehnke, D. Schlessinger, K. L. Mohlke, and G. R. Abecasis. 2008. Newly identified loci that influence lipid concentrations and risk of coronary artery disease. *Nature Genetics* 40(2):161-169.

Yang, Q., J. Cui, I. Chazaro, L. A. Cupples, and S. Demissie. 2005. Power and type I error rate of false discovery rate approaches in genome-wide association studies. *BMC Genetics* 6(Supl 1):S134.

Yeager, M., N. Orr, R. B. Hayes, K. B. Jacobs, P. Kraft, S. Wacholder, M. J. Minichiello, P. Fearnhead, K. Yu, N. Chatterjee, Z. Wang, R. Welch, B. J. Staats, E. E. Calle, H. S. Feigelson, M. J. Thun, C. Rodriguez, D. Albanes, J. Virtamo, S. Weinstein, F. R. Schumacher, E. Giovannucci, W. C. Willett, G. Cancel-Tassin, O. Cussenot, A. Valeri, G. L. Andriole, E. P. Gelmann, M. Tucker, D. S. Gerhard, J. F. Fraumeni, Jr., R. Hoover, D. J. Hunter, S. J. Chanock, and G. Thomas. 2007. Genome-wide association study of prostate cancer identifies a second risk locus at 8q24. *Nature Genetics* 39(5):645-649.

Yusuf, S. 2004. Randomized clinical trials: Slow death by a thousand unnecessary policies? *Canadian Medical Association Journal* 171(8):889-892; discussion 892-883.

Yusuf, S., J. Bosch, P. J. Devereaux, R. Collins, C. Baigent, C. Granger, R. Califf, and R. Temple. 2008. Sensible guidelines for the conduct of large randomized trials. *Clinical Trials* 5(1):38-39.

Zareparsi, S., K. E. Branham, M. Li, S. Shah, R. J. Klein, J. Ott, J. Hoh, G. R. Abecasis, and A. Swaroop. 2005. Strong association of the Y402H variant in complement factor H at 1q32 with susceptibility to age-related macular degeneration. *American Journal of Human Genetics* 77(1):149-153.

Zeggini, E., M. N. Weedon, C. M. Lindgren, T. M. Frayling, K. S. Elliott, H. Lango, N. J. Timpson, J. R. Perry, N. W. Rayner, R. M. Freathy, J. C. Barrett, B. Shields, A. P. Morris, S. Ellard, C. J. Groves, L. W. Harries, J. L. Marchini, K. R. Owen, B. Knight, L. R. Cardon, M. Walker, G. A. Hitman, A. D. Morris, A. S. Doney, M. I. McCarthy, and A. T. Hattersley. 2007. Replication of genome-wide association signals in UK samples reveals risk loci for type 2 diabetes. *Science* 316(5829):1336-1341.

4

Organizing and Improving Data Utility

INTRODUCTION

An enormous untapped capacity for data analysis is emerging as the research community hones its capacity to collect, store, and study data. We are now generating and have access to vastly larger collections of data than have been available before. The potential for mining these robust databases to expand the evidence base is experiencing commensurate growth. New and emerging design models and tools for data analysis have significant potential to inform clinical effectiveness research. However, further work is needed to fully harness the data and insights these large databases contain. As these methods are tested and developed, they are likely to become an even more valuable part of the overall research arsenal—helping to address inefficiencies in current research practices, providing meaningful complements to existing approaches, and offering means to productively process the increasingly complex information generated as part of the research enterprise today.

This chapter aims to (1) characterize some key implications of these larger electronically accessible health records and databases for research, and (2) identify the most pressing opportunities to apply these data more effectively to clinical effectiveness research. The papers that follow were derived from the workshop session devoted to organizing and improving data utility. These papers identify technological and policy advances needed to better harness these emerging data sources for research relevant to providing the care most appropriate to each patient.

From his perspective at the Geisinger Health System, Ronald A. Paulus describes successful applications of electronic health records (EHRs) and point-of-care data to create delivery-based evidence and make further steps in transforming clinical practice. These data present the opportunity to develop data useful for studies needed to complement and fill gaps in randomized controlled trial (RCT) findings. In the next paper, Alexander M. Walker from Worldwide Health Information Science Consultants and the Harvard School of Public Health discusses approaches to the development, application, and shared distribution of information from large administrative databases in clinical effectiveness research. He describes augmented databases that include laboratory and consumer data and discusses approaches to creating an infrastructure for medical record review, implementing methods for automated and quasi-automated examination of masses of data, developing "rapid-cycle" analyses to circumvent the delays of claims processing and adjudication, and opening new initiatives for collaborative sharing of data that respect patients' and institutions' legitimate needs for privacy and confidentiality. In the context of the ongoing debate about the relative value of observational data (e.g., as provided by registries) versus RCTs, Alan J. Moskowitz from Columbia University argues that registries provide data that are important complements to randomized trials (including efficacy and so-called pragmatic randomized trials) and to analyses of large administrative datasets. In fact, Moskowitz asserts, registries can assess "real-world" health and economic outcomes to help guide decision making on policies for patient care.

Complicated research questions increasingly need current information derived from a variety of sources. One promising source is distributed research models, which provide multi-user access to enormous stores of highly useful data. Several models are currently being developed. Speaking on that topic was Richard Platt, from Harvard Pilgrim Health Care and Harvard Medical School, who reports on several complex efforts to design and implement distributed research models that derive large stores of useful data from a variety of sources for multiple users.

THE ELECTRONIC HEALTH RECORD AND CARE REENGINEERING: PERFORMANCE IMPROVEMENT REDEFINED

Ronald A. Paulus, M.D., M.B.A.; Walter F. Stewart, Ph.D., M.P.H.; Albert Bothe, Jr., M.D.; Seth Frazier, M.B.A.; Nirav R. Shah, M.D., M.P.H.; and Mark J. Selna, M.D.; Geisinger

Introduction

The U.S. healthcare system has struggled with numerous, seemingly intractable problems including fragmented, uncoordinated, and highly variable care that results in safety risks and waste; consumer dissatisfaction; and the absence of productivity and efficiency gains common in other industries (The Commonwealth Fund Commission on a High Performance Health System, 2005). Multiple stakeholders—patients and families, physicians, payors, employers, and policy makers—have all called for order of magnitude improvements in healthcare quality and efficiency. While many industries have leveraged technology to deliver vastly superior value in highly competitive environments over the last several decades, healthcare performance has, on a comparative basis, stagnated. In the absence of the ability to transform performance, health care "competition" has too often focused on delivering more expensive services promoted by better marketing and geographic presence; true outcomes-based competition has been lacking (Porter and Olmsted-Teisberg, 2006). Implications of these failures have been profound for the care delivery system and for all Americans.

Recently, one area of hope has emerged: the adoption of electronic health records. EHRs, if successfully deployed, have tremendous potential to transform care delivery. Despite a primary focus on benefits derived from practice standardization and decision support, diverse uses of EHR data including enhanced quality improvement and research activities may offer an equal or even greater potential for fundamental care delivery transformation. Limits of guideline-based evidence have produced a growing recognition that observational data may be essential to complement gaps in randomized controlled trial data needed to fulfill this transformation potential. Despite serious challenges, EHR data may offer an invaluable look into interventions and outcomes in clinical practice and offer promise as a complementary source of evidence directly relevant to everyday practice needs.

EHR data also may provide an essential complement to clinical performance improvement initiatives. Healthcare performance improvement activities are defined here as an ongoing cycle of positive change in organization, care process, decision management, workflow, or other components of care, regardless of methodology (collectively PI) (Hartig and Allison, 2007). Despite the underlying logic and history of success in other business sectors, the impact of healthcare performance improvement activities is often negligible or unsustainable. As with the evidence gap, EHR data offer promise as a transformation resource for PI. The inability to achieve broad and systematic quality and operational improvements in our delivery system has left all stakeholders deeply frustrated.

This paper explores a potentially powerful new approach to leverage the latent synergy between EHR-based PI efforts and research and presents a vision of how PI at the clinical enterprise level is being transformed by the EHR and associated data aggregation and analysis activities. In that context, we describe a revision to the classic Plan-Do-Study-Act (PDSA) cycle that reflects this integration and the development of a Performance Improvement Architecture (PI Architecture), a set of reusable parts, components, and modules along with a process methodology that focuses relentlessly on eliminating all unnecessary care steps, safely automating processes, delegating care to the lowest cost, competent caregiver, maximizing supply chain efficiencies and activating patients in their own self-care. Early Geisinger Health System (Geisinger) experience suggests that use of such a PI Architecture in creating change is likely to provide guidance on what to improve, an enhanced ability to implement and track initiatives and to specifically link discrete elements of change to meaningful outcomes, a simultaneous focus on quality and efficiency, improved utilization of scarce healthcare resources and personnel, dramatic acceleration of the pace of change, and the capacity to maintain and grow that change over time.

Delivery-Based Evidence—A New EHR Role

When doctors care for patients, the very essence of the interaction requires extrapolation from knowledge and experience to tailor care for the particular circumstances at hand (i.e., bridging the "inferential gap") (Stewart et al., 2007). No two patients are alike. While a certain level of "experimentation" is a part of good care, the knowledge base required for such experimentation is growing at a pace that far exceeds the ongoing learning capacity of primary care providers and even most specialists. Hence, the nature of care provided is dated or experimental, venturing beyond what is known or is optimal.

How do providers move beyond the limits of what they can learn or "trials where n = 1"? Although the RCT serves as the "gold standard" design for making causal inferences from data, there are practical limits to the utility of RCT-based evidence (Brook and Lohr, 1985; Flum et al., 2001; Krumholz et al., 1998). Today, RCTs are largely guided by the Food and Drug Administration (FDA) and related regulatory needs, not necessarily by the most important clinical questions. They are frequently performed in specialized settings (e.g., academic medical centers or the Veterans Administration) that are not representative of the broader arena of care delivery. RCTs are used to test drugs and devices in highly selected populations (i.e., patients with relatively low co-morbid disease burdens), under artificial conditions (i.e., a simple, focused question) that are often unrelated to usual clinical care (i.e., managing complex needs of patients with multiple co-morbidities), and are focused on outcomes that may be incomplete (e.g., short-term outcomes leading to changes in a disease mediator). Efficacy equivalence with existing therapies rather than comparative effectiveness is the dominant focus of most trials, with little or no thought given to economic constraints or consequences. RCTs are not usually positioned to address fundamental questions of need for subgroups with different co-morbidities, and results rarely translate into the clinical effectiveness hoped for under real-world practice conditions (Hayward et al., 1995). As the population continues to age and the prevalence of co-morbidities increases, the gap between what we know from RCTs and what we need to know to support objective clinical decisions is increasing, despite the pace at which new knowledge is being generated. Furthermore, decisions based primarily on randomized trial data do not incorporate local values, knowledge, or patient preferences into care decisions.

From a distance, EHR data offer promise as a complementary source of evidence to more directly address questions relevant to everyday practice needs. However, a closer look at EHR data reveals challenges. Compared to data collection standards established for research, EHR data suffer from many limitations in both quality and completeness. In research settings, specialized staff follow strict data collection protocols; in routine care, even simple measures such as blood pressure or smoking status are measured with many more sources of error. For example, the wording of a question may differ, and responses to even identical questions can be documented in different manners. In routine care, the completeness of data may vary significantly by patient, being directly related to the underlying disease burden and the need for care. Furthermore, physicians may select a particular medication within a class based on the perceived severity of a patient's disease, resulting in a complex form of bias that is difficult to eliminate (i.e., confounding by indication) (de Koning et al., 2005). In the near term, these and other limitations will raise questions about the credibility of evidence derived from EHR data. However, weaknesses inherent to EHR data as a source of evidence (e.g., false-positive associations) and to the current practice of PI (e.g., initiatives confined to guideline-based knowledge) can be mitigated through replication studies using independent EHRs and by using PI to test and validate EHR-based hypotheses.

Healthcare Quality Improvement

Since the early observations of Shewart, Juran, and Demming, quality improvement has become routine in most business sectors and has been formalized into a diverse set of methodologies and underlying philosophies such as Total Quality Management, Continuous Quality Improvement, Six Sigma, Lean, Reengineering and Microsystems (Juran, 1995). While late-comers, healthcare organizations have increasingly adopted these practices in an attempt to optimize outcomes. Healthcare PI involves an ongoing cycle of change in organization, care process, decision management, workflow, or other components of care, evolving from a culture often previously dominated by blame and fault finding (e.g., peer and utilization review) to devising evidence-based "systems" of care.

In general, healthcare PI relies on "planning" or "experimentation" approaches to improve outcomes. These models employ a diversity of philosophies including a commitment to identifying, meeting, and exceeding stakeholder needs; continuously improving in conjunction with escalating performance standards; applying structured, problem-solving processes using statistical and related tools such as control charts, cause-and-effect diagrams, and benchmarking; and empowering all employees to drive quality improvements. Experimentation-based PI typically relies on the PDSA model (Shewhart, 1939), as recently refined by the Institute for Healthcare Improvement (IHI) for the healthcare community (see Box 4-1) (Institute for Healthcare Improvement). Most approaches involve analysis that begins with a "diagnosis" of cause(s), albeit with limited data, followed by new data collection (frequently manual) to validate that the new process improves outcomes. Deployment of these models is often labor-intensive (e.g., evidence gathering, workflow observation), and effectuating change may take months, in part due to lack of dedicated support resources as well as a historical lack of focus on scalability. As a result, each successive itera-

---

BOX 4-1
IHI PDSA Cycle

Step 1: Plan—*Plan the test or observation, including a plan for collecting data.*
- State the objective of the test.
- Make predictions about what will happen and why.
- Develop a plan to test the change. (Who? What? When? Where? What data need to be collected?)

Step 2: Do—*Try out the test on a small scale.*
- Carry out the test.
- Document problems and unexpected observations.
- Begin analysis of the data.

Step 3: Study—*Set aside time to analyze the data and study the results.*
- Complete the analysis of the data.
- Compare the data to your predictions.
- Summarize and reflect on what was learned.

Step 4: Act—*Refine the change, based on what was learned from the test.*
- Determine what modifications should be made.
- Prepare a plan for the next test.

tion may be performed without the ability to reuse previously developed tools, datasets, or analytics.

Limitations to Healthcare Performance Improvement

Despite the underlying logic and history of success in other business sectors, the impact of healthcare PI has too frequently been negligible or unsustainable (Blumenthal and Kilo, 1998). The gap between the potential for PI and results from actual practice has been substantial, as have the consequences of historical failures to improve outcomes. A number of factors explain this gap.

First, PI initiatives are commonly motivated by guideline-based evidence and, as such, are subject to the same limitations as RCT data discussed above. Second, the PI-focused outcome may be only distantly or indirectly related to meaningful change in patient health or to a concrete measure of return on investment (ROI), largely because of the limits to available data and how such initiatives are organizationally motivated and executed. For example, there may not be the organizational will to make change happen or to support change efforts to sustainability. Even when PI is applied to an important problem (e.g., slowing progression of diabetes) in a manner that improves a chosen metric (e.g., ordering a HbA1c lab test), the effort may have only an incomplete or a delayed effect on more relevant outcomes (e.g., fewer complications, reductions in hospital admissions or improved quality of life). Third, outcomes are usually not evaluated in real time or at frequent intervals, limiting the timeliness, ease, and speed of innovation, as well as the dynamism of the process itself. When change and the associated process unfold in slow motion, participants' (or their authorizing leaders') commitment may not rise to or maintain the threshold required to institutionalize new standards of practice. Fourth, validation that a PI intervention actually works may be lacking altogether or lacking in scientific or analytic rigor, leaving inference to the realm of guesswork. Fifth, when human or labor-intensive processes are required to maintain change, performance typically regresses to baseline levels as vigilance wanes. Lastly, without a broad strategic framework, PI can be perceived as the "initiative of the month," leading to temporary improvements that are quickly lost due to inadequate hardwiring, support systems, vigilance, or PI integration across an organization.

The Geisinger Health System Experience

At Geisinger, PI is evolving to become a continuous process involving data generation, performance measurement, and analysis to transform clinical practice, mediated by iterative changes to clinical workflows by elimi-

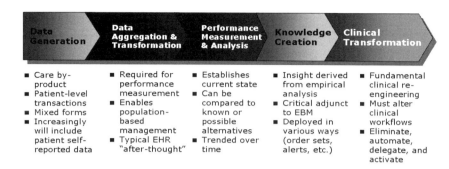

Data Generation	Data Aggregation & Transformation	Performance Measurement & Analysis	Knowledge Creation	Clinical Transformation
■ Care by-product ■ Patient-level transactions ■ Mixed forms ■ Increasingly will include patient self-reported data	■ Required for performance measurement ■ Enables population-based management ■ Typical EHR "after-thought"	■ Establishes current state ■ Can be compared to known or possible alternatives ■ Trended over time	■ Insight derived from empirical analysis ■ Critical adjunct to EBM ■ Deployed in various ways (order sets, alerts, etc.)	■ Fundamental clinical re-engineering ■ Must alter clinical workflows ■ Eliminate, automate, delegate, and activate

FIGURE 4-1 Transformation infrastructure.

nating, automating, or delegating activities to meet quality and efficiency goals (see Figure 4-1).

By way of background, Geisinger is an integrated delivery system located in central and northeastern Pennsylvania comprised of nearly 700 employed physicians across 55 clinical practice sites providing adult and pediatric primary and specialty care; 3 acute care hospitals (one closed, two open staff); several specialty hospitals; a 215,000 member health plan (accounting for approximately one-third of the Geisinger Clinic patient care revenue); and numerous other clinical services and programs. Geisinger serves a population of 2.5 million people, poorer and sicker than national benchmarks, with markedly less in- and out-migration. Organizationally, Geisinger manages through clinical service lines, each co-led by a physician-administrator pair. Strategic functions such as quality and innovation are centralized with matrixed linkage to operational leaders. A commercial EHR platform adopted in 1995 is fully utilized across the system (Epic Systems Corporation, 2008). An integrated database consisting of EHR, financial, operational, claims, and patient satisfaction data serves as the foundation of a Clinical Decision Intelligence System (CDIS).

At Geisinger, data are increasingly viewed as a core asset. A very heavy emphasis is placed on the collection, normalization, and application of clinical, financial, operational, claims, and other data to inform, guide, measure, refine, and document the results of PI efforts. These data are combined with other inputs (e.g., evidence-based guidelines, third-party benchmarks) and leveraged via decision support applications as schematically illustrated below (see Figure 4-2).

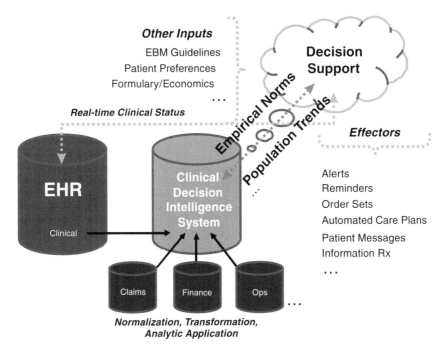

FIGURE 4-2 Clinical decision intelligence system design.

Transforming Performance Improvement: From a Human Process to a Scalable Performance Improvement Architecture

Early Geisinger experience supports the view that a PI Architecture, including EHR data and associated data warehousing capabilities can transform healthcare PI, as well as how an organization behaves.

Data, System, and Analytic Requirements

Most performance improvement efforts lack the rich data required to validate outcomes (i.e., test the initial hypothesis) or the integrated data infrastructure required for rapid feedback to refine or modify large-scale interventions. When available at all, data are often limited in scope and consist of simple administrative and/or manually collected elements that may not be generated as part of the routine course of care. By contrast, robust EHRs inherently provide for extensive, longitudinal data (i.e., clinical test results, vital signs, reason for order or other explicit information regarding the intent of the provider, etc.). When used in conjunction with an integrated data warehouse and normalized, searchable electronic data,

EHRs can motivate a quantum shift in the PI paradigm. As a core asset, this new PI Architecture is used to ask questions, pose hypotheses, refine understanding, and ultimately develop improvement initiatives that are directly relevant to current practice with a dual focus on quality and efficiency.

Natural "experiments" are intrinsic to EHR data. Patients with essentially the same or similar disease profiles receive different care. For example, one 60-year-old diabetic patient may be prescribed drug A, while a similar diabetic patient may be described drug B because of formulary or practice style differences. When repeated hundreds or thousands of times, routinely collected EHR data offer a unique data mining resource for important clinical and economic insights. When combined with health plan claims and other information, additional questions may be answered such as: Is there a difference in drug fill/refill rates between drugs A and B identified above?

In addition to the need for an EHR, an integrated, normalized data asset simplifies the logistics and cycle time for exploration, development of an ROI argument (e.g., forecasting, simulating), planning and implementation, and performance analysis. While data aggregation, standardization, and normalization are often centralized activities, data access should be as decentralized, simple, and low cost as possible (i.e., no incremental barrier to review). Providing clinical and business end-users with direct, unrestricted access helps to motivate a cultural shift toward identifying opportunities for improving care quality and access and for reducing the cost of care. In this way, everyday clinical hunches (e.g., a patient who used drug X subsequently shows impaired renal function) can be formulated into questions (e.g., "has this phenomenon been observed in the last X hundred patients that we cared for here?"), rapid analysis, and "answers." This capability to rapidly place in context both the individual patient and the broader population is routinely missing in nearly all healthcare delivery organizations. This frame of reference is important for physicians who have been shown to be overly sensitized by recent patient experience (Greco and Eisenberg, 1993; Poses and Anthony, 1991).

The PI Architecture should be capable of answering previously imponderable questions such as "How many patients with chronic kidney disease do we care for?" and in so doing, compare the results from operationally identified patients (e.g., derived from the Problem List) versus biologically identified patients (e.g., via calculations from laboratory creatinine measurements). This level of data interrogation enables PI teams to be fully grounded in the reality of what actually happens, rather than guided by impressions, selective or hazy memories, or idyllic desires. Similarly, when using benchmarks to compare performance, hypothesis-driven data mining asks "Why are we different?," regardless of whether that difference is positive or negative. As such, it enables even a benchmarking leader to continue to innovate and improve (Gawande, 2004). This approach parallels Berwick's recent call to *"equip the workforce to study the effects of their efforts, actively and objectively, as part of daily work"* and creates a "culture of empirical review" as a critical determinant of success (Berwick, 2008).

Organizational Requirements

Global and local organizational requirements are essential to institutionalizing a culture of improvement using a PI Architecture. First, Board and CEO level support for transformation is required to support adoption. PI Architecture investment is not trivial, and several years are required to reach peak output. Stable resourcing and strategic investment is essential to achieve success. Control and responsibility of the PI process (e.g., selection of issues, control of implementation, and evaluation of outcomes and ongoing feedback) must be entrusted to leaders held accountable for results. Where PI is centralized, local clinical and operational leaders must be engaged from the beginning to be part of and motivated by the opportunities inherent to the care process change. In addition, staff (or teams) should be experienced in change management, workflow analysis, health information technology (HIT) integration, and performance management skills and orientation. The extent to which this group has aligned goals and is free to innovate beyond usual organizational constraints, policies, and practices will dictate the breadth of possible change. Finally, passion for success is a powerful force. We believe that an entrepreneurial approach to PI, a well-established motivation in other business sectors, produces sustainable change, especially when balanced with appropriate skepticism on defining success and the "permission" to fail but with the expectation of ultimately persevering.

At Geisinger, this culture is embedded through formal links between the traditional silos of Innovation, Clinical Effectiveness, Research, and the Clinical Enterprise along with critical underlying support from Information Technology. Innovation's role is to support a broad range of change initiatives that are designed to fundamentally challenge historical assumptions. Innovation typically reaches for large successes with a focus on knowledge transfer across the organization and on creating a reusable, scalable transformation infrastructure. Clinical Effectiveness often takes a complementary approach to change across a broader swath of the organization with a focus on process redesign and skill development. The Clinical Enterprise represents the "front line" of patient care; its "sources of pain" provide a strong indication of opportunity; its ideas, clinical hunches, and feedback on innovation are essential for success.

At Geisinger, research has a multi-year horizon. Adoption of a traditional research and development model, used in other business sectors, leads to a translation-focused process to bring value to the clinical enterprise, rather than a focus on traditional "knowledge creation." This model leads to ongoing interactions, where research leverages the insights of Innovations, Clinical Effectiveness, the Clinical Enterprise, the ROI model, and the tactics of implementation. To some degree, PI initiatives serve as the preliminary work for research to pursue a product-oriented process for extending and scaling the PI architecture that moves beyond the tactics of initiatives, relies less on organizational vigilance and individual learning, and can more easily be scaled within Geisinger and potentially exported elsewhere. The continuum of activities among collaborating divisions offers a unique potential for broader commercial application via Geisinger Ventures, which seeks to capture fundamental breakthrough technologies, techniques, or approaches to care that represent a sensible and more certain means of translating knowledge to practice (i.e., through the commercial marketplace) in a manner that cannot be achieved rapidly by publications, speaking, or collaboratives.

Building a Performance Improvement Architecture

The core feature of the PI Architecture (and associated analytics and process methodology) is to support the following key goals: (1) to rank-order PI initiatives for the largest ROI; (2) to support a simultaneous focus on quality and efficiency; (3) to require the development or refinement of reusable parts, components, and modules from each PI initiative to support future efforts; and (4) to ensure that practitioners evaluate the opportunity to eliminate any unnecessary steps in care, automate processes when safe and effective to do so, delegate care to the least-cost, competent caregiver, and activate the patient as a participant in her own self-care.

Using this model, care processes selected for improvement can be identified proactively via a thoughtful rank-ordering of problems based upon ROI criteria (whether clinical, business, or both). Example ROI-based approaches include selecting those processes with outcomes farthest from benchmark performance; those with the largest impact by patient population or resource consumption; or those with the most significant variation. The absence of an ROI-based selection process often precludes the development of a "clinical business plan" that can meet the requirements of skeptical observers, an activity routine in other industries and one where if skipped makes post-intervention value determination problematic. As Berwick noted, when evaluating areas for PI intervention one must *"reconsider thresholds for action on evidence"* (Berwick, 2008). In this context an appropriate threshold may be far below the traditional research standard of significance where $p < 0.05$. Less restrictive interpretations of data and "evidence" are commonplace in other industries, where in the absence of better information, a p-value < 0.5 is often indicative of a reasonable idea for change, and p-values < 0.25 would routinely create sustained success.

Of course, evidence at this level may not indicate a true need to change care, but rather the need to more formally study a partially validated question in a more rigorous manner.

Once selected, attractive areas for more detailed PI intervention tend to fall into two broad categories: (1) what should we be doing systematically that we are not? and (2) what should we stop doing that is causing harm or simply not adding value? These questions are fundamentally related to whether or not some aspect of provider-delivered care (e.g., the treatment plan, flow, caregivers, timing, or setting such as inpatient versus outpatient, nursing unit versus nursing unit, etc.) improves the value of healthcare delivery. One structured way to perform this analysis is to review at least the following:

1. *Missing Elements of Care.* Is something missing that seems to provide benefit (e.g., beta blockers post MI, statins for CAD)?
2. *Potential Diagnostic or Therapeutic Substitutions.* Does something (or someone) seem to work better than another (e.g., breast MRI versus mammography in high-risk patients)?
3. *Excess Diagnostic or Treatment Intensity.* What care patterns persist but appear to add no apparent value (e.g., plain film + CT + MRI + PET)?
4. *Flow Impediments.* Does the sequence of care and/or settings seem to make a difference (e.g., weekend care, getting to the right inpatient unit)?
5. *Supply Chain Inefficiencies.* Is care standardized enough to generate maximum supply chain economies and familiarity (e.g., implant devices or benefits of silver-impregnated versus standard foley catheters relative to UTI)?
6. *Provider Care Team Variation.* Are there different outcomes with different providers and/or provider teams (e.g., physician–physician, physician–NP, etc.)?

Box 4-2 defines an update of the PDSA cycle to reflect the availability of a PI Architecture.

Benefits of a Performance Improvement Architecture

Several important benefits from our recent experience evolving this approach are noteworthy as potentially generalizable findings.

BOX 4-2
Performance Improvement Architecture Cycle

Step 1: Document Focus—*Document the current state using local data.*
- Identify settings and circumstances from which the PI is most likely to be generalizable, scalable, and sustainable; choose high-ranking opportunities where stakeholder support is evident or predictable.
- Define current practice and variation level and measure gap between current and desired state.
- Confirm all needed data are available for review, minimum documentation: flow, diagnostic and treatment intensity, supply chain, accountable clinicians, safety.

Step 2: Simulate—*Confirm hypothesis via electronic review and simulate results if desired state is achieved.*
- Establish what benefits the minimal, maximum, and expected change would yield.
- Translate those benefits into clinical, financial, and satisfaction metrics and targets.
- Compare different avenues for change to allow for rank-ordering of the most likely approach to yield the largest return.

Step 3: Iterate—*Try out the test on a small scale, but with a strategy for rapid escalation.*
- Carry out the test, documenting both expected and unexpected observations relative to the simulation.
- Compare performance to previously established metrics in near real time; confirm or deny ROI.
- Iterate for success or shut down, and move on if results are below threshold expectations.

Step 4: Accelerate—*Leverage reusable parts from past initiatives and build core infrastructure for future work.*
- Always use prior components and off-the-shelf content whenever available.
- Resist the temptation for "one-off" solutions that are inherently unscalable.
- Ensure that solutions implemented for a given initiative are incorporated into the overall transformation architecture for future use and scalability.

Reduced Cycle Time

First, much of the historical PDSA cycle can be performed electronically. For example, opportunities for improvement can be automatically rank-ordered according to specified criteria (e.g., systematically screening care relative to evidence-based guidelines, with deviations used as objective input for ranking). Also, "clinical hunches," comparisons of actual performance to guidelines, evaluation of new medical literature findings for local practice, and other comparisons can be tested via database queries in a matter of minutes, rather than taking days, weeks, or months using traditional human-based assessments. If designed appropriately, the impact of hopeful interventions can be simulated. Such simulations can provide insight into the need for change and also can help to establish the clinical-business case and anticipate the ROI from any given intervention, again with only limited resource commitments. As a result, those hypotheses that actually make it to a real test of change are much more likely to be important and to have a greater chance for success. Once tests are underway, real-time data access supports rapid change cycles, where sequentially refined hypotheses can be tested and refined in increasingly shorter short periods of time.

Increased Quality of Hypothesis Generation and Relevance of Initiatives

Second, the purview of inquiry moves beyond guidelines, encompassing questions more directly relevant to practice and the related business case, as well as what an organization should stop doing, recognizing that many components of care are embedded by tradition and offer little or no value. Importantly, metrics can be focused on measures that are directly relevant to patient health (e.g., actual low density lipoprotein levels rather than lab orders) and downstream impact (e.g., cardiac events or visits avoided), substantially improving the saliency of feedback to guide productive change that yields tangible value, holds the attention of organizational leaders, and motivates continued vigilance.

Increased Sustainability

EHRs can be used to "hard wire" process changes, to automatically track and trend important metrics after an intervention has been made, to watch for regression, and to learn of unexpected consequences (whether good or bad). Further, dashboards can serve to link PI efforts to strategic objectives and gain the attention of a much broader community to provide additional incentive to maintain gains from change.

Increased Focus on Return on Investment

Because resources are always constrained, it is critical to focus PI efforts on those interventions that can deliver the most clinical and business return. Under this framework, PI is strongly focused on ROI as evidenced by empirical data. As those data allow for more thoughtful clinical-business planning, more leaders are engaged (e.g., CFO, clinic directors), thereby enabling PI to rapidly evolve its purview to a much broader and more refined set of measurable outcomes that are likely to impact quality and efficiency in a material way.

Enhanced Research Capabilities

A PI Architecture can augment research. First, PI informs opportunities for success. Interventions that appear to be important, impactful, and sustained, guide researchers on opportunities that are likely to be successful for more complete testing via a robust study and for development and testing of tools to replace labor-intensive workflows and processes. Second, the data asset can be used to quickly "confirm or deny" results from newly published trials, whether randomized or observational. Further, when performed proactively, data mining for unintended consequences of new drugs can be an important adjunct to current forms of postmarketing surveillance. Similarly, one can mine such databases (which include reason codes for medication orders) for off-label usage patterns, risks, and benefits. All of these data-driven opportunities would be enhanced even further if disparate health systems using common data standards pooled their data (or results) for such purposes. Finally, EHRs can be used to identify patients who meet criteria for research studies and to capture data elements relevant for analysis.

Summary and Conclusion

Many health systems are experimenting with new approaches to quality improvement that leverage EHR capabilities. In addition to practice standardization and decision support, EHR data provide a new source of hypotheses and evidence for both PI and research. When complimented by a broader data aggregation, analysis infrastructure, and process to create a PI Architecture, the potential is significant. While there are numerous limitations yet to be overcome, the latent potential between EHR (and other electronic) data, performance improvement and research is both significant and exciting. The next decade of work will be transformative; this is an exciting time for health care.

ADMINISTRATIVE DATABASES IN CLINICAL
EFFECTIVENESS RESEARCH

Alexander M. Walker, M.D., Dr.P.H.
Harvard School of Public Health
World Health Information Science Consultants, LLC

Background

The most exigent demands for large-scale integration of medical data have come from healthcare administrators and payors. Their needs to create effective payment schemes and basic monitoring of medical resource utilization have been susceptible to ready standardization and have provided immediate financial returns that have in turn justified the investment in the requisite data systems. The many-to-many relations between insurers and providers in the United States, in which an insurer may deal with hundreds of thousands of providers and a provider may deal with tens of insurers, has meant that the only functioning systems are highly standardized and internally consistent.

The resulting progress in the development of administrative databases stands in marked contrast to the world of electronic health records, which capture far more complex clinical and laboratory data, and for which there has been the growth of many competing local standards. While the advantages in patient care with a well-functioning electronic record are evident to practitioners, the cost and complexity of these systems still poses a barrier to implementation. Implemented systems that follow different standards pose even more formidable barriers to standardization.

For all the advantages that a research-enabled electronic health record will one day offer, it is administrative databases that form the heart of large-scale population research for most medical applications. The purpose of this report is to touch on the key features of these resources.

Insurance Claims Data

The most widespread technique for distributing healthcare funds in industrial countries involves some form of fee-for-service reimbursement, in which providers of services turn to private or governmental insurance programs for payment for specified services. Insurance schemes have been advocated as the most effective way to pay for services even in societies with limited medical resources (Second International Conference on Improving Use of Medicines, 2004).

The population definition for an insurance database is contained in the eligibility file, which identifies all covered individuals and basic demographic data such as date of birth, sex, and address. This file will include dates of coverage and may contain some family information in the form of an identified primary contract holder, along with dependents.

The service claims in a typical insurance database include identities of both the provider and recipient of services, the nature and date(s) of services, and presumptive diagnoses that motivated the services. Services may be visits, diagnostic tests, or procedures. The results of laboratory procedures, as opposed to the fact of the test having been performed, are not part of the insurance claims system.

Hospitalizations are a special form of service, typically accompanied by more detailed information, including dates, procedures, and primary and secondary diagnoses. In the United States, physician charges that do not flow through the hospital billing system appear as individual provider claims during a period of hospitalization and can be used to flesh out events during hospitalization.

Pharmacy insurance claims arise for each dispensing, with identities of the pharmacy, the prescribing physician, and the recipient and details on the product supplied, substance, manufacturer, form, dose, quantity, and days supply. The indication for treatment is not typically part of the claim and must typically be inferred from diagnoses recently assigned in conjunction with visits to the prescribing physician.

Insurers may use these data internally for administrative purposes. Researchers in the United States operate under rules set by HIPAA (the Health Insurance Portability and Accountability Act), which circumscribes their permitted activities in order to safeguard individual's medical privacy. Under HIPAA, personally identifying data, termed PHI (protected health information) includes both obvious identifiers, such as name and address, and data from which persons might be identifiable with the supplementary use of other publicly identifiable information. This includes for example exact date of birth. HIPAA provides standards for creating "deidentified" data, which can be exchanged and analyzed without further oversight. If PHI is required, researchers must obtain the permission of a Privacy Board, which is typically constituted under an Institutional Review Board (IRB). The researcher needs to provide details of methods by which the minimum necessary amount of PHI will be employed for the minimum time required and which will safeguard that PHI during its period of use.

Currently available insurance claims databases with full information range in size of up to about 20 million persons cross-sectionally, with substantially larger numbers of cumulative "lives" and for data that may omit one or more of the elements above. U.S. Medicare data, not yet widely available, include claims information on over 40 million persons over the age of 65, with drug data from 2007 forward.

Though well suited to studies of health services utilization, insurance data serve clinical research only with substantial further processing and with caution even at that. Drug use is inferred from dispensing data. Medical conditions must be inferred from patterns of claims for services, treatments, and diagnostic procedures. Thus a recently used algorithm for venous thromboembolism included the occurrence of a suitable diagnosis associated with a physician visit, emergency room or hospital claim, performance of an appropriate imaging procedure, and at least two dispensings of an anticoagulant (Jick et al., 2007; Sands et al., 2006). Algorithms for more subtle conditions may be more complex still. Conditions for the pattern of care attendant on a "rule out" diagnosis resembles that for a confirmed diagnosis may be impossible to identify with any specificity.

The advantages of pure insurance claims data include easy access to data on very large numbers of individuals, detailed drug information, and the absence of reporting biases related to knowledge of exposure or outcome. There are substantial drawbacks. There is a lag in the creation of research-ready insurance files that runs from months to a year. The lack of medical record validation means that crucial cases may be missed and that others may be incorrectly ascribed to a condition under study. For nonemergency conditions, it may be very difficult to pinpoint the date of onset and the distinction between recurring, recrudescent, and new-onset conditions may be elusive. Apart from special circumstances involving serious acute outcomes and drug or vaccine exposures, insurance claims data may typically be insufficient for clinical research purposes.

Augmented Claims Data

Research groups within the insurance organizations that generate data have begun to systematically augment these files. Increasingly insurers are negotiating arrangements with independent laboratories under which the analyte results must be submitted with the claim for reimbursement. These are outpatient files and do not represent complete laboratory histories. Since the arrangements are made between the insurer and the laboratory, an individual's record will contain repeated measures to the extent that he/she returns to the same site for testing. These have been used for example to relate cardiovascular disease to severe anemia (Walker et al., 2006).

Marketing databases contain self-report data on ethnicity and income, which have been linked to insurance data. In the United States there are available files that link postal code information to detailed census data on income and ethnicity as well.

Far more important than laboratory values and income has been the ability to return to providers and patients for direct information. With Privacy Board approval, researchers can approach physicians and institutions holding patients' medical records to verify diagnoses and treatments, and to eke out information on lifestyle, chronic risk factors, and family history that is not available in the insurance claims history. With IRB approval, they can approach patients themselves for information, biometric data, and even tissue samples. These studies permit analyses carried out with a reasonable certainty that the underlying elements are correct.

A good example of the multifaceted work that augmented claims databases permit is an FDA-mandated program of surveillance of the oral contraceptive Yasmin. The progestational agent in Yasmin is drospirenone, which is functionally related to the potassium-sparing diuretic spironolactone. Though no problems of potassium handling had been seen in clinical trials, the analogy was sufficient to bring the FDA to have the sponsor initiate a program that (1) followed hospitalization and mortality in over 20,000 Yasmin initiators and a two-fold larger comparison group; (2) monitored contraindicated dispensing to patients with adrenal, renal, and hepatic dysfunction; (3) quantified the use of potassium monitoring in certain indicated patients; and (4) ascertained the outcomes of breakthrough pregnancies. Chart reviews, physician interviews, and even interventions with doctors prescribing to contraindicated patients rounded out a clinically useful surveillance program (Eng et al., 2008; Mona Eng et al., 2007; Seeger et al., 2007).

Enhanced claims studies include the insurance claims database advantages of large numbers of subjects, detailed drug exposure information, and lack of reporting bias, and add to these much greater confidence in the nature of events being studied and knowledge of timing. Like insurance claims studies, research programs in augmented databases may still be hindered by a lag in adjudication of claims on the order of months to a year. These data resources serve well for observational studies of outcomes that are highly likely to result in medical care.

Automated and Quasi-Automated Database Review

Many of the research and surveillance activities that take place in insurance files take advantage of repeatedly implemented computer routines, which offer the hope that some of these programs could be automated as decision support tools for both clinical safety and efficacy.

The core idea for creating such tools is to simplify the welter of claims data into manageable units. In part this can come about through routine implementation of algorithms, such as the one described above for venous thromboembolism, into standard units for off-the-shelf programming or routine tabulation. A number of data holders have taken this concept even further, with the concept of "episode groupers," programs that recast a broad range of related claims into single clinical entities, such as for example "community acquired pneumonia."

A second element of routine surveillance computer programs is a standard way for handling the confounding that is so prevalent in observational studies of the outcomes medical regimens. One approach is to take the wealth of data represented in insurance claims into a multivariate prediction of therapeutic choice, called a *propensity score*. These models can be rich because they draw on thousands or ten of thousands of observations and can incorporate claims history items that collectively represent strong proxies for confounding factors (Seeger et al., 2005). Propensity-matched groups can be created routinely in advance for new, commonly used therapies, or scores can be calculated and stored with individual records for future use.

The final *sine qua non* of automated surveillance is a plan for dealing with multiplicity of outcomes. Some investigators have proposed restricting attention to a smallish number of disease outcomes previously associated with drug effects, such as hepatitis, rashes, or ocular toxicity. This may be a strategy with little marginal gain, as these will be precisely the drug outcomes for which clinicians are most sensitive and likely to report adverse effects already. Another option is to apply a formal Bonferroni correction to thousands of possible combinations of drugs and outcomes being tested, much in the same way that whole-genome scans are subjected to radical statistical attenuation to reduce false positives. This approach has the drawback of curtailing power to detect true association in proportion to the reduction in risk of false positives (Walker and Wise, 2002).

A more productive approach to multiplicity in large database is to apply both statistical and medical logic to the problem of pruning false-positive results. Does the timing look right? Is the outcome plausible in light of the mechanism of action, or perhaps the route of administration of a drug? Are there analogies to be drawn from the experience with similar products?

Decision support tools do not have a promising history. Perhaps the technology for creating them tends to lag the decision-maker needs, or it may be that the enthusiasm required to generate development funding inevitably raises expectations beyond what the technologists can reasonably achieve. It may be that comprehensive indexing, retrieval, and counting functions, and not sophisticated analysis, are the proper goal of massive, automated data integration.

Distributed Processing

Part of the push for greater sensitivity and speed in drug safety surveillance is taking the form of programs to include large numbers of automated databases in common surveillance mechanisms. At the level of database amalgamation, the large U.S. insurance databases would seem to be ideal candidates, as they already operate under common rules for coding and

242 REDESIGNING THE CLINICAL EFFECTIVENESS RESEARCH PARADIGM

have similar structures, imposed by the common format of the component data items.

There are however major institutional barriers to having holders of large datasets contribute them to a common pool. Giving up the ability to approve of the analyses done in one's own data underlies some of the reluctance, and it may be that the details of pricing and reimbursement contained in the data are considered sensitive and proprietary.

The most promising solution to both computational and institutional obstacles to very large database research may lie in distributed processing, discussed by Richard Platt in more detail elsewhere in this volume. Under distributed processing models, data holders create standard views of their databases, or even standardized extracts. A central office then distributes computer code to pull out key information from each database, for trans-mittal back, where the statistical coordinating center assembles the elements into a common analysis.

A Note of Caution

Observational data, no matter how assembled, require special care in clinical effectiveness research. The likelihood that persons undergoing compared therapies will different with respect to fundamental predictors of outcome is large and needs to be addressed head-on. There is a growing family of research methodologies, including propensity techniques (mentioned above), proxy variable analysis, and instrumental variables that are the objects of vigorous methodological research (Schneeweiss, 2007). While these necessary efforts continue, science-based skepticism of non-randomized studies remains highly appropriate, even though unthinking rejection may properly belong to the past.

CLINICAL EFFECTIVENESS RESEARCH:
THE PROMISE OF REGISTRIES

Alan J. Moskowitz, M.D., and Annetine C. Gelijns, Ph.D.
Mount Sinai School of Medicine

Introduction

In comparison to other sectors of the economy, modern health care is a technologically highly innovative field. New drugs, devices, procedures, and behavioral interventions continuously emerge from the research and development (R&D) pipeline and then get established into clinical practice. The R&D process in medicine generally involves "premarketing" clinical trials, particularly in the case of drugs, biological products, and devices.

The development process of these new technologies as well as procedures, however, does not end with their introduction and adoption into practice. Over time as these interventions diffuse into widespread use, the medical profession tends to further modify and extend their application—by finding new populations, indications, and long-term effects. These dynamic patterns of adaptation and evolution underscore the importance of measuring the health and economic outcomes of clinical interventions in everyday practice and drive the renewed interest in developing a robust clinical effectiveness research enterprise.

There are various ways of measuring the clinical effectiveness of diagnostic and therapeutic interventions, including so-called pragmatic randomized trials, large administrative dataset analyses, and observational studies using clinical registries (Gliklick and Dreyer, 2007; Tunis et al., 2003). In this paper, we focus on the role and potential of registries in capturing information about "real-world" health and economic outcomes. We also highlight their potential value for assessing quality of care; for instance, through studies of risk-adjusted volume–outcome relationships. Finally, we address an often under-examined benefit of clinical registries; that is, their potential to accumulate information that, in turn, can increase the efficiency of randomized clinical trials, and premarketing studies in general. As such, clinical registries can be an important tool to help to guide decision making for patient care and health policy.

Obviously, clinical registries have their methodological and practical vulnerabilities, and we will review some analytical, organizational, and financial measures to strengthen them. In particular, we will discuss the incentives of stakeholders to support these data collection efforts and new models of public-private partnerships. But first, we will provide a more in-depth rationale for investing in clinical registries, most of which can be found in the dynamics of the medical innovation process itself.

Importance of Downstream Innovation and Learning

Over time, we have seen a move toward more rigorous and well-controlled premarketing studies for all therapeutic and diagnostic modalities. Despite this move, there are practical constraints that limit how much we will learn in the premarketing setting. Randomized trials involve a sampling process and typically minimize heterogeneity of the target population to facilitate the efficient testing of hypotheses. Clinical trials have limited timeframes and usually are underpowered for secondary end-points. Moreover, the skill of the participating centers may be specialized, raising questions about generalizability of trial results to a broader set of health-care institutions and practitioners. Regulatory (premarket approval) and clinical decisions, therefore, are made in the context of uncertainty and limited information about the ultimate outcomes of an intervention. Dispelling such uncertainties requires measuring outcomes in widespread clinical use (Gelijns et al., 2005).

The focus on general practice allows us to capture outcomes of a broader set of providers and to detect long-term and low-frequency events, such as serious adverse events. In addition to the spreading of a new technology throughout the healthcare system, and its attendant change in outcomes, clinical practice is the locus of much downstream learning and innovation. First, after a new technology is introduced into practice, the medical profession typically expands and shapes the targeted patient population within a particular disease category. A case in point is coronary artery bypass grafting (CABG) surgery. Only 4 percent of patients, who were treated with such surgery a decade after its introduction, would have met the eligibility criteria of the trials that determined its initial value (Hlatky et al., 1984). These trials excluded the elderly, women, and patients with a range of co-morbidities, all of whom are recipients of CABG surgery today.

Second, the process of postmarketing innovation also includes the discovery of totally new, and often unexpected, indications of use. The history of pharmaceutical innovation is replete with such discoveries (see Table 4-1). A case in point are the alpha blockers, which were first introduced for hypertension and only 20 years later were found to be an important agent in the treatment of benign prostate hyperplasia. We found that the discovery of such new indications of use is an important public health and economic phenomenon, accounting for nearly half of the overall market for blockbuster drugs (Gelijns et al., 1998).

A third dimension of downstream learning is that physicians gain

TABLE 4-1 Original and New Indications for Pharmaceuticals

Drug	Original Indications	New Indications
Beta-blockers	Angina pectoris, arrhythmias	Hypertension, anxiety, migraine headaches
Aspirin	Pain	Stroke, coronary artery disease
Anticonvulsants	Seizure disorders	Mood stabilization
Alpha blockers	Hypertension	Benign prostatic hyperplasia
RU-486	Abortive agent	Endometriosis, fibroid tumors, benign brain tumors
Fluoxetine (Prozac)	Depression	Bulimia, obsessive compulsive disorder
Thalidomide	Anti-emetic and tranquilizer	Leprosy; graft-vs-host, Bechet's, AIDS, ulcers

further know-how about integrating a technology into the overall management of particular patients. Consider, for example, left ventricular assist devices (LVADs). These devices were FDA approved in 1998 to support end-stage heart failure patients awaiting cardiac transplant as a bridge to transplantation. Subsequently, LVADs were approved for marketing by the FDA in 2002 and for reimbursement by Medicare in 2003 for those patients who were ineligible for transplantation. This indication is also referred to as "destination therapy," or intended life-long implantation of the LVAD. Whereas LVAD destination therapy was shown to provide a clear survival, functional status, and quality-of-life benefit over medical management, LVADs were plagued by significant serious adverse events, especially bleeding, infections, and thromboembolic events (Rose et al., 2001). Following approval of the device, the expanding experience of clinicians further highlighted shortcomings in its use and safety, which led to subsequent incremental device improvements by the manufacturing community. At the same time, clinicians improved their management of LVAD patients by modifying the operative procedure, developing new ways to prevent driveline infections, and changing anticoagulation regimens, among others. These changes in patient management techniques led to a reduction in the adverse event profile associated with the therapy. Beyond changing clinical outcomes, these changes affected economic outcomes as well. Over time, for example, there has been a 25 percent reduction in the length of stay for the implant hospitalization from an average of 44 days in the pivotal FDA trial (with a mean cost of $210,187) to 33 days within 3 years of dissemination—the most costly part of the care process (Miller et al., 2006; Oz et al., 2003). The dissemination to the broader healthcare system, and the changes in technologies, patients, and management techniques over time, argue for ongoing monitoring of health outcomes.

What Can We Learn from Registries?

Clinical registries, as mentioned, are an important means to capture use and outcomes in everyday practice. A recent Agency for Healthcare Research and Quality (AHRQ) report defined registries as an "organized system using observational study methods to collect uniform data to evaluate specified outcomes for a population defined by a particular disease, condition or exposure, and that serves a predetermined scientific, clinical or policy purpose" (Gliklick and Dreyer, 2007). Table 4-2 depicts some registries and their different objectives.

An important objective of registries is to collect data on long-term outcomes and rare adverse events. This is especially the case, where outcomes and adverse events take a long time to manifest themselves; a dramatic example can be found in diethylstilbestrol (DES), where clear cell carci-

TABLE 4-2 Existing Registry Content and Sponsor Descriptions

Name	Content	Sponsor
INTERMACS	National registry of patients receiving mechanical circulatory support device therapy to treat advanced heart failure. (Membership required for Medicare clinical site approval)	Joint effort: National Heart, Lung and Blood Institute (NHLBI), Centers for Medicare & Medicaid Services (CMS), and FDA
Cardiac Surgery Reporting System	Detailed information on all CABG surgeries performed in New York State for tracking provider performance. (Reporting mandated for all hospitals in New York State performing CABG)	New York State Department of Health
ICD Registry (Implantable Cardioverter Defibrillator Registry)	Detailed information on implantable cardoverter defibrillator implantations. (Meet CMS coverage with evidence development policy)	The Heart Rhythm Society & American College of Cardiology Foundation
ICG G (International Collaborative Gaucher Group)	Information on clinical characteristics, natural history, and long-term treatment outcomes of patients with Gaucher Disease, a rare disorder.	Genzyme Corporation
CASE S-PMS (Carotid Artery Stenting with Emboli Protection Surveillance Post-Marketing Study)	Evaluation outcomes of carotid artery stenting in periapproval setting.	Cordis Coporation
Alpha-1 Antitrypsin Deficiency Research Registry	Regsitry of patients with alpha-1 antitrypsin deficiency for purposes of recruiting them to clinical trials.	Alpha-1 Foundation

noma of the vagina only appeared in daughters of the women taking the drug to prevent premature birth. The realization of its side effects subsequently led to a registry for those exposed to DES.

Another important use of registries is to gather information on the outcomes achieved as a technology spreads to a wide range of practitioners and institutions. As such, registries can measure the quality of care provided. Administrative datasets, which are less costly in terms of data collection, also lend themselves to this purpose. Using the Medicare dataset, for exam-

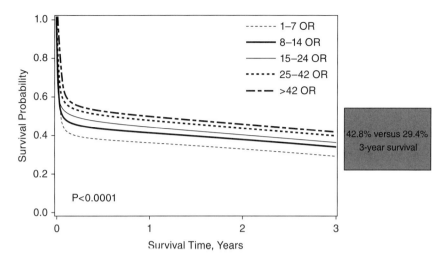

FIGURE 4-3 Survival after open ruptured AAA by hospital volume quintiles (1995–2004, Medicare, n = 41,969).
SOURCE: Reprinted from the *Journal of Vascular Surgery*, Vol. 48/No. 5, Egorova et al. 2008. National outcomes for the Treatment of ruptured abdominal aortic aneurysm: Comparison of open versus endovascular repairs, pp. 1092-1100, with permission from Elsevier.

TABLE 4-3 Endovascular Repair AAA Patients (2000–2004, Medicare, n = 39,815)

Risk Factor	Parameter	Odds Ratio and 95% CL	P-Value
Renal Failure w/ Dialysis	1.95	7.06 [5.23–9.53]	<.0001
LE Ischemia	1.27	3.55 [2.65–4.75]	<.0001
Age ≥85	1.13	3.10 [1.57–2.37]	<.0001
Liver Disease	0.93	2.52 [1.54–4.12]	0.0002
CHF	0.80	2.23 [1.89–2.64]	<.0001
Renal Failure w/o Dialysis	0.65	1.91 [1.45–2.51]	<.0001
Age 80–84	0.65	1.92 [1.56–2.36]	<.0001
Female	0.52	1.68 [1.42–1.99]	<.0001
Neurological	0.45	1.59 [1.29–1.94]	0.0001
Chronic Pulmonary	0.45	1.57 [1.35–1.83]	<.0001
Hospital Annual Vol <7	0.37	1.45 [1.18–1.80]	0.0005
Age 75–79	0.34	1.40 [1.14–1.71]	0.001
Surgeon EVAR Vol <3	0.26	1.30[1.04–1.62]	0.002

NOTE: AAA = abdominal aortic aneurysm; CL = confidence limit.
SOURCE: Reprinted from the *Journal of Vascular Surgery*, Vol. 50/Issue 6, Egorova, Giacovelli et al. 2009. Defining high-risk patients for endovascular aneurysm repair, pp. 1271-1279, with permission from Elsevier.

ple, we found a significant volume–outcome relationship for open repair in about 42,000 ruptured abdominal aortic aneurysm (AAA) patients treated between 1995 and 2004 (Figure 4-3; Egorova, 2008). AAA patients now increasingly receive an endovascular repair, which was approved for reimbursement in 2000. The same volume–outcome relationship holds for high-risk AAA patients treated by an endovascular approach between 2000 and 2006 (Table 4-3). Again, low volume, less than 7 procedures per year, is an independent predictor of mortality, increasing risk by 45 percent (Egorova, 2009). In comparison to administrative datasets, however, registries are able to offer the clinical details needed to create richer statistical models that better characterize patient risk factors and process of care variables to predict outcomes. To expand on our aneurysm case, for example, a clinical registry would have been able to provide important information about the anatomical features of the aneurysm, which are not captured in administrative datasets and yet may have an important influence on outcomes. Moreover, in administrative datasets, it is often hard to distinguish between baseline co-morbidities and adverse events (e.g., myocardial infarction or heart failure) during the hospitalization of interest. Registries do not have this problem, and if they capture the whole population they are an important tool for measuring quality of care. If registries are used to measure quality of care among providers than it is obviously important that they appropriately adjust for differences in risk of the populations among these providers, and risk-adjustment techniques are improving (see below).

Just as registries are able to capture a broadening of providers, they also can capture the use and outcomes of a technology in a broader set of patients. To return to the LVAD case, the pivotal trial for destination therapy patients demonstrated a significant survival and quality-of-life benefit of the HeartMate (HM) XVE LVAD over optimal medical management. In fact, Kaplan-Meier survival analysis showed a 48 percent reduction in the hazard of all-cause mortality in the LVAD group (hazard ratio = 0.52; 0.34–0.78; p = 0.001). In the 2 years following CMS approval (2003) for reimbursement, an analysis of an industry-sponsored postmarketing registry showed that the overall survival rate of LVAD patients remained similar to the trial. However, a multivariable regression analysis of the larger population captured by the registry (n = 262) identified that baseline risk factors, such as poor nutrition, hematological abnormalities, and markers of end-organ dysfunction, distinguish patient risk groups (Lietz et al., 2007). Stratification of destination therapy candidates into low, medium, high, and very high risk on the basis of a risk score corresponded with very different 1-year survival rates (81 percent, 62 percent, 28 percent, and 11 percent, respectively; see Figure 4-4). The broader experience of clinical registries, as such, can provide important information to stratify patients on the basis of baseline risk factors, and, thereby, help to refine patient selection criteria.

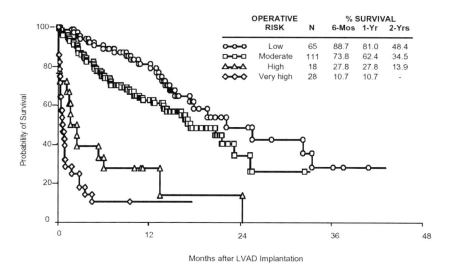

FIGURE 4-4 Probability of survival after LVAD implantation.

Finally, an important objective for clinical registries is their ability to provide comparative effectiveness information. In New York State, for example, registries exist for all patients undergoing CABG surgery (Cardiac Surgery Reporting System) or interventional cardiac procedures (Percutaneous Coronary Intervention Reporting System). Over time, numerous randomized trials have compared CABG surgery to percutaneous transluminal coronary angioplasty (PTCA). However, both procedures have been characterized by a high level of ongoing incremental change (e.g., most trials pre-dated the use of stents) as well as ongoing changes in patient selection criteria, raising questions about the clinical effectiveness of these approached in particular patient groups. An analysis of nearly 60,000 patients captured by the above-mentioned New York State registries showed that for patients with two or more diseased coronary arteries CABG is associated with higher adjusted rates of survival than stenting (Hannan et al., 2005).

Strengthening Registries

Enhancing the value of registries for clinical effectiveness research requires obtaining "trial quality" data at low cost and low burden, and here we will review some opportunities for strengthening data elements and data collection.

Target Population

The target patient population needs to be clearly defined, and data should capture its characteristics in terms of medical history and severity of illness. In the case of LVADs, for example, the National Institutes of Health (NIH) provided financial support for the creation of a registry, with close involvement of CMS, FDA, the clinical community and industry, called INTERMACS. This registry targets patients who receive durable mechanical circulatory assist devices (either for bridge to transplantation or destination therapy). The data elements were designed to capture important baseline characteristics of LVAD patients and have resulted in patient profiles that are useful for clinical communication and treatment planning that correlate with mortality risk (INTERMACS, 2008). Even though registries are more apt to capture broader populations than randomized efficacy trials, there is always a risk that patients are entered selectively. Statewide hospital discharge datasets (such as SPARCS in New York State) may offer a means for monitoring the completeness of patient population capture. Linking payment for patient care to data entry is another way to improve capture. By participating in INTERMACS, for example, clinical centers can meet CMS and Joint Commission on the Accreditation of Healthcare Organizations (JCAHO) reporting requirements, necessary for certification, which stipulate that centers submit data to a nationally audited registry that tracks life-time outcomes of all destination LVAD patients (INTERMACS, 2008).

Outcomes

In terms of outcome measures, mortality is a relatively unambiguous end-point, but adverse events (AEs) require standardization of definitions that should not be unique to a registry but should be more generally accepted in the clinical community. INTERMACS, for example, offered much needed standardization of AE definitions, and facilitated the comparisons of different circulatory support devices, which until recently defined important events differently, including stroke and major bleeding. Registries can improve data quality by adjudicating adverse events and implementing a monitoring process to ensure data integrity. Functional status and quality of life are critical end-point measures, but difficult to capture and analyze longitudinally, even in randomized trials. But as with randomized trials, using instruments that are self-administered or administered by phone, such the Rankin scale in stroke, can increase feasibility. For some diseases, such as heart failure, there is a correlation between patient-derived measures of functional status and hospitalizations, which facilitates using hospitalizations as a proxy measure.

Control Group

Critical for measuring comparative effectiveness is defining the control group, which optimally will be internal to the registry being analyzed. While device registries, for example, may facilitate comparing the effectiveness of alternative devices, such registries are unlikely to provide a medical therapy control group needed for evaluating new indications for device use. Such questions are better addressed in a broader disease-based registry; for example, defining the appropriate role of LVADs in managing slightly less sick heart failure patients would require a comparison to patients receiving optimal medical management and expansion of the LVAD registry to an overall heart failure registry. One weakness of observational studies (i.e., nonrandomized studies) is that clinical judgment is the basis for treatment assignment and clinical characteristics of the comparison groups may differ substantially, affecting the ability to make fair comparisons. Rigorous techniques to adjust for these differences, such as propensity score-based analyses, have become more common over time. However, our ability to create such adjustment models requires that we have an understanding of the prognostic factors that affect treatment outcomes. With newer forms of treatment, this is not always the case. If there is very rapid technological change, the evolution to major new patient populations and/or little know-how about prognostic factors, observational studies may no longer be sufficient and randomized trials may be in order.

Data Collection Burden and Cost

Improving the efficiency of data collection for registries is crucially dependent on advances in the use of informatics. With the growth and improvement of electronic health records, institutions have the capability of automated transfer of patient, process of care, and outcome data into registries, which may address some of the data collection and cost burden. In the same manner, administrative datasets can be linked to patient record, which would improve their usefulness for clinical effectiveness studies.

The Role of Registries in Improving the Clinical Trials Process

An under-examined benefit of registries may be their potential to increase the efficiency of conducting RCTs. First, registry data can provide a prior estimate of the success distribution in the control group that gets updated by prospectively collected data in a randomized trial (through Bayesian analysis), or concurrent control data can be directly pooled with randomized data. The benefit of either approach could be to allow a higher likelihood of randomization into the experimental group, say a 3:1 or 4:1 randomization ratio (Neaton et al., 2007). This is especially important when there are strong physician and patient preferences for an experimental therapy. This is often the case with major surgical interventions for life-threatening diseases and may constitute a major deterrent to enrollment in a randomized trial.

Registries also may offer a means to eliminate the need for collecting a new control group altogether, which has relevance to premarketing efficacy trials for orphan diseases and small populations. Here registries can provide an empirically derived performance goal or objective performance criterion to facilitate a single arm study. The use of LVADs for bridge to transplantation, for instance, is a so-called orphan indication, with around 500 patients being implanted in the United States annually. INTERMACS is now providing data to establish a performance goal in terms of "survival to transplantation or being alive at 180 days and listed for transplantation" for newer generation devices that are seeking approval for use in Bridge-to-Transplant (BTT) patients. More recently, INTERMACS has been the source for providing a matched control arm.

Finally, the existence of a robust postmarketing infrastructure can balance the acceleration of premarketing trials. This is especially important if drugs or devices are approved under the FDA fast track mechanism. For example, of the 60 cancer drugs that have been approved between 1995 and 2004, a third of these compounds received accelerated approvals based on surrogate measures of clinical benefit (Roberts and Chabner, 2004).

Concluding Observations

In conclusion, the often underappreciated dynamics of medical innovation, where much of innovation and downstream learning takes place in actual clinical practice itself, argues for capturing the changing outcomes throughout the lifecycle of medical interventions. Registries offer the means to do so, and recently, new opportunities for addressing their traditional weaknesses have emerged in the realm of informatics, analytical techniques, and new models of financing. With the expansion and enhancement of electronic health records comes the possibilities of utilizing the clinical encounter to directly populate research registries and decreasing the burden of primary data collection. Moreover, efforts to address the traditional weaknesses of observational registry-based studies have led to the increased use of propensity score techniques to adjust for differences in baseline differences between nonrandomized comparison groups. Finally, an important issue concerns the financial support for clinical registries. Traditionally, registries have been supported either by the public and non-for-profit sectors, such as foundations, or the private sector (especially the device, biotech, and drug industries). The information generated by registries, in many respects, can be characterized as a public good. Public–private partnerships offer an interesting new model for registry support. A case in point is the recently created INTERMACSs registry for LVAD therapy, which brings together three major government agencies, the NIH, which provides funding for an independent coordinating center as well as oversight, Medicare, and the FDA, which are involved in planning and oversight as well. The participating hospitals provide in-kind support for data collection and analysis efforts. Industrial firms are heavily involved in the design and implementation of the registry, and the expectation is that over time these firms will assume the financial responsibility for the registry.

There has been a long and often heated debate about the value of randomized versus observational, registry-based studies. In this paper, we argue that the data of registries tend to be not only complementary to, but also, in some circumstances, alternative to randomized trials. Moreover, clinical registries offer many untapped opportunities for improving the efficiency of the randomized trials enterprise itself, both of premarketing trials as well as so-called pragmatic trials of diagnostic or treatment modalities. Registries, as such, are, and will remain, critical to the conduct of clinical effectiveness research, particularly if we capitalize on emerging opportunities in the informatics, analytical, and financial realms.

DISTRIBUTED DATA NETWORKS

Richard Platt, M.D., M.S.
Harvard Medical School, Harvard Pilgrim Health Care

The Case for Distributed Networks

The information created by the delivery of medical care—about individuals, their health status, the treatment they receive, and their health outcomes—also can teach us a great deal about how well treatments work, the risks they entail, and the cost of better health. This information also can provide information about the health of the population and the adequacy of healthcare delivery, illuminate gaps in care, and support clinical research. Additionally, it will be possible to assess the quality of health care if we add information about providers and the organizations that deliver care.

This information exists for a substantial fraction of the U.S. population, although it takes many forms and is held by many organizations. Examples include ambulatory practices' and hospitals' separate electronic medical records, health plans' and insurers' membership and administrative claims systems, pharmacy benefits managers' dispensing records, and, increasingly, individuals' personally controlled health records. Additional information like public health agencies' birth, death, and cancer registries and research organizations' special purpose datasets also may play an important role.

This discussion focuses on distributed data networks to allow the secondary use, i.e., not direct patient care, of different organizations' data. "Distributed data network" is used here to mean a collection of separate data repositories that can function as if they were linked in a single combined dataset by executing and responding to electronic queries posed in a standard format. The critical notion is that it is not necessary to create a large pooled dataset containing enough information to answer a wide range of potential questions, since nearly all of the goals described above can be accomplished by having the separate data sources provide limited amounts of information on a just-in-time basis to answer specific questions. This makes an important distinction between the data, e.g., all of a person's drug dispensings and diagnoses, and the answer to a question, such as whether a specific drug is associated with a specific adverse outcome among individuals with various characteristics. A fully developed distributed data network will be able to address efficiently essentially any question that could be answered by a pooled dataset.

Maintaining the information in a distributed network has advantages over a pooled dataset with regard to protection of confidential and proprietary information, local decision making regarding participation in specific activities, and the ongoing involvement of individuals with expertise in interpretation of the data. With regard to privacy, the distributed approach minimizes, and often eliminates, sharing of confidential personal information that is increasingly difficult to fully de-identify without compromising its utility. Because of this privacy concern, avoiding creation of large pooled datasets conforms to widely held public views about the use of personal information (The Markle Foundation, 2006). It is also easier to satisfy the privacy requirements of the Health Insurance Portability and Accountability Act (HIPAA) (U.S. Department of Health and Human Services, 2008). For data owners, a network structure in which the data originators maintain physical control over the data reduces the barrier to participation. For private organizations, it allows them to weigh any risk associated with sharing of proprietary value against the public health utility of participation. Private organizations are more likely to participate in networks that allow them to decide on a case-by-case basis whether to join a specific activity, e.g., assessment of postmarketing drug safety. Such organizations are more likely to assent to such uses than to uses that will be determined after a pooled dataset is created. Keeping the data in the possession of the data developers also means there will be better ability to interpret the information. Both clinical and administrative data systems are evolving rapidly in ways that may not be apparent but which can profoundly influence the interpretation of the information they contain. For example, an undocumented increase in the number of diagnoses that a clinical data system stored per encounter led to a spurious signal of an influenza outbreak (Buehler et al., 2007). There is thus a need for ready access to local expertise to interpret content. Finally, centralized data systems entail greater risks of catastrophic security breaches.

Initiatives to Build Large Distributed Research Networks

Several initiatives are currently underway to develop distributed networks that are intended eventually to have access to the health information of a substantial fraction of the U.S. population.

The Institute of Medicine stimulated current efforts to develop a network to assess postmarketing experience with drugs by recommending that the FDA develop an active postmarketing surveillance program (IOM, 2006). The Food and Drug Administration Amendments Act (FDAAA) of 2007 (FDA, 2007b) mandated the FDA to develop a postmarketing evidence system that can evaluate the experience of 100 million people. The FDA announced plans for a Sentinel Network (FDA, 2007a, 2008), which it describes as a distributed network, rather than a single database.

The Agency for Healthcare Research and Quality is supporting development of a prototype for a scalable national network to support research on the comparative effectiveness and safety of therapeutics (Agency for Healthcare Research and Quality, 2008). This initiative is part of the Agency's Developing Evidence to Inform Decisions about Effectiveness (DEcIDE) program and is led by the HMO Research Network Center for Education and Research on Therapeutics (CERT) and the University of Pennsylvania. It builds on the HMO Research Network's experience in using distributed data methods for therapeutics research (Andrade et al., 2006; Raebel et al., 2007; Wagner et al., 2006).

The Robert Wood Johnson Foundation has funded an initiative to create a distributed data capability to provide national information about the quality and cost of health care (Robert Wood Johnson Foundation, 2007). One of the components of this activity involves development of a distributed data network, led by America's Health Insurance Plans.

Models for Organizing Distributed Networks

Existing distributed networks provide some idea about approaches that may be successful as larger networks are developed. Each of these examples relied on several common features: (1) the organizations that developed the data (HIPAA's "covered entities") extracted a common set of data elements from their information systems, transformed them into a common format, and stored the data so they could access it easily for repeated queries; (2) to function as a distributed network, they executed identical computer programs that were developed by an agreed-upon process to which all participants provided input; (3) they typically shared summary data with a coordinating center, rather than person-level analysis files; and (4) they provided detailed, patient-level data, sometimes to a health department, only in the event of a specific need to know more about the individual.

The National Bioterrorism Syndromic Surveillance Demonstration Program used a distributed network approach to surveillance for bioterrorism events and clusters of naturally occurring illness, in five HMO Research Network health plans (Lazarus et al., 2006; Yih et al., 2004). This demonstration program used a fully distributed automated method to identify clusters of illness. It accomplished this by having the health plans execute computer programs that created daily extracts of the preceding days' encounters, put them into a standard format, and identified new episodes of illness that met Centers for Disease Control and Prevention's (CDC's) criteria for syndromes of interest, such as influenza-like illness or lower gastrointestinal illness. The programs assigned the new episodes to the patients' zip codes of residence, and then each site automatically communicated the daily totals of new episodes for each syndrome in each zip codes to a coordinating center that used a space and time scan statistic to identify unusual clusters of illness. Notice of these clusters was sent from the coordinating center back to the originating site and to the relevant health department. If the health department wanted more information about the individuals who were part of the cluster, it contacted the health plan, which retained full information about the individuals and could provide identifying information as well as the full clinical detail available in the patients' electronic medical records (Figure 4-5). This program illustrates the ability of a distributed system to provide immediate information to support public health needs. Although the health plans used information from their entire populations, they only shared person-level information about individuals in whom the health department was specifically interested.

The CDC-sponsored Vaccine Safety Datalink (VSD), founded in 1991, has operated since 2000 as a distributed data network in eight health plan members of the HMO Research Network. The VSD's distributed network operates a real-time active postmarketing surveillance system for new vaccines. It relies on weekly automated submission to a coordinating center of counts of vaccine exposures and prespecified outcomes of interest in a total analyzable population of approximately 8 million individuals. It uses sequential analysis methods to identify signals of excess risk, which are validated by review of full text medical records (Lieu et al., 2007). This dis-

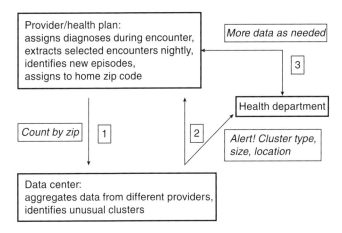

FIGURE 4-5 Schematic view of data flow for the National Bioterrorism Syndromic Surveillance Demonstration Program.

tributed method of active surveillance recently identified a signal of excess seizures associated with a quadrivalent measles-mumps-rubella-varicella vaccine, prompting a change in the Advisory Committee for Immunization Practice's recommendation for use of the vaccine (Centers for Disease Control and Prevention, 2008). The Vaccine Safety Datalink's general approach to real-time postmarketing surveillance also should be applicable to drugs, although additional development will be required (Brown et al., 2007).

An ad hoc distributed network assembled to evaluate the risk of Guillain-Barré syndrome, a potentially life-threatening neurologic condition following meningococcal conjugate vaccine (ClinicalTrials.gov, 2008) is notable both because of the size of the covered population and because it uses a hybrid data model that incorporates both distributed and pooled data methods. Five health plans with a combined membership exceeding 50 million people—half the number required by the FDAAA—are collaborating in this study. The health plans operate as a distributed network insofar as they create standard data files and execute shared computer programs that perform the large majority of the analyses, which are shared in tabular form and then pooled. The health plans also obtain detailed clinical information about potential cases of Guillain-Barré syndrome identified through diagnosis codes by obtaining full text medical records. Final case status is determined by an expert panel that reviews these records after the health plans redact personal identifying information. The study includes both an analysis of the full cohort, which is performed in a fully distributed fashion, plus a nested case control study that uses multivariate methods requiring creation of a pooled dataset involving 0.2 percent of the entire cohort (12,000 individuals). To support the case control study health plans create analysis-level files containing one record for each case or control. The only protected health information that the covered entity shares with the coordinating center is the month and year in which individuals were immunized.

These examples of distributed networks illustrate the potential for distributing much of the data processing as well as the data storage. Distributed processing minimizes the need to create pooled person-level datasets, and is thus an important contributor to minimizing the amount of patient level data that must leave the covered entities.

Organizational Models for Distributed Networks

Distributed networks can operate in several ways. Figure 4-6 shows a schematic of the network design that is planned as part of the AHRQ prototype distributed network mentioned above. The system will accommodate

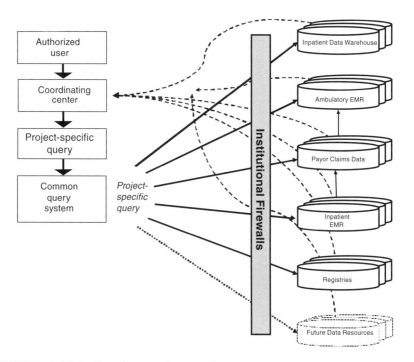

FIGURE 4-6 Distributed research network prototype using central coordinating center.

different kinds of data and is planned eventually to include claims data, inpatient and outpatient EMR data, registry data, and other information that are not part of the current prototype. It also will be able to integrate information in personally controlled health records (Mandl and Kohane, 2008), to the extent that these become widespread and that both individuals and the organizations that hold the records make them available.

In this system, a common query system will send queries to participating organizations. Queries go to participating sites through their firewalls, as much processing as possible takes place behind the firewalls, and then responses to the queries are sent back from participating organizations. As noted above, the network will emphasize the sharing of results of analyses, rather than patient-level datasets.

Another organizational model is the peer-to-peer design used by the Shared Pathology Information Network (SPIN) (Drake et al., 2007). This model has been generalized to apply to other uses, including public health surveillance and clinical research (McMurry et al., 2007). The peer-to-peer approach also underlies the planned Shared Health Research Information Network (SHRINE) (Brigham and Women's Hospital, Harvard Medical School, 2008), developed at Harvard to support research uses of separate data warehouses maintained by different healthcare institutions. This networking capability is an extension of software created for Informatics for Integrating Biology and the Bedside (i2b2), to support clinical research using health care institutions' clinical data warehouses (Partners Healthcare, 2008).

Governance

Developing effective governance models for distributed networks to improve population health and healthcare delivery will be a major challenge. Figure 4-7 illustrates a potential governance model for a multipurpose network that accommodates participation by multiple users. In this model the development and maintenance of infrastructure is largely separate from, though informed by, the users. Governance of infrastructure would focus on the creation of data standards and infrastructure that allow the same resources to support separate user groups and uses. In such a model, decisions about the availability of the network's information to public and private users would rest most naturally with the holders of the data, who could choose as individual organizations whether or not to participate in individual activities or categories of activities on a case by case basis. However, since certain types of uses are likely to recur, individual data holders or groups of data holders may develop standards that apply generally to their participation. Such standards might address issues such as the amount of participation of data holders in the development and execu-

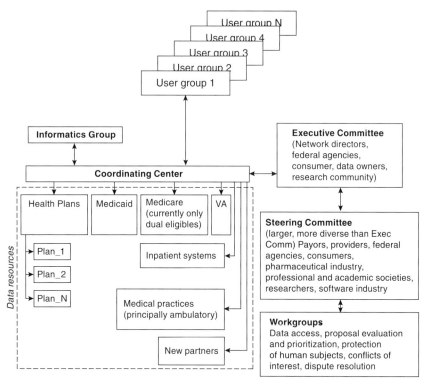

FIGURE 4-7 Potential schema for organization and governance of a multipurpose national distributed network. In this arrangement, the distributed network serves multiple users, which would include both public agencies, such as the FDA, CDC, NIH, or AHRQ, and private organizations, such as academic research organizations or industry. Different priorities and rules of access would apply depending on the use and the user.

tion of studies, ensuring confidentiality of personal information, secondary use of data, transparency regarding the specific studies being performed, and commitments to dissemination of results.

Specific examples of activities the network might support include the following. The FDA might use relevant parts of the network to support postmarketing surveillance, CDC might use the same or other parts to support prevention initiatives, AHRQ might use it to support comparative effectiveness research, and the NIH might use it to support clinical research. Private organizations would also be logical users of the network to support a wide range of inquiries. Each activity, or category of activity, could be led by the separate user groups, usually in collaboration with the data holders, and have separate governance mechanisms and funding models.

Summary

We will need distributed networks to assess medical care and its outcomes because this is almost certainly a more realistic way to develop and maintain these data than large pooled databases. Experience to date makes clear that it is technically feasible to build and use distributed networks, although considerable investment will be needed to develop additional resources and to create more efficient methods of using the networks. Furthermore, it appears feasible to develop distributed networks so that a common infrastructure can support an array of different uses in the public interest. Creation of effective governance mechanisms will be a considerable challenge, as will development of a sustainable mechanism to fund development and maintenance of infrastructure for both technical issues and governance.

REFERENCES

Agency for Healthcare Research and Quality. 2008. *Developing a Distributed Research Network to Conduct Population-based Studies and Safety Surveillance.* http://effectivehealth care.ahrq.gov/healthInfo.cfm?infotype=nr&ProcessID=54 (accessed March 30, 2008).
Andrade, S. E., M. A. Raebel, A. N. Morse, R. L. Davis, K. A. Chan, J. A. Finkelstein, K. K. Fortman, H. McPhillips, D. Roblin, D. H. Smith, M. U. Yood, R. Platt, and J. H. Gurwitz. 2006. Use of prescription medications with a potential for fetal harm among pregnant women. *Pharmacoepidemiology and Drug Safety* 15(8):546-554.
Berwick, D. M. 2008. The science of improvement. *Journal of the American Medical Association* 299(10):1182-1184.
Blumenthal, D., and C. M. Kilo. 1998. A report card on continuous quality improvement. *Milbank Quarterly* 76(4):511, 625-648.
Brigham and Women's Hospital. Harvard Medical School. 2008. *Decision Systems Group, Weekly Seminars.* http://www.dsg.harvard.edu/index.php/Main/Seminars2007#d51 (accessed April 19, 2008).
Brook, R. H., and K. N. Lohr. 1985. Efficacy, effectiveness, variations, and quality. Boundary-crossing research. *Medical Care* 23(5):710-722.
Brown, J. S., M. Kulldorff, K. A. Chan, R. L. Davis, D. Graham, P. T. Pettus, S. E. Andrade, M. A. Raebel, L. Herrinton, D. Roblin, D. Boudreau, D. Smith, J. H. Gurwitz, M. J. Gunter, and R. Platt. 2007. Early detection of adverse drug events within population-based health networks: Application of sequential testing methods. *Pharmacoepidemiology and Drug Safety* 16(12):1275-1284.
Buehler, J. W., Sosin, D. M., and R. Platt. 2007. *Evaluation of Surveillance Systems for Early Epidemic Detection, in Infectious Disease Surveillance.* Edited by N. M. M'ikanatha, R. Lynfield, C. A. Van Beneden, and H. de Valk. Malden, MA: Blackwell Publishing.
Centers for Disease Control and Prevention. 2008. *Vaccines and Immunizations: Recommendations and Guidelines.* http://www.cdc.gov/vaccines/recs/ACIP/slides-feb08.htm#mmrv (accessed March 31, 2008).
ClinicalTrials.gov. 2008. *Safety Study of GBS Following Menactra Meningococcal Vaccination.* http://clinicaltrials.gov/ct2/show/NCT00575653?term=NCT00575653&rank=1 (accessed March 31, 2008).

The Commonwealth Fund Commission on a High Performance Health System. 2005. *Framework for a High Performance Health System for the United States.* New York: The Commonwealth Fund.

de Koning, J. S., N. S. Klazinga, P. J. Koudstaal, A. Prins, G. J. Borsboom, and J. P. Mackenbach. 2005. The role of 'confounding by indication' in assessing the effect of quality of care on disease outcomes in general practice: Results of a case-control study. *BMC Health Services Research* 5(1):10.

Drake, T. A., J. Braun, A. Marchevsky, I. S. Kohane, C. Fletcher, H. Chueh, B. Beckwith, D. Berkowicz, F. Kuo, Q. T. Zeng, U. Balis, A. Holzbach, A. McMurry, C. E. Gee, C. J. McDonald, G. Schadow, M. Davis, E. M. Hattab, L. Blevins, J. Hook, M. Becich, R. S. Crowley, S. E. Taube, and J. Berman. 2007. A system for sharing routine surgical pathology specimens across institutions: The shared pathology informatics network. *Human Pathology* 38(8):1212-1225.

Egorova, N., et al. 2008. National outcomes for the treatment of ruptured abdominal aortic aneurysm: Comparison of open versus endovascular repairs. *Journal of Vascular Surgery* 48(5):1092.e2-1100.e2.

Egorova, N., J. Giacovelli, A. Gelijns, L. Mureebe, G. Greco, N. Morrissey, R. Nowygrod, A. Moskowitz, J. McKinsey, and K. C. Kent. 2009. Defining high risk patients for endovascular aneurysm repair. *Journal of Vascular Surgery* 50(6):1271-1279.

Eng, P. M., J. D. Seeger, J. Loughlin, C. R. Clifford, S. Mentor, and A. M. Walker. 2008. Supplementary data collection with case-cohort analysis to address potential confounding in a cohort study of thromboembolism in oral contraceptive initiators matched on claims-based propensity scores. *Pharmacoepidemiology and Drug Safety* 17(3):297-305.

Epic Systems Corporation. 2008. *EpicCare.* http://www.epicsystems.com/ (accessed July 8, 2008).

FDA (Food and Drug Administration). 2007a. *Food and Drug Administration Sentinel Network Public Meeting.* http://www.fda.gov/oc/op/sentinel/transcript030707.html (accessed March 30, 2008).

———. 2007b. *Law Strengthens FDA.* http://www.fda.gov/oc/initiatives/advance/fdaaa.html (accessed March 30, 2008).

———. 2008. *Sentinal Network.* http://www.fda.gov/oc/op/sentinel/ (accessed March 30, 2008).

Flum, D. R., A. Morris, T. Koepsell, and E. P. Dellinger. 2001. Has misdiagnosis of appendicitis decreased over time? A population-based analysis. *Journal of the American Medical Association* 286(14):1748-1753.

Gawande, A. 2004. The bell curve: What happens when patients find out how good their doctors really are? *The New Yorker.* December 6, 2004.

Gelijns, A. C., N. Rosenberg, and A. J. Moskowitz. 1998. Capturing the unexpected benefits of medical research. *New England Journal of Medicine* 339(10):693-698.

Gelijns, A. C., L. D. Brown, C. Magnell, E. Ronchi, and A. J. Moskowitz. 2005. Evidence, politics, and technological change. *Health Affairs (Millwood)* 24(1):29-40.

Gliklich, R. E., and N. Dreyer. 2007. AHRQ Registries for Evaluating Patient Outcomes: A User's Guide. AHRQ Publication 07-EHCOO1-1. Rockville, MD: U.S. Department of Health and Human Services, Public Health Service, Agency for Healthcare Research and Quality.

Greco, P. J., and J. M. Eisenberg. 1993. Changing physicians' practices. *New England Journal of Medicine* 329(17):1271-1273.

Hannan, E. L., M. J. Racz, G. Walford, R. H. Jones, T. J. Ryan, E. Bennett, A. T. Culliford, O. W. Isom, J. P. Gold, and E. A. Rose. 2005. Long-term outcomes of coronary-artery bypass grafting versus stent implantation. *New England Journal of Medicine* 352(21):2174-2183.

Hartig, J. R., and J. Allison. 2007. Physician performance improvement: An overview of methodologies. *Clinical and Experimental Rheumatology* 25(6 Supl 47):50-54.

Hayward, R. S., M. C. Wilson, S. R. Tunis, E. B. Bass, and G. Guyatt. 1995. Users' guides to the medical literature. VIII. How to use clinical practice guidelines. A. Are the recommendations valid? The evidence-based medicine working group. *Journal of the American Medical Association* 274(7):570-574.

Hlatky, M. A., K. L. Lee, F. E. Harrell, Jr., R. M. Califf, D. B. Pryor, D. B. Mark, and R. A. Rosati. 1984. Tying clinical research to patient care by use of an observational database. *Statistics in Medicine* 3(4):375-387.

Institute for Healthcare Improvement. *Testing Changes.* http://www.ihi.org/IHI/Topics/Improvement/ImprovementMethods/HowToImprove/testingchanges.htm (accessed July 8, 2008).

INTERMACS (Interagency Registry for Mechanically Assisted Circulatory Support). 2008. http://www.intermacs.org/ (accessed July 9, 2008).

IOM (Institute of Medicine). 2006. *The Future of Drug Safety.* Washington, DC: The National Academies Press.

Jick, S., J. A. Kaye, L. Li, and H. Jick. 2007. Further results on the risk of nonfatal venous thromboembolism in users of the contraceptive transdermal patch compared to users of oral contraceptives containing norgestimate and 35 microg of ethinyl estradiol. *Contraception* 76(1):4-7.

Juran, J. M. 1995. *Managerial Breakthrough: The Classic Book on Improving Management Performance.* 30th anniversary ed. New York: McGraw-Hill.

Krumholz, H. M., M. J. Radford, Y. Wang, J. Chen, A. Heiat, and T. A. Marciniak. 1998. National use and effectiveness of beta-blockers for the treatment of elderly patients after acute myocardial infarction: National cooperative cardiovascular project. *Journal of the American Medical Association* 280(7):623-629.

Lazarus, R., K. Yih, and R. Platt. 2006. Distributed data processing for public health surveillance. *BMC Health Services Research* 6:235.

Lietz, K., J. W. Long, A. G. Kfoury, M. S. Slaughter, M. A. Silver, C. A. Milano, J. G. Rogers, Y. Naka, D. Mancini, and L. W. Miller. 2007. Outcomes of left ventricular assist device implantation as destination therapy in the post-rematch era: Implications for patient selection. *Circulation* 116(5):497-505.

Lieu, T. A., M. Kulldorff, R. L. Davis, E. M. Lewis, E. Weintraub, K. Yih, R. Yin, J. S. Brown, and R. Platt. 2007. Real-time vaccine safety surveillance for the early detection of adverse events. *Medical Care* 45(10 Supl 2):S89-S95.

Mandl, K. D., and I. S. Kohane. 2008. Tectonic shifts in the health information economy. *New England Journal of Medicine* 358(16):1732-1737.

The Markle Foundation. 2006. *The Common Framework: Overview and Principles. Connecting for Health.* http://www.connectingforhealth.org/commonframework/docs/Overview.pdf (accessed March 19, 2008).

McMurry, A. J., C. A. Gilbert, B. Y. Reis, H. C. Chueh, I. S. Kohane, and K. D. Mandl. 2007. A self-scaling, distributed information architecture for public health, research, and clinical care. *Journal of the American Medical Informatics Association* 14(4):527-533.

Miller, L. W., K. E. Nelson, R. R. Bostic, K. Tong, M. S. Slaughter, and J. W. Long. 2006. Hospital costs for left ventricular assist devices for destination therapy: Lower costs for implantation in the post-rematch era. *Journal of Heart and Lung Transplantation* 25(7):778-784.

Mona Eng, P., J. D. Seeger, J. Loughlin, K. Oh, and A. M. Walker. 2007. Serum potassium monitoring for users of ethinyl estradiol/drospirenone taking medications predisposing to hyperkalemia: Physician compliance and survey of knowledge and attitudes. *Contraception* 75(2):101-107.

Neaton, J. D., S. L. Normand, A. Gelijns, R. C. Starling, D. L. Mann, and M. A. Konstam. 2007. Designs for mechanical circulatory support device studies. *Journal of Cardiac Failure* 13(1):63-74.

Oz, M. C., A. C. Gelijns, L. Miller, C. Wang, P. Nickens, R. Arons, K. Aaronson, W. Richenbacher, C. van Meter, K. Nelson, A. Weinberg, J. Watson, E. A. Rose, and A. J. Moskowitz. 2003. Left ventricular assist devices as permanent heart failure therapy: The price of progress. *Annals of Surgery* 238(4):577-583; discussion 583-585.

Partners Healthcare. 2008. *Informatics for Integrating Biology and the Bedside.* http://www.i2b2.org/ (accessed April 19, 2008).

Porter, M. E., and E. Olmsted-Teisberg. 2006. *Redefining Health Care—Creating Value-based Competition on Results.* Boston, MA: Harvard Business School Press.

Poses, R. M., and M. Anthony. 1991. Availability, wishful thinking, and physicians' diagnostic judgments for patients with suspected bacteremia. *Medical Decision Making* 11(3):159-168.

Raebel, M. A., D. L. McClure, S. R. Simon, K. A. Chan, A. Feldstein, S. E. Andrade, J. E. Lafata, D. Roblin, R. L. Davis, M. J. Gunter, and R. Platt. 2007. Laboratory monitoring of potassium and creatinine in ambulatory patients receiving angiotensin converting enzyme inhibitors and angiotensin receptor blockers. *Pharmacoepidemiology and Drug Safety* 16(1):55-64.

Robert Wood Johnson Foundation. 2007. *National Effort to Measure and Report on Quality and Cost-effectiveness of Health Care Unveiled.* http://www.rwjf.org/pr/product.jsp?id=22371&typeid=160 (accessed March 30, 2008).

Roberts, T. G., Jr., and B. A. Chabner. 2004. Beyond fast track for drug approvals. *New England Journal of Medicine* 351(5):501-505.

Rose, E. A., A. C. Gelijns, A. J. Moskowitz, D. F. Heitjan, L. W. Stevenson, W. Dembitsky, J. W. Long, D. D. Ascheim, A. R. Tierney, R. G. Levitan, J. T. Watson, P. Meier, N. S. Ronan, P. A. Shapiro, R. M. Lazar, L. W. Miller, L. Gupta, O. H. Frazier, P. Desvigne-Nickens, M. C. Oz, and V. L. Poirier. 2001. Long-term mechanical left ventricular assistance for end-stage heart failure. *New England Journal of Medicine* 345(20):1435-1443.

Sands, B. E., M. S. Duh, C. Cali, A. Ajene, R. L. Bohn, D. Miller, J. A. Cole, S. F. Cook, and A. M. Walker. 2006. Algorithms to identify colonic ischemia, complications of constipation and irritable bowel syndrome in medical claims data: Development and validation. *Pharmacoepidemiology and Drug Safety* 15(1):47-56.

Schneeweiss, S. 2007. Developments in post-marketing comparative effectiveness research. *Clinical Pharmacology and Therapeutics* 82(2):143-156.

Second International Conference on Improving Use of Medicines. 2004. *Recommendations on Insurance Coverage.* http://mednet3.who.int/icium/icium2004/Documents/Insurance%20coverage.doc (accessed July 8, 2008).

Seeger, J. D., P. L. Williams, and A. M. Walker. 2005. An application of propensity score matching using claims data. *Pharmacoepidemiology and Drug Safety* 14(7):465-476.

Seeger, J. D., J. Loughlin, P. M. Eng, C. R. Clifford, J. Cutone, and A. M. Walker. 2007. Risk of thromboembolism in women taking ethinylestradiol/drospirenone and other oral contraceptives. *Obstetrics and Gynecology* 110(3):587-593.

Shewhart, W. A. 1939. *Statistical Method from the Viewpoint of Quality Control.* Dover Publications, December 1, 1986.

Stewart, W. F., N. R. Shah, M. J. Selna, R. A. Paulus, and J. M. Walker. 2007. Bridging the inferential gap: The electronic health record and clinical evidence. *Health Affairs (Millwood)* 26(2):w181-w191.

Tunis, S. R., D. B. Stryer, and C. M. Clancy. 2003. Practical clinical trials: Increasing the value of clinical research for decision making in clinical and health policy. *Journal of the American Medical Association* 290(12):1624-1632.

U.S. Department of Health and Human Services. 2008. *Medical Privacy—National Standards to Protect the Privacy of Personal Health Information.* http://www.hhs.gov/ocr/hipaa/ (accessed March 30, 2008).

Wagner, A. K., K. A. Chan, I. Dashevsky, M. A. Raebel, S. E. Andrade, J. E. Lafata, R. L. Davis, J. H. Gurwitz, S. B. Soumerai, and R. Platt. 2006. FDA drug prescribing warnings: Is the black box half empty or half full? *Pharmacoepidemiology and Drug Safety* 15(6):369-386.

Walker, A. M., and R. P. Wise. 2002. Precautions for proactive surveillance. *Pharmacoepidemiology and Drug Safety* 11(1):17-20.

Walker, A. M., G. Schneider, J. Yeaw, B. Nordstrom, S. Robbins, and D. Pettitt. 2006. Anemia as a predictor of cardiovascular events in patients with elevated serum creatinine. *Journal of the American Society of Nephrology* 17(8):2293-2298.

Yih, W. K., B. Caldwell, R. Harmon, K. Kleinman, R. Lazarus, A. Nelson, J. Nordin, B. Rehm, B. Richter, D. Ritzwoller, E. Sherwood, and R. Platt. 2004. National bioterrorism syndromic surveillance demonstration program. *Morbidity and Mortality Weekly Report* (53 Supl):43-49.

5

Moving to the Next Generation of Studies

INTRODUCTION

Scientific information today is expanding much faster than our ability to effectively translate and process knowledge in ways that improve patient care. To expedite the development of information—and to address both existing gaps in the evidence base and newly emerging research challenges—innovation is needed in how we use existing research tools, strategies, and study design methodologies to produce reliable knowledge. Furthermore, new approaches are needed, with special attention to using new tools, techniques, and data resources. Workshop participants discuss the potential of a next generation of studies that complement and possibly supplant those already employed in clinical effectiveness research. In that regard, decisive efforts are need to support the development of new approaches and to nurture their inclusion in research. Papers included in this chapter examine opportunities to take better advantage of emerging resources to plan, develop, and sequence studies that are more timely, relevant, efficient, and generalizable. Also considered are approaches that better account for lifecycle variation of the conditions and interventions in play. Current opportunities and needed advancements also are discussed.

A variety of innovations are presented as important components of a redesigned research paradigm as well as immediate opportunities to build toward a next generation of studies. These innovations include new approaches to observational and hybrid studies; tools for collecting and using information captured at the point of care, including those relevant to genetic variation; cooperative research networks; and possible incentives.

Presenting a vision for new inferential and statistical tools, Sharon-Lise T. Normand from Harvard Medical School discusses opportunities to increase the efficiency with which information is produced through improved use of large data streams from a variety of sources, including clinical registries, billing databases, electronic health records, preclinical research, and trials. New tools are needed to develop and implement data pooling algorithms and inferential tools. In addition, study designs not used to their full potential—including hybrid designs, preference-based designs, and quasi-experimental designs—are well suited to exploit features of the new information sources.

Findings of observational studies are intrinsically more prone to uncertainty than those from randomized trials; however, Wayne A. Ray from Vanderbilt University contends that this methodology has great value in its capacity to address the dilemma presented by the logistical difficulties and slow pace of randomized controlled trials (RCTs). Perhaps more importantly, they also enable research on many important clinical questions that RCTs are not appropriate to answer. To exploit the wealth of data becoming available, researchers will need to become more familiar with and adhere to fundamental clinical and epidemiological principles that define state-of-the-art use of observational data.

Giving clinicians information on how, for whom, and in what settings specific treatments are best used is essential to improving clinical care. John Rush from the University of Texas Southwestern Medical Center proposes that researchers widen the breadth of study designs that they employ. Rush illustrates how certain clinically important questions can be addressed with observational data obtained when systematic practices are employed, or with new study designs (e.g., hybrid studies and equipoise stratified randomized designs) or posthoc analyses. Additional challenges will be to identify key questions and develop infrastructure to conduct the needed studies.

Echoing Rush's call for a reengineered practice system to better facilitate research, Isaac Kohane from Harvard Medical School discusses opportunities to instrument the health delivery system for research. While speaking specifically to the potential of high-throughput genotyping, phenotyping, and sample acquisition to accelerate genomic research, Kohane emphasizes the additional benefit to quality and performance improvement efforts. Needed for progress are increased investments in information technology (IT), increased transparency in regulation and patient autonomy, continued development of an informatics-savvy healthcare research workforce, and creation of a safe harbor for methodological experimentation.

Citing the experience of the Center for Medical Technology Policy (CMTP) in attempting to facilitate private-sector coverage with evidence development, the CMTP's Wade M. Aubry argues that "coverage with evidence development" should complement, not compete with, traditional research enterprises. Aubry proposes that in order to draw from and expand on the experience of existing models, researchers must formalize ground rules for workgroups and separate evidence gap identification, prioritization, and selection for study design and funding. He discusses coverage with evidence development and outlines concepts for phased introduction and payment for interventions under protocol. Eric B. Larson from the Group Health Cooperative concludes the chapter by suggesting that emerging research networks, such as the development of programs funded by the National Institutes of Health (NIH) under the Clinical and Translational Science Awards, offer opportunities to contribute to a learning healthcare system in ways that produce relevant results that can be generalized.

LARGE DATA STREAMS AND THE POWER OF NUMBERS

Sharon-Lise T. Normand, Ph.D.
Harvard Medical School & Harvard School of Public Health

Abstract

This paper describes the rationale for integrating information from multiple and diverse data sources in order to efficiently produce information. Key statistical challenges involved in integrating and interpreting information are described. The fundamental issue underpinning the use of large data streams is the *poolability* of the data sources. New statistical tools are required to integrate the multiple and diverse data streams in order to produce valid scientific findings.

Introduction and Background

We are witnessing the rapid growth in the quantity, the type, and the quality of health data that are collected. These data derive from many different information sources: preclinical data obtained from the bench, clinical trial data, registries maintained by professional societies such as the American College of Cardiology, electronic health record data, administrative billing data such as those maintained by the Centers for Medicare & Medicaid Services, hospital discharge billing data maintained by state departments of public health, and population-based surveys data such as the Medical Expenditure Panel Survey maintained by the Agency for Healthcare Research and Quality (AHRQ).

We also are collecting more information than ever before about outcomes in both the clinical trial and observational settings. This increasingly frequent strategy has been adopted for several reasons: A single outcome may not adequately characterize a complex disease; there may be a lack of consensus of the most important outcome; or there may be a desire to demonstrate clinical effectiveness on multiple outcomes. The consequence of the proliferation of these databases is an unprecedented demand to combine and use diverse data streams.

What circumstances have led to the proliferation of databases? First, technology and innovation are evolving rapidly, producing a plethora of new medical devices, biologics, drugs, and combination products. Scientists have made medical devices smaller, smarter, and more convenient for patients. Miniaturization techniques have allowed pacemakers to weigh less than one ounce and are the size of a quarter; biological medical devices, such as microarray-based diagnostic tests for detection of genetic variation to select medication and doses of medications, are promoting personalized medicine; and combination products, such as antimicrobial catheters and drug-eluting stents, have changed the way diseases are diagnosed and treated. Moreover, in the fast-paced device environment, technologies become quickly outdated as designs are rapidly improved. Consequently, at market introduction, the next-generation devices are already under development and under study.

Second, information technology has revolutionized medicine. The design, development, and implementation of computer-based information systems have permitted major advances in our understanding of the consequences of medical treatments through access to large data streams. Similarly, the excitement in bioinformatics of discovery of new biological insights has resulted in the development of tools to enable access to and use and management of these computer-based information systems. New initiatives to develop technologies and resources to advance the handling of larger and diverse datasets and to assist interpretation have been established in the fields of proteomics, genomics, and glycomics.

Third, rising healthcare costs have prompted stakeholders to assess the value of health care through *measurement*. Using administrative billing data, early research funded by the AHRQ documented substantial variations in the use of medical therapies across geographic units such as states as well as across patient subgroups such as race/ethnicity and sex. The corresponding lack of geographic variation in patient outcomes prompted research using administrative data enhanced with clinical data to assess the quality of medical care. The number and type of quality measures reported on healthcare providers, such as hospitals, nursing homes, physicians, and health plans, have grown substantially over the past decade (Byar, 1980). A second and related line of research related to rising healthcare costs is the comparative effectiveness of therapeutic options. Information obtained from comparative randomized trials, systematic reviews of randomized trials, decision analyses, or large registries are used to quantitatively assess effectiveness of competing technologies.

The availability of many large and diverse data sources presents an opportunity and a challenge to the scientific community. Under the current paradigm of assessing evidence, we continue to waste information by adhering to historical analytical and inferential procedures. Data sources relating to the same topic are treated as silos of information rather than as well-integrated information when assessing new technologies; information contained in multiple outcomes and multiple patient subgroups is ignored; and treatment heterogeneity in randomized trials is overlooked. The scientific community is not producing information efficiently. New tools, beyond those that expedite the mechanics of searching and accessing information, are required.

Using Diverse Data Streams

A fundamental problem of using diverse data sources is that of *poolability*. Combining data from multiple data sources is not new. At a practical level, for example, zip code level sociodemographic information from census data is often merged with patient-level information in administrative claims data to supplement covariate information. Estimates of treatment effects from diverse studies are commonly combined in the context of meta-analyses in order to learn about adverse events. The next generation of studies need to combine data sources for other reasons, however: to enhance results when the data source from which the information is based is different from the population of interest; to bridge results when transitioning from one definition to another (changing the definition from single to multiple race and ethnicity reporting); and to enhance small area estimation (see Schenker and Raghunathan, 2007, for a summary for combining survey data). Meta-analysis methods for combining information for assessing the relative effectiveness of two treatments when they have not been directly compared in randomized trials but have each been compared to other treatments have recently emerged (Lumley, 2002).

When is it *sensible* to combine data sources? While this is not a new statistical problem, it is increasingly more frequent and more complex. A familiar setting of combining data sources is that of meta-analysis in which the data sources are estimates obtained from multiple studies. In the typical meta-analysis setting, researchers consider whether the study populations are adequately similar, whether the treatments are defined similarly, and whether the clinical outcomes are similar. These decisions are *subjective*.

Once the decision is made to combine data, how should the information be *pooled*? Even if the patient-level data from each study were available, it would not be sensible to treat the observations from each patient across all of the studies as completely exchangeable. *Exchangeability* implies that we have no systematic reason to differentiate between the outcomes of patients participating in different studies. There are numerous methodological issues to consider, such as whether data are missing and the reason for missingness, the quality of the data, the completeness of follow-up, type of measurement error, etc, and are beyond the scope of this paper. In looking forward, however, increasing data pooling should provide more information.

Using Observational Data to Enhance Clinical Trial Data

The use of observational data to supplement a randomized trial is not a new idea, and there exists a large literature describing advantages and disadvantages. There has been much discussion, for example, on the use of historical controls in clinical trial (Byar, 1980). Viewing data sources as a continuum, at one extreme, we could *ignore* concurrent observational data but clearly that would be wasteful and inefficient (Figure 5-1). When collecting data from participants in a clinical trial, obtaining parallel information from non-trial participants at study sites will enhance inferences. At the other end of the continuum we could use all available data and treat information obtained from the observational subjects on an equal footing (that is, exchangeable) with the information obtained from the clinical trial participants. This strategy involves a heroic assumption that will typically be unmet in practice. Between these extremes, there are many options available but rarely utilized. Neaton and colleagues summarize strategies for pooling information in the context of designs for circulatory system devices (Neaton et al., 2007).

The Mass COMM trial[1] is a randomized trial comparing percutaneous coronary intervention (PCI) between Massachusetts hospitals with cardiac surgery-on-site (SOS) and community hospitals without cardiac surgery-on-site. The primary objective of the trial is to compare the acute safety and long-term outcomes between sites with and without cardiac SOS for patients with ischemic heart disease treated by elective PCI. The trial involves a 3:1 (sites without SOS: sites with SOS) randomization scheme that permits community hospitals to keep their volume given the substantial infrastructure investment they have made and the knowledge that volume is important. The recruitment strategy for the randomized study involves only patients presenting to community hospitals[2] (it would be very difficult to randomize patients arriving at tertiary hospitals to community hospitals).

---

[1] A randomized trial to compare percutaneous coronary intervention between Massachusetts hospitals with cardiac surgery-on-site and community hospitals without cardiac surgery-on-site (see http://www.mass.gov/Eeohhs2/docs/dph/quality/hcq_circular_letters/hospital_mdph_protocol.pdf).

[2] Massachusetts law permits elective angioplasty only at hospitals with cardiac surgery-on-site.

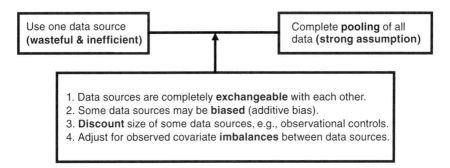

FIGURE 5-1 Options for pooling data in the context of a randomized trial.
SOURCE: Spiegelhalter, D. J., K. R. Abrams, J. P. Myles. 2004. Bayesian approaches to clinical trials and health-care evaluation. West Sussex, England: John Wiley & Sons, Ltd. Reproduced with permission of John Wiley & Sons, Ltd.

To bolster inferences and increase efficiency, the Mass COMM investigators adopted a *hybrid* design that borrows information from patients presenting at tertiary hospitals (concurrent observational controls). Figure 5-2 diagrams the hybrid design of this study, a randomized controlled trial using observational data.

How will the data sources (the randomized subjects and the observational subjects) be pooled? From a practical standpoint, it is not sensible to assume the observational patients arriving at tertiary hospitals and the patients randomized from community to tertiary hospitals are completely exchangeable. One strategy is to assume some differences in the outcomes of the observational controls ("additive bias") compared to patients randomized to the tertiary hospitals. The Mass COMM investigators assumed that the observational controls either over- or under-estimate the trial end-point by a factor of two. This decision was made prior to the enrollment of any patients.

Using Multiple Data Sources to Enhance Inference

Drug-eluting stents (DES) are combination products that have largely prevented the problem of restenosis. The critical path for approval of DES, like all first-in-class therapies, included several phases, each of which involved a pass or fail score: basic research, prototype design, preclinical development including bench and animal testing, clinical development, and Food and Drug Administration (FDA) filing. Sharing of knowledge in each of these domains rather than a pass or fail grade should enhance the

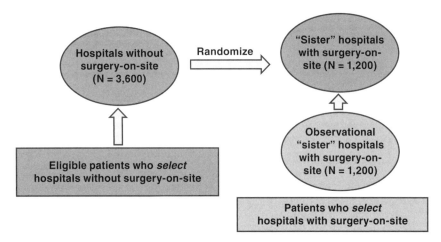

FIGURE 5-2 Schematic of Mass COMM Trial: One-way randomization with observational arm.

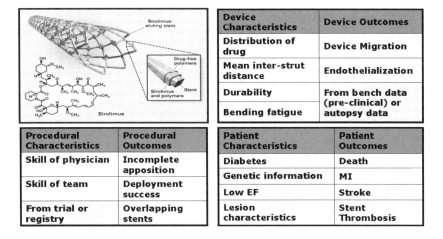

FIGURE 5-3 Integrating information: New ontologies (variations to consider in designing processes that link data in the case of drug-eluting stents).
SOURCE: Image appears courtesy of the Food and Drug Administration.

estimates of effectiveness and safety. A selection of types of data streams for DES includes device, procedure, patient characteristics and outcomes, as displayed in Figure 5-3. It seems sensible to assume that the device characteristics would impact the device, procedural, and patient outcomes and that the procedural characteristics would impact the procedural and patient outcomes, etc. By linking together all of these data streams through pooling, we will make more efficient use of information.

How should we pool these data sources? It is clear that there should be some probability model that links together the various silos of information. Statistical models for networks of information like that for DES exist but their practical applications have been limited.

Concluding Remarks

A key issue in the next generation of studies involves the development and implementation of pooling algorithms. The appropriateness of any pooling algorithm depends on the structure of the data, the data collection tools, and the completeness, maintenance, and documentation of data elements. Expanding our experience with pooling different data sources is the next step. New study designs are needed that exploit features of diverse information sources. There is some experience in pooling observational data with clinical trial data. These designs, such as hybrid designs, preference-based designs, and quasi-experimental designs, while available, have not been exploited to their full potential. Little experience exists for pooling data beyond the historical or concurrent observational control setting. The diverse data streams, such as that illustrated by the DES problem, are increasingly common. More focus on the development of inferential tools that will enable combining data appropriately and assessing the relationships among the streams in large databases is needed.

With the increasing number of registries, approaches for building the infrastructure to enable data sharing must be developed. Very little attention and money have been allocated for sufficient data documentation and for quality control. An additional consideration is how to best validate findings. What is the correct strategy for combining preclinical, clinical, and bench data? How do we minimize false discovery rates and determine which hypotheses are true and which are false.

Finally, we need to educate researchers, regulators, and policy makers in the interpretation of results from more diverse study designs, and the assumptions made and limitations with these designs. The availability of large data streams does not guarantee valid results—thoughtful use of data sources and innovative analytical strategies will help produce valid information.

OBSERVATIONAL STUDIES

Wayne A. Ray, M.D., M.P.H.
Vanderbilt University

Observational studies of therapeutic interventions are critical for protecting the public health. However, high-profile, misleading observational studies, such as those of hormone replacement therapy (HRT), have materially undermined confidence in this methodology. While findings of observational studies are intrinsically more prone to uncertainty than those from randomized trials, at present many of these investigations have suboptimal methodology, which can be corrected. Common problems include elementary design errors; failure to identify a clinically meaningful t_0, or start of follow-up; exposure and disease misclassification; use of overly broad end-points for safety studies; confounding by the healthy drug user effect; and marginal sample size. If observational studies are to play their needed role in clinical effectiveness studies, better training of epidemiologists to recognize and address these key issues is essential.

New technologies and expanding innovations in therapeutic interventions have led to an urgent need for expansion of safety and efficacy studies. The logistical difficulties and slow pace of randomized controlled trials limit its use in many cases; but the RCT is also not appropriate for all research questions. The value of observational studies to address this dilemma and to enable research on many important clinical questions is illustrated by a number of findings regarding safety and efficacy that have been made in the past through observational designs. Prominent examples include the high risk of endometrial cancer associated with unopposed estrogen therapy and the mortality benefit of colonoscopy in colorectal cancer.

However, observational studies have been criticized as inadequate for this purpose, having yielded several controversial and misleading findings, such as HRT and vitamin E associated with cardiovascular disease and dementia protection, findings later shown to be inaccurate by randomized controlled trials. The HRT findings led to millions more women using these therapies without the expected benefits. The same pitfalls are present in efficacy and safety studies based on observational data, as illustrated by findings that demonstrated a protective effect of non-steroidal anti-inflammatory drugs (NSAIDs) on dementia.[3] The outcome of these well-publicized inaccurate findings is to lead researchers to discount the value of observational studies without exploring the source or analyzing the meth-

---

[3] Thal, L. J., S. H. Ferris, L. Kirby, G. A. Block, C. R. Lines, E. Yuen, C. Assaid, M. L. Nessly, B. A. Norman, C. C. Baranak, S. A. Reines. Rofecoxib Protocol 078 Study Group. 2005. A randomized, double-blind, study of rofecoxib in patients with mild cognitive impairment. *Neuropsychopharmacology* 30(6):1204-1215.

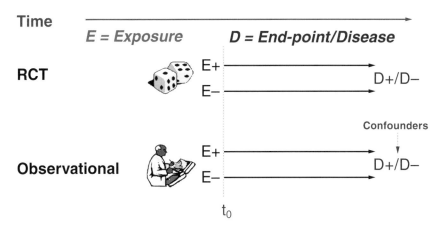

FIGURE 5-4 Notation used for observational studies in this paper.

odology. A closer look reveals that these errors are really the predictable result of ignoring some basic pharmaco-epidemiologic principles.

Figure 5-4 lays out the notation that will be followed throughout this paper. Consider a medication under study. Exposure (E) to a medication is either present (E+) or absent (E–) for various patients. In a clinical trial, individuals are randomized and starting at t_0, these individuals are followed forward in time where occurrence and end-points of a disease under-study are recorded for both E+ and E– groups. Observational studies also have E+ and E– groups, follow-up commences at a certain t_0, and individuals are followed forward in time to determine end-points; however, there are some important differences. First, the exposure group (E) is determined not by randomization but by measurement, and, secondly, choice by providers and patients in an observational study will lead to differences based on self-selection, some of which may present as confounders of real associations. Other potential problems that frequently surface during pharmaco-epidemiology studies include suboptimal t_0, immortal person-time with respect to follow-up, misclassification of exposure (both at baseline and time-dependent), misclassification of disease end-points—including overly broad or narrow designations. Potential confounders include the health user effect and variables that are time dependent, unavailable, or misclassified. Finally, the study may be powered inadequately—particularly in situations with infrequent end-points or chronic exposure.

The issue of suboptimal t_0, or beginning of follow-up, is best illustrated by first considering evaluation of a surgical intervention such as coronary artery bypass graft (CABG). An evaluation that started following patients 90 days after surgery—perhaps to wait for patients to stabilize

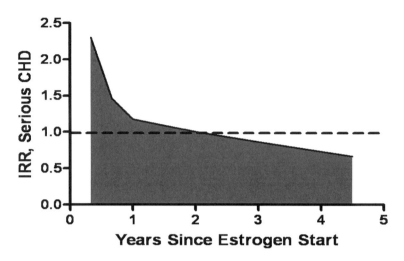

Years Since Estrogen Start

FIGURE 5-5 Risk of developing serious CHD in women using HRT therapy.
SOURCE: Derived from Hulley, S., D. Grady, T. Bush, et al. 1998. Randomized trial
of estrogen plus progestin for secondary prevention of coronary heart disease in
postmenopausal women. Heart and Estrogen Replacement Study (HERS) Research
Group. *Journal of the American Medical Association* 280:605-613; Ray, W. A.
2003. Evaluating medication effects outside of clinical trials: new-user designs.
American Journal of Epidemiology 158(9):915-920.

post-op—would conveniently exclude perioperative mortality. With these
data excluded, CABG would appear much better than actual results.
Although this type of t_0 is an obvious error for surgical interventions,
studies of medication often make this error with disastrous results. For
example consider a woman who starts HRT. Studies suggest that as shown
in Figure 5-5, there is an initial period of high risk for occurrence of coronary heart disease (CHD) and that this period of high risk abates with time
(Ray, 2003). However, most of the epidemiologic studies of HRT began
follow-up after this initial period, leading to a distortion of these studies'
results. Simply ensuring that follow-up initiates immediately following the
start of therapy would greatly improve confidence in study findings.

Another common problem is the failure to consider drug exposure that
changes over time. This commonly will lead to underestimation of drug
risk. For example, attrition and dosing changes can obscure true effects. For
example in an examination of benzodiazepine use, in just 1 month, fewer
than 60 percent of patients on the drug at baseline were still using it and
by 1 year this was less than 40 percent. Figure 5-6 illustrates the point that
if this single-point-in-time measurement of drug exposure is used to deter
mine relative risk for falls, no effect is observed (1.02); whereas, if we take

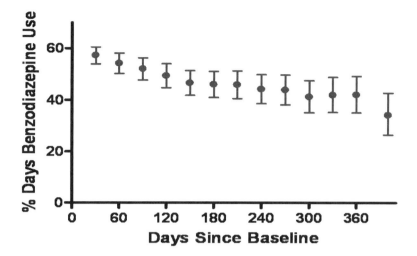

FIGURE 5-6 Relative risk of benzodiazinepine determined through a single-point-in-time measurement of drug exposure.
SOURCE: Ray, W. A., P. B. Thapa, and P. Gideon. 2002. Misclassification of current benzodiazepine exposure by use of a single baseline measurement and its effects upon studies of injuries. *Pharmacoepidemiology and Drug Safety* 11(8):663-669. Reproduced with permission of John Wiley & Sons, Ltd.

into account time-dependent changes, a 44 percent increased risk of falls is observed (Ray et al., 2002). Although some advocate the use of intention to treat as in the conduct of clinical trials, in observational studies, there is not necessarily an intention to treat, maintain treatment, or promote adherence as in an RCT, so adherence rates may be low and discontinuation rates may be very high.

A third common issue is the use of overly broad end-points. The choice of end-points should differ between the two designs, although RCT design often uses broad end-points appropriately to assess safety and efficacy, it may not be as useful in larger observational trials. A pitfall of the broad approach in analyzing safety end-points is obscuring more serious events by including them under less serious categories, such as classifying torsades-de-pointes as an "arrhythmia." In addition, all-cause mortality, which is an important indicator in closely defined, homogeneous populations of RCTs, is much more difficult to assess in the more heterogeneous and less controlled setting of observational studies. This makes certain therapies associated with death or general functional health appear to have mortality benefits when in fact none exist. For example, NSAID use has been shown statistically to confer a mortality benefit in observational studies that cannot be reproduced in randomized trials.

A final but important source of bias in observational studies is the healthy drug user effect. People who seek preventive interventions and take medications regularly are different from those who do not. This effect will bias results in favor of medications via healthier status of those who will consistently take medication. For example, a study of antiotensin receptor blockers (ARBs) in heart failure demonstrated a 30–50 percent reduction in cardiovascular mortality for persons that were "good compliers," but with placebo. These data showed medication adherence to be better predicted by adherence than therapy.

Given these potential problems, designing a "false-negative safety study" would include the following: a marginally adequate sample size and the use of an exposure that is not time dependent or includes substantial nonuser person time. The end-points should be broad and perhaps detected by invalidated computerized date. Similarly, one can create a "false-positive efficacy study" by focusing on an exposure that people seek, whether it is one used for prevention, sought out by informed consumers, or requires patient reporting of symptoms. Second, the cohort is a large group of prevalent users who are survivors of the period of prior drug therapy. This cohort is compared to a group of nonusers of drugs. Finally we use an end-point—such as cardiovascular disease or mortality—that is strongly influenced by behavior.

The design of observational studies is a complex subject but the previous discussion has outlined some starting points for the way forward. A first step is to separate observational analyses looking at safety from efficacy. For safety, the limitations that lead to false results are fairly easy to identify and counteract. A more difficult challenge is the need for infrastructure changes to reduce conflicts of interest by those who conduct safety studies. For efficacy, RCTs should generally be a required first step to ensure the expected benefits of therapy exist for the population as a whole if not for the individual. Third, it is necessary to challenge the assumption that because observational data often already exists in a database, study design and analysis will be fast or easy. There is an enormous amount of work involved in thinking through the particular question at hand, how various biases might apply, and how study design might effectively avoid these pitfalls. Finally, it is time to train a generation of epidemiologists to be more familiar with the clinical and pharmacological principles that affect the use of observational data. This expertise will allow clinicians to better exploit the wealth of available observational data and will lead to improve study designs. These efforts also will improve the reviews of grants and manuscripts, two additional forces critically important to improving the quality of studies of healthcare interventions.

ENHANCING THE EVIDENCE TO IMPROVE PRACTICE: EXPERIMENTAL AND HYBRID STUDIES

A. John Rush, M.D.
Departments of Clinical Sciences and Psychiatry
The University of Texas Southwestern Medical Center at Dallas

Abstract

Efficacy studies establish treatments as safe, effective, and tolerable. Clinicians, however, need to know how, for whom, when (in the course of illness or in the course of multiple treatment steps), and in what settings specific treatments are best used. Variations in treatment tactics (e.g., dose, duration) are often required for patients with different ages or co-morbid conditions, for example. Alternatively, treatments are sometimes combined to enhance outcomes, but for which patients is a particular combination better? At what treatment step(s) is/are particular treatment(s) best? When should a treatment be switched if patients are not responding? Is there a preferred sequence of treatments for specific patient groups?

This report illustrates how some of these clinically important questions can be addressed with observational data obtained when systematic practices are employed, or with new study designs (e.g., hybrid studies, equipoise stratified randomized designs) or post hoc (e.g., moderator) analyses. Suggestions for advancing this type of T_2 translational research are provided.

Introduction

In the pursuit of new treatments, basic science focuses on elaborating our understanding of how the human organism works—often relying on nonhuman experiments to elucidate biological processes and functions. As this understanding grows, one attempts to determine what diseases might be better understood with this basic knowledge. For example, new "drugable" targets may be identified. Then, new molecules are developed and tested preclinically to define their effects on the targets, their effects in animal models of disease, and their safety.

Once these hurdles are passed, these potential treatments are tested in man. If successful, one has established efficacy and safety of the new drug in one or another condition. FDA approval ensues, and the new treatment is announced.

The primary outcome of this process—sometimes called T_1 translational research or "bench to bedside" research—is the development of a new treatment (Woolf, 2008). This process entails the "effective translation of the new knowledge, mechanisms, and techniques generated by advances in basic science research into new approaches for prevention, diagnosis, and treatment of disease" (Fontanarosa and DeAngelis, 2002).

Alternatively, an established treatment for one disease may be found in clinical practice (or by additional basic laboratory testing) to be of potential utility in another condition (e.g., the use of selected antiepileptic medications in the treatment of bipolar disorder) (for example, Emrich, 1990).

Once a new treatment is defined as safe enough and effective, many issues remain. Specifically, how to apply the treatment in practice— sometimes called T_2 translational research (Sung et al., 2003)—must be addressed. T_2 translational research has several components: (1) At the patient/clinician level: How, when, for whom, and in what settings or contexts should the new treatment be provided; (2) How can the new treatment be implemented widely (disseminated); and (3) If widely implemented, what is the cost, cost efficiency, and cost consequences of properly using the treatment.

I suggest that T_1 translational research should be called Translational Research and that T_2 research be renamed to Applications Research and divided into Clinical Implementation, Dissemination, and Systems/Policy research to further specify these different research enterprises, as implied by Woolf (2008).

This paper focuses on Clinical Implementation Research at the clinician/patient level. The following discussion attempts to identify the knowledge gaps that exist when a new treatment becomes available (i.e., it has established efficacy, safety, and regulatory approval). Major depressive disorder (MDD) (American Psychiatric Association, 2000) is used to illustrate the principles discussed and the issues that need to be addressed in this type of research.

Depression as a Case Example

Clinical depression is prevalent, typically chronic or recurring, disabling, and amenable to treatment with a wide range of interventions (Practice guideline for the treatment of patients with major depressive disorder [revision]. American Psychiatric Association, 2000; U.S. Department of Health and Human Services et al., 1993). Similar to other medical syndromes, it is heterogeneous in terms of pathobiology, course of illness, genetic loading, and response to various treatments. It typically requires longer-term, not simply brief, acute management. These properties are common to other major medical disorders (e.g., congestive heart failure, cancer, hypertension, migraine headaches, epilepsy, etc.). Therefore, the following will use depression as an example to illustrate the principles proposed.

Conceptualizing Clinical Applications Research

When a new antidepressant is released, it is known to be: (1) more effective than placebo; (2) as effective as other available medications; (3) safe and well-enough tolerated to be a sensible option; and (sometimes) (4) to have established longer term efficacy based on randomized, placebo-controlled discontinuation trials.

What is unknown (Figure 5-7) are answers to a plethora of clinically relevant questions in addition to how well it works overall in practice. Specifically, how, when, for whom, and in what settings is the new treatment best used? Historically, answers to these questions have been relegated to the "art of medicine"—meaning that they are never empirically answered. These evidence deficits in turn lead to a high variance in how treatments are used and in the outcomes obtained.

Why are these questions unanswered? Perhaps it is assumed that clinicians will learn on their own how best to dispense the treatment. Alternatively, this type of research may be viewed as too simple or of little public health significance to merit funding. Or perhaps systems of care will decide these issues based on bottom line, short-term costs. In fact, without answers to these questions, far from optimal outcomes are likely with the treatment, and the cost efficiency is reduced.

Figure 5-7 suggests a conceptual map of the key factors that affect

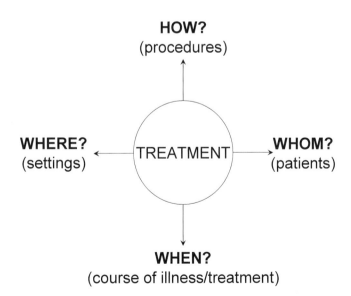

FIGURE 5-7 T_2 Translational research.

outcomes of any treatment. The treatments are sometimes called treatment strategies. The remaining factors (how, whom, when, where) inform the treatment tactics (Crismon et al., 1999; Rush and Kupfer, 1995).

Treatment guidelines often provide what strategies are reasonable options at various steps in treatment (e.g., what medications are best used in the first, second, or subsequent steps). Guidelines also may recommend tactics about delivering the treatment (Rush, 2005; Rush and Prien, 1995). These recommendations more often than not rest largely or entirely on clinical consensus rather than on definitive evidence.

The "How" Factors. How treatment is delivered clearly affects the outcome. If the dose is too low, efficacy is low. If it is too high, either efficacy is again reduced and/or side effects ensue such that poor outcomes result. Other "how" factors include visit frequency, rate of dose escalation, and the diligence with which the dose and duration are managed such that an optimal chance of benefit can be achieved. These "how" factors, as with the other factors, affect outcomes and patient retention or attrition.

To illustrate the importance of how a treatment is delivered, consider Figure 5-8. Greater depressive symptom reduction than achieved by treatment as usual was obtained with a treatment algorithm (which provided both strategic and tactical recommendations and included the routine measurement of symptoms and tolerability to inform dose adjustments) (Trivedi et al., 2004a), despite the availability of the same antidepressant medications for both the algorithm and treatment as usual groups. Thus, a systematic approach that enhanced the quality of care resulted in better outcomes than more widely varying routine practice.

As further evidence of the importance of how a treatment is delivered, consider recent results from the National Institute of Mental Health (NIMH) multisite Sequenced Treatment Alternatives to Relieve Depression (STAR*D) trial (Fava et al., 2003; Rush et al., 2004). Typical practice entails a 2–4 week trial of an antidepressant, after which, when little effect is seen, the treatment is switched. The STAR*D trial revealed that one-third of those who ultimately responded after up to 14 weeks of treatment did so *after* 6 weeks of medication (Trivedi et al., 2006a). These new data argue for longer trials that are likely to improve response rates.

The "When" Factors. When to use a new treatment is also unclear. "When" refers to either when *in the course* of an illness (e.g., earlier or later) or when in the course of multiple treatment steps, or when in the context of treatment that has produced only a partial response. To illustrate the importance of these "when" factors, Figure 5-9 shows that remission is least likely and slowest in depressed patients with a recurrent course and

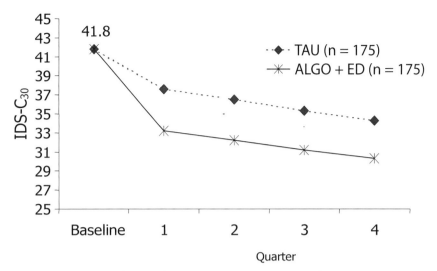

FIGURE 5-8 Adjusted mean depressive symptom scores on the IDS-C$_{30}$.
NOTE: IDS-C$_{30}$ = 30-item Inventory of Depressive Symptomatology–Clinician-rated.
SOURCE: Trivedi, M. H., A. J. Rush, M. L. Crismon, T. M. Kashner, M. G. Toprac, T. J. Carmody, T. Key, M. M. Biggs, K. Shores-Wilson, B. Witte, T. Suppes, A. L. Miller, K. Z. Altshuler, and S. P. Shon. 2004 (July). Clinical results for patients with major depressive disorder in the Texas Medication Algorithm Project. *Archives of General Psychiatry* 61(7):669-680. Copyright © 2004 American Medical Association. All rights reserved.

a chronic (≥2 year) index episode, while it is most rapid and effective in nonchronic, nonrecurrent patients (Rush et al., 2008). This previously unavailable information tells clinicians that a longer treatment trial is especially needed for more chronic and recurrent depressive illnesses (e.g., 9–12 weeks). Furthermore, relapse is most likely for those with chronic and recurrent depressions (Figure 5-10).

In addition, when a treatment is used in the course of multiple treatment steps, it can affect outcomes. Often new treatments are used only after several prior standard treatments. Is this preferred? In STAR*D, remission rates were lower if any treatment was used later in the step sequence. Only 33 percent remitted after the first treatment, 30 percent after the second, and 14 percent after the third and fourth treatment steps, respectively (Rush et al., 2006).

The "For Whom" Factors. The third domain that affects outcome involves patient groups for whom the treatment is best. Since depression is hetero-

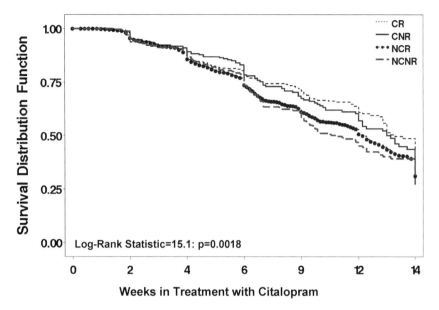

FIGURE 5-9 Time to remission by prior course of illness.
NOTE: CNR = chronic and nonrecurrent; CR = chronic and recurrent course;
NCNR = neither chronic nor recurrent; NCR = non chronic but recurrent.

geneous with regard to response, no one treatment works for all. While some evidence suggests that medication responses run in families (Stern et al., 1980), the "for whom" question is never addressed in efficacy trials, perhaps in part because efficacy trials enroll symptomatic volunteers with little or no co-morbid psychiatric or general medical pathology, with minimal chronicity and treatment resistance (i.e., prior failed treatment trials) (Table 5-1).

Narrowly defined efficacy samples arguably enhance internal validity by excluding subjects with concurrent co-morbid disorders that could affect efficacy or tolerability. Such samples, however, cannot address the "for whom" question. To illustrate this point, consider the results of our recent finding (Wisniewski et al., 2007) that only 635 of 2,855 depressed STAR*D participants (22 percent) would have qualified for typical efficacy trials conducted for registration purposes. Remission rates were 35 percent for efficacy trial–eligible patients and 25 percent for efficacy trial–ineligible patients. Similarly, for depressed outpatients with three to four concurrent general medical conditions (GMCs), the odds ratio of remission was

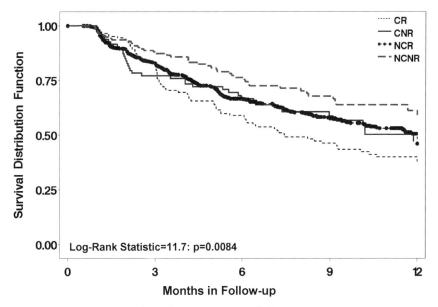

FIGURE 5-10 Time to relapse by prior course of illness.
NOTE: CNR = chronic and nonrecurrent; CR = chronic and recurrent course; NCNR = neither chronic nor recurrent; NCR = non chronic but recurrent.

TABLE 5-1 Population Gaps

Parameter	Symptomatic Volunteers	Typical Patients
Chronically ill	–	+++
Concurrent Axis I	+	+++
Concurrent Axis III	+	+++
Treatment-resistant	±	++
Suicidal	–	++
Substance abusing	–	++
Will accept placebo	+	±

0.47 (for three) and 0.52 (for four or more), as compared to 1.0 for no co-morbid GMCs and 0.83 for one to two co-morbid GMCs (Trivedi et al., 2006b). Similar results were found if depression was accompanied by several anxiety disorders (Fava et al., 2008; Trivedi et al., 2006b). These findings question the value of antidepressant medication in those with more GMCs—a fact that could not be learned from efficacy trials.

The "In What Settings" Factor. Finally, practice setting or context may well affect outcome. Different settings are associated with different kinds of patients, with different degrees of treatment resistance, different co-morbidities, different levels of social support or stress, different treatment procedures (e.g., visit frequency, dose escalation profiles, etc.), and different prior history. Thus, setting itself is likely a highly relevant outcome parameter as it encompasses several factors that can affect outcomes.

The above conceptual model (illustrated by case examples from depression) is applicable to treatment of most diseases. The answers to the "how?," "who?," "for whom?," and "in what setting?" questions will better define the best (safest, most effective) treatment for particular patients, treated under specific conditions. To develop Clinical Implementation Research, two key issues must be resolved: (1) designing cost-efficient, rapidly executed studies to obtain the answers and (2) developing a consensus by which to prioritize the questions to be answered.

Trial Design Options

Efficacy

Efficacy trials carefully control the parameters of how, whom, when, and in what settings so that when treatments are randomly assigned, should a treatment difference (e.g., drug versus placebo or drug versus drug) be found, one can ascribe the differences in outcomes to the treatments with high certainty. A classic effectiveness trial can be seen as allowing all four parameters to vary. In fact, variance is sought, as are large samples, so that post hoc moderator analyses might be conducted to generate hypotheses about for which patient group a treatment is clearly better than another (Kraemer et al., 2002). Alternatively, one can ask whether between-treatment differences are greater in one (e.g., primary care) versus another (e.g., psychiatric care) setting. Such effectiveness studies require large samples and simple outcomes—so-called Practical Clinical Trials (March et al., 2005; Tunis et al., 2003). They usually entail randomization and are most easily conducted across sites with common electronic records and clinicians who routinely use the same primary outcome measures (e.g., blood pressure, a common depression rating scale like the 16-item Quick Inventory of Depressive Symptomatology—Self-report or QIDS-SR$_{16}$ (Rush et al., 2003; Trivedi et al., 2004b).

Effectiveness

These effectiveness trials have the advantage of "generalizability" and the potential for identifying target populations, settings, preferred treatment procedures, or optimal timing (the "when" issue) on the use of a treatment. Once these moderators are identified, they must be prospectively tested to be valid (Kraemer et al., 2002). If differences between treatments A and B are found in an effectiveness trial, the cause of the difference could be due to patient subgroups, different treatment procedures in use, the timing of the use of the treatment, etc., or a combination. If the sample is large, the randomization should usually guard against these parameters being causally related to outcomes, however.

Hybrid

An alternative to a full effectiveness trial is a "hybrid trial" (Rush, 1999). Hybrid trials allow variance in one or more of the above four Treatment Outcome Relevant Parameters (TORPs) while controlling some or all of the remaining parameters. One can randomize to treatments, to different treatment procedures, or to different populations, etc.

The STAR*D trial (Fava et al., 2003; Rush et al., 2004) was a hybrid trial. The primary question in STAR*D was "what is the next best treatment if the initial, second, or third treatment steps have failed?" In essence, what are the best treatments for treatment-resistant depressions (i.e., depressions that have not benefited from one or several prior treatments)? Results had to be applicable to primary and psychiatric care settings, and generalizable to typical patients in practice (i.e., with common co-morbidities and a level of depression for which medications would typically be used as a first step). Thus, a full range of variance in patients ("for whom") was allowed, but settings were restricted to primary and psychiatric care (public and private).

We wanted to know what the next best treatment is for depressions that did not benefit after one or several prior adequate treatment trials—not poorly delivered treatment. We, therefore, controlled both for the "how" and "when" parameters. In terms of the "how" parameters, we had to ensure that treatment was well delivered (i.e., to ensure that sufficient doses and durations were used in each treatment step) so that a failure to benefit from a treatment was likely due to the failure of the treatment and not to the failure to deliver the treatment.

We had to control for the "when" parameter to define the number of prior failed treatments and to enroll nonresistant (i.e., no prior treatment failures) in the first step. Thus, at enrollment eligible patients were defined as *not* treatment resistant. The first step was a single Selective Seratonin Reuptake Inhibitor (SSRI). Then, by using randomized treatment assignment in the second, third, and fourth treatment steps, we could isolate which of several different treatment options would be best for patients for whom one, two, or three prior treatments (each provided in the study itself) had failed.

Since both primary and psychiatric care settings were involved in the study, there was a risk that setting could affect outcome. We found, however, that both the types of patients and the fidelity to protocol-recommended, guideline-based treatment was similar across the two types of settings. Consequently, we found outcomes to be comparable across settings throughout all four treatment steps in the study.

This sort of hybrid design allows rather clear causal attribution to be made when between-treatment differences occur. For example, some advantage to bupropion-SR versus buspirone augmentation of citalopram was found in the second step. This difference was not due to setting, differences in treatment procedures, or when in the course of treatment these two treatments were used. In addition, hybrid trials of sufficient size can be subjected to moderator analyses (Rush et al., 2008).

Registries

Registries also can provide important information about the how, whom, when, and what setting parameters noted above. Since STAR*D patients received a single, well-delivered SSRI (citalopram) in the first step, for those who did not need the second step, we had a large population that was followed for up to a year after this first step. These sorts of registry-like data help to define the long-term course of treated depression, and such registry cohorts also provide safety and tolerability data. For example, Figure 5-10 shows that among depressed patients who do well enough to enter long-term treatment, those with a more chronic or recurrent prior course have the worst prognosis, even in treatment. They also may suggest genetic features relevant to side effects (Laje et al., 2007) or longer term outcomes. As with any observational study, replication is essential, however.

Other Designs

Finally, a comment about other study designs is in order—in particular adaptive designs (Murphy et al., 2007; Pineau et al., 2007) and equipoise stratified randomized designs (Lavori et al., 2001). Both designs attempt to mimic practice and allow prospective evaluation of common practice procedures about which there is controversy. For example, adaptive designs can determine whether continuing the same treatment longer, switching to a different treatment, or adding a second treatment to the first is preferred overall for certain patient subgroups. As a further illustration, when depressed patients have a worsening following months of a good response on treatment, does one raise the dose, hold and wait, or add an augmenting agent? We have no idea now. While a registry without randomization may identify the common practices for these cases, without randomization we cannot be sure of the next best step.

Another attempt to mimic practice while retaining randomization entails the equipoise stratified randomized design (ESRD) (Lavori et al., 2001), which was used in STAR*D. It allowed patients with an inadequate benefit from the first treatment step (citalopram) to eliminate certain treatment strategies in the second step, while accepting the remaining treatment strategies, all of which entailed randomization to various treatment options. To illustrate, the second step provided both (1) a switch strategy (randomization to one of four new treatments after the first step was discontinued) (i.e., citalopram was stopped; the new treatment was begun) and (2) an augmentation strategy (to one of three new treatments to be added to continuing citalopram). Patients could decline one of these strategies (e.g., eliminate augmentation) while accepting the switch strategy and the subsequent randomization to one of four treatments. This design was based on clinical experience, which suggested that patients who were substantially better with the first treatment—but not entirely well so that additional treatment would be needed—would decline switching (to avoid losing the benefit from the step 1 treatment). On the other hand, we expected that those with little benefit and/or high side effects from the first treatment would prefer to switch and decline augmentation. This is, in fact, what we found (Wisniewski et al., 2007). This ESRD allowed participants to be randomized to the specific second step treatments that they were more likely to receive in practice, so that results are generalizable to practice.

Our conclusion is that effectiveness, hybrid, registry adaptive treatment, and other designs all can inform practice. The key issue is to identify the most important questions to be addressed in Clinical Implementation Research.

Defining the Key Clinical Implementation Questions

The discussion above illustrates that a host of clinically critical questions remain once a new treatment becomes available. These questions can be grouped into four conceptual domains (how, for whom, when, what setting). A range of study designs (registry/cohort studies, effectiveness, hybrid, adaptive, and ESRD) are available. The most important issue, however, is how to identify the most important questions to be addressed by Clinical Implementation Research.

Ideally, all stakeholders would have the same question in mind at the outset, but this is often not the case. In fact, the key questions likely vary based on the disease and the available knowledge about treatment of the disease. For example, for STAR*D we wanted to know the next best treatment if the first (or a subsequent one) failed. For Parkinson's disease, it could be how to manage the depression or prevent the dementia. For HIV, it could be how to manage lipodystrophy or when to use specific combination treatments.

In addition, the perspective of various stakeholders are different. Patients may be more concerned with side effects, adherence, or quality of life. For clinicians, it may be symptom control. For payers, it may be cost recovery or defining the best way to implement procedures. For family members, it could be how to reduce care burden.

Other parameters that affect selection of the key questions for study include (1) Will the answer change practice?, (2) Will the answer change our understanding of the disorder?, (3) Will the answer have an enduring shelf life?, and (4) Will the answer reduce wide practice variations or resolve common controversies about how to manage the disease? If the procedure is commonly used but supported with little evidence, the importance of evaluating the new procedure may be particularly high—especially if it is a more or less costly procedure (e.g., a diuretic versus an ACE inhibitor for hypertension).

One way to define the key questions is to use disease focus groups, which could be accomplished by Web meetings or in-person meetings or perhaps by convening task forces that report to Councils of specific NIH Institutes. Based on registries or large healthcare use databases or literature reviews—perhaps commissioned by AHRQ—one could identify common practices for which there is wide practice variation (or uncommon practices for which there is great promise), with little evidence for which of these alternatives is most effective, safe, or cost-efficient.

Other information sources that could help to define these key questions could include secondary analyses of available large trials, data from current registries, development of registries to identify common practices or potential changes in practice, and data mining large databases (e.g., HMOs).

I would suggest that each NIH Institute select one to three disease targets based on the public health impact of the diseases and the potential for better prevention or treatment, given current practice, practice variation, cost impact, and knowledge about and availability of the interventions. This could be accomplished by the Institute with a consensus conference to identify the key one to two questions that are the highest priority to diverse stakeholder participation. From this consensus, requests for application (RFAs) could be released and contracts let to address these questions in a timely and focused fashion. A significant annual financial commitment from the relevant institutes should be made to Clinical Implementation Research (T_2) as well as System Implementation Research (T_2).

Reengineering Practice for T_2 Research

Not only must the key questions for specific diseases be identified, but also the practice "system" needs to be reengineered to facilitate such efforts. By such efforts, the cost of such research should go down, the system can learn as it goes, and answers can be provided much more rapidly. Obvious suggestions include (1) registries for difficult-to-treat diseases to raise hypotheses about treatment for whom and when or to identify safety/tolerability EMRs, (2) agreement on common outcome measures that have both research *and* clinical relevance, (3) payment to providers to obtain these measures if not part of current care (e.g., function at work, absenteeism, role function as parent, student, etc.), (4) training of clinicians who could participate in the basics of clinical research so that collaboration is facilitated, and (5) payment to clinics in the system for research time and effort if needed.

Conclusion

While major treatment advances have been realized from basic research, it is clear that simply making a new treatment available to clinicians is not sufficient to ensure its optimal, appropriate, and safe use. How, for whom, when, and in what context it is best to use the treatment, and the cost implications of these decisions, deserves higher emphasis in funding and prioritization than previously. A variety of design options are available. With systems of care now using electronic medical records, large practical clinical trials are feasible. One major hurdle remains: how to select the most important questions for prospective study to ensure results will change practice, enhance outcomes, improve cost efficiency, and/or make treatments safer.

To define these key questions, one must engage key stakeholders, focus on particular diseases, and engage care systems or develop specialized networks in which the research can be conducted. Finally, once the questions are defined, designs must be identified or developed to obtain the answers.

Institute leadership from across the NIH with critical input and collaboration from clinicians, patients, investigators, and payers is a prerequisite. Finally, either additional funding targeted at these questions or a shift in already very restricted resources is called for. Without these commitments, how, when, for whom, and in what setting a treatment is best will remain the "art of medicine," rather than the science it could be.

ACCOMMODATING GENETIC VARIATION AS A
STANDARD FEATURE OF CLINICAL RESEARCH

Isaac Kohane, M.D., Ph.D.
Harvard Medical School

Large numbers of subjects are needed to obtain reproducible results relating disease characteristics to rare events or weak effects such as those measured for common genetic variants. These numbers appear to be much higher than the 3,000–5,000 that was characteristic of such studies only 5 years ago. The costs of assembling, phenotyping, and studying these large populations are substantial, estimated at $3 billion for 500,000 individuals. Fortunately, the informational by-products of routine clinical care can be used to bring phenotyping and sample acquisition to the same high-throughput, commodity price-point as is currently true of genotyping costs. The National Center for Biomedical Computing, Informatics for Integrating Biology to the Bedside (i2b2), provides a concrete and freely available demonstration of how such efficiencies in discovery research can be delivered today without creating an entirely parallel biomedical research infrastructure and at an order of magnitude lower cost.

Although genomics is poised to have a significant impact on clinical care, the medical system is relatively ignorant about genetics. A classic example is the surprising result of a recent survey that showed that although 30–40 percent of primary care practitioners had ordered a genetic test for cancer screening in the prior year, this was not due to expected predictors such as a patient's family history or the education of the practitioner, but rather due to patient requests for the test (Wideroff et al., 2003). The interesting thing about the genomic era is that it poses all of the questions that we are asking about secondary use of data in sharper fashion and as such it is a useful lens to look at these problems of secondary use of data. Even when you go beyond the genetics and genomics the same issues come back again and again. Nonetheless, this brief overview will address how we might instrument the healthcare system for discovery research in the genomic era.

Determining true genetic associations is difficult as illustrated by a meta-analysis done by Hirschhorn of 13 studies of a single nucleotide polymorphism (SNP) that results in an amino acid substitution in the protein PPAR-gamma. This substitution has long been suspected as implicated with Type 2 diabetes susceptibility. The odds ratio reported by each of these individual studies is all over the map, and only when these data are considered in total, is it clear that their polymorphism is actually slightly protective for Type 2 diabetes (Figure 5-11) (Altshuler et al., 2000). This finding illustrates two key issues: (1) research on common variants will need

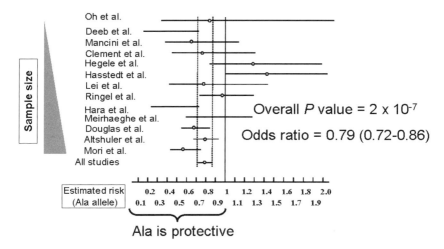

FIGURE 5-11 Comparison of studies for PPARγ Pro12Ala and Type 2 diabetes susceptibility.
SOURCE: Adapted by permission from Macmillan Publishers, Ltd. *Nature Genetics* 26(1):76-80. Copyright © 2000.

to include the appropriate sample size. Rather than sample sizes such as 100 or even 1,000 patients, as in these 13 underpowered studies, research will require populations on the order of 10,000 patients; (2) the large number of SNP (current tests incorporate 500,000 SNPs) coupled with relatively inexpensive and fast analyses will likely result in an overwhelming number of misleading findings and associations. The commercialization of genomic sequencing and screenings will likely compound these issues.

A significant threat to genomic medicine therefore, is the phenomenon of the "incidentalome," in which the dangers of a large N and small p(D) contribute to the discovery of multiple abnormal genomic findings. If all of these findings are pursued without thought, ramifications for clinicians, patients, and the health system will bring into question the overall societal benefit of genomic medicine (Kohane et al., 2006). For example, testing 100,000 individuals with a genetic test that is 100 percent sensitive and 99.99 percent specific, will lead to 10 false positives. If a commercially available DNA chip has 10,000 independent gene tests, 60 percent of the population would be falsely positive. Although current genetic tests have lower specificity and sensitivity (perhaps 80 percent and 90 percent, respectively) because their utilization in practice is limited and clinicians tend to order them when there is a clinical indication (thereby increasing the prior likelihood that the patient has the disease), we have fortunately not yet been assaulted by the tsunami of false-positive results. However, the emerging commercial approach to enable broad population screens and conduct many tests in parallel without enriching first for risk, threatens to greatly increase the number of spurious findings. And, because it no more difficult to get a 100,000 SNP chip approved by the FDA as it is for a 100 SNP chip, pressures towards the incidentalome (the universe of all possible false-positive findings) are very substantial and will increasingly present significant challenges to providers, patients, and insurers.

To overcome these problems, the field should focus on approaches and opportunities to garner a large number of appropriate patients (N). The three prongs of instrumentation that are needed to efficiently reach a large N include high-throughput genotyping, high-throughput phenotyping, and high-throughput sample acquisition. The emphasis on efficiency is paramount given resource constraints. In the U.S. Department of Health and Human Services for example, the Secretary's Advisory Committee on Genetics, Health and Society (SACGHS) recognizes the significant health value of having a 500,000 to 1 million subject study to understand the interaction between genes and environment; however, this study is estimated to cost about $3 billion. Likewise, the cost of a pediatric study launched by the NIH for merely 100,000 individuals will cost an estimated $1–$2 billion over the next two decades. Given the number of similar large-scale genomic studies that could be initiated in the coming decades, developing efficient and inexpensive approaches to obtain data of needed quality and quantity is of utmost importance.

With respect to the three prongs of instrumentation, only high-throughput genotyping is in place and with commoditization the price is rapidly dropping—currently $250–$500 for 500,000 SNPs. The remainder of my discussion will focus on efforts to bring greater efficiency and affordability to the processes of phenotyping and sample acquisition and, in particular, on several new open source tools that aim to help the healthcare enterprise better capture the information and bioproducts produced during the course of clinical care such that they can be used effectively for discovery research.

An important component of any analysis is being able to obtain the "right" populations though phenotyping. To develop an appropriate approach, we have collaborated with computer scientists and software engineers and are working to assess a wide range of phenotypes and diseases—from asthma to major depression, rheumatoid arthritis, essential hypertension, and other common diseases. The following example focuses on efforts to translate genetic findings to improve clinical outcomes in the treatment of asthma. Several colleagues had identified a collection of SNPs in populations in Costa Rica and China that were moderately distinguishing between asthmatics that were responders or nonresponders to glucocorticoid therapy. To determine the relevance of these findings to clinical practice in Boston required the identification of the appropriate set of patients to study. How could we identify these patients through our computerized health records? Because for this type of analysis, billing codes are too coarse grained and biased, we used automated natural language processing to evaluate text of doctors' notes in online health records. Improving this technique to the point that it was useful was quite challenging; but, ultimately we were able to quickly, reproducibly, and accurately stratify 96,000 out of 2.5 million patients for disease severity, pharmaco-responsiveness, and exposures. Now with cases and controls (from extrema) re-consented and biomaterials obtained, we were able to identify responders and nonresponders to glucocorticoid therapy. If this type of system can be implemented and successfully used across many systems, high-throughput phenotyping may be achievable at the national level. Indeed, over 15 large academic centers have adopted the i2b2 software (freely available under open source license) so there is some reason for optimism in this regard.

Another significant barrier is in obtaining the biosamples for any phenotyped population. That is, how do we find the samples to match the phenotyped patients just identified through natural language processing? Initial efforts to obtain samples and consent entailed outreach through primary care practitioners to patients, a process that was resource and time intensive. The newly developed Crimson system, pioneered by Dr. Bry at the Brigham and Women's Hospital in Boston, is being tested as an alternative and more efficient way to unite patient phenotype with genotype data. This system takes advantage of the many biosamples collected by laboratories in the routine course of care but ultimately discarded after use. Crimson is able to identify when these samples match up with phenotyped populations (such as the 96,000 asthmatics identified in our previous example). The end result is efficient acquisition of real biological samples—that can be used for a number of genomic tests and biological assays—matched with a rich set of known phenotypes. We have obtained 8,000 samples to date, with over 5,000 released for analysis. The opportunities presented by these richly annotated biospecimens is substantial, whether through DNA analysis by gene array, genomewide association studies, or SNP analyses; the identification of new serum/plasma markers; auto-antibody studies; testing of new antibiotics or antiviral compounds; or metabolism studies of clinical isolates.

If these advances lead to high-throughput phenotyping and sample acquisition, within the decade, we can decrease costs of large-scale genomic studies significantly. In contrast to the estimated $3 billion needed for the SACGHS study of 1 million patients, in 3 years we might expect such a study to less than $150 million and take less than one-tenth of the time to execute. These order of magnitude changes will significantly change the number of studies that can or cannot be done.

Instrumenting the health enterprise has important implications outside of genomic research as well. Existing databases such as the data mart maintained by Partner's Health Care can be used for analyses aimed at detecting safety or risk signals such as the increased cardiovascular risk in patients taking Vioxx (Brownstein et al., 2007). As we move forward, it is therefore important to consider how the healthcare enterprise can be used for both discovery research and for surveillance. Finally it is worth noting that health is not limited to the provision of healthcare, and personally controlled health records (Kohane and Altman, 2005; Riva et al., 2001; Simons et al., 2005) may provide us with the tools that will instrument the rest of the health care that occurs outside the provider-based healthcare system.

In summary, several specific actions will help to accelerate progress. The first is the increased investment in healthcare IT; these tools will not only will improve the quality of delivered health care but also will increase the quality of secondary uses of electronically captured data. Second, increased transparency in both regulation and patient autonomy is needed to resolve the many worries (often unjustified) about HIPAA that prevent the broader implementation of these systems and approaches. With appropriate education, HIPAA should not present an obstacle to research. Third, we need the continued development of an informatics-savvy healthcare research workforce that understands relationships between health information, genomics, and biology. And finally, the most important step is to create a safe harbor for methodological "bake-offs" that challenge researchers to experiment with large datasets analysis. For example, the protein-folding community has for nearly a decade sponsored contests that pit various methodologies against one another to see which can best predict, computationally, how a given protein sequence will fold. This type of safe harbor has led to innovation in computational methodologies. Yet these types of challenges and safe harbors do not exist for equally complex areas in clinical medicine— such as predicting risk of recurring breast cancer (e.g., the Oncotype or MammaPrint gene expression tests) and/or improving natural language processing approaches to phenotyping of patients. To have an open and transparent discussion about methodological strengths and weaknesses, data should be made available and these biomarkers and studies tested. However, there is no such test bed available for methodologists around the world seeking to improve the state of the art. For the safe and meaningful conduct of biomedical research, particularly in genomics, it is essential that we start testing our data, our methodologies, and our findings.

PHASED INTRODUCTION AND PAYMENT FOR
INTERVENTIONS UNDER PROTOCOL

Wade M. Aubry, M.D.
Senior Advisor
Health Technology Center

Coverage of health interventions has historically been a binary decision by Medicare and commercial health plans. Over the last two decades, however, the concept of phased introduction and payment for emerging technologies under protocol, or "coverage with evidence development (CED)" has evolved as a flexible or conditional alternative to a complete denial of coverage. An important early example of this approach from the 1990s was the support of commercial payers such as Blue Cross Blue Shield Plans for patient care costs of high-priority National Cancer Institute (NCI)-sponsored randomized clinical trials evaluating high-dose chemotherapy with autologous bone marrow transplantation (HDC/ABMT) compared to conventional-dose chemotherapy for the treatment of metastatic breast cancer. Importantly, the financial support for this investigational treatment was contractually facilitated by the Blue Cross Blue Shield Association (BCBSA) as a "Demonstration Project" operating outside of the usual medical necessity provisions in the health plan "evidence of coverage (EOC)" documents. Accrual of patients to the RCTs was slow because of the widespread availability of HDC/ABMT outside of research protocols, delaying the trials which would eventually report no benefit from the more toxic high-dose chemotherapy.

Other examples of CED can be found in the Medicare program (IOM, 2000) and include the Health Care Financing Administration (HCFA) (now Centers for Medicare & Medicaid Services [CMS])/FDA interagency agreement from 1995 allowing for coverage of Category B investigational devices (incremental modification of FDA-approved devices), coverage of lung volume reduction surgery (LVRS) for bullous emphysema under an NIH protocol (1996) (Mckenna, 2001), and the Medicare Clinical Trials Policy (CMS, 2000), under which qualifying clinical trials receive Medicare coverage for patient care costs under an approved research protocol. Over the past 4 years, Medicare CED has been formalized by CMS with a guidance document, a CED policy for implantable cardioverter defibrillators (ICDs) for the prevention of sudden cardiac death, and a Position Emission Tomography (PET) oncology registry for indications not previously covered by Medicare. In addition, the Medicare federal advisory committee established in 1999 for developing national coverage decisions (NCDs) was renamed the Medicare Evidence Development and Coverage Advisory Committee

(MedCAC), emphasizing the importance to CMS of developing better evidence to inform Medicare coverage decisions.

The concept of applying CED to commercial health plans has grown in interest over the past 2 years due to the Medicare CED experience but also as part of the debate over whether a national comparative effectiveness (CER) institute should be established. Under this idea, which has been advanced by Wilensky, prospective comparative studies generating new evidence would be included as well as systematic reviews or technology assessments of existing research (Wilensky, 2006). However, as per the experience of the Center for Medical Technology Policy (CMTP) over the past 2 years and of others interested in creating better evidence for decision makers, significant barriers remain in regard to further development of CED in the private sector. These include (1) health plan contracts (EOCs) defining medical necessity as not experimental or investigational, (2) ethical issues such as whether CED is really research, whether it is coercive, and whether it is fair (Pearson et al., 2006), (3) the difficulty in achieving multistakeholder consensus when funding depends on vendors such as medical device companies for research costs and health plans for patient care costs, (4) lack of a clear definition of what constitutes "adequate" evidence compared to what constitutes "ideal evidence" when designing the study protocol and end-points, (5) timing of CED in regard to existing coverage without restrictions (lack of incentives for sponsors of new technologies if coverage is already widespread), and (6) limitations of the number of studies that can be implemented under CED.

The story of HDC/ABMT for the treatment of breast cancer provides a good starting point to understand how similar phased introduction and payment for interventions under protocol might be used to facilitate next-generation studies of clinical effectiveness. HDC/ABMT emerged in the 1980s as a combination therapy for breast cancer that combined high-dose chemotherapy and autologous (self-donated) bone marrow transplantation based on the observation that higher doses of chemotherapy resulted in more complete and partial tumor response rates. Various factors led to a fateful branching of this procedure's use. The two pathways or "systems" of use that emerged can be characterized as a (1) a "rational system" of evaluation—emphasizing systematic evaluation of evidence by technology assessments, clinical practice guidelines, and randomized clinical trials—and (2) a "default system" of clinical use—one that reflects uncoordinated action driven by Phase II studies, patient demand, physicians seeking better treatments for seriously ill patients while building financially successful bone marrow transplant programs, lawyers, media, entrepreneurs, and state and federal governments (Figure 5-12). Approximately 1,000 patients were treated "on protocol" in the evaluation of HDC/ABMT for breast cancer, in high priority NCI randomized controlled trials; whereas, simultaneously an

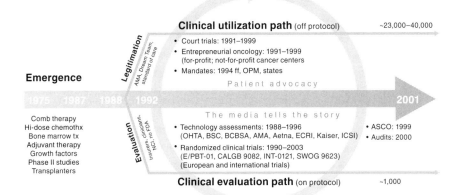

FIGURE 5-12 The timeline of the branching of the HDC/ABMT experience in breast cancer.

estimated 23,000–40,000 patients were treated off-protocol. After 10 years, the results of the on-protocol trials demonstrated that while HDC/ABMT positively affected surrogate outcomes such as response rates, these early markers did not translate into improved survival and ultimately conferred no benefit to patients (Jacobson et al., 2007).

Key issues in the HDC/ABMT story were access to new treatments—how innovations in medicine and promising treatments are made available to patients, what type of evaluations are necessary to demonstrate evidence of benefit for various circumstances, and what role the health insurers could play when patients demand access to treatments that do not meet evidence criteria. In this specific example, BCBSA created a mechanism or Demonstration Project outside of coverage that would allow its plans to participate in randomized trials evaluating the effects of HDC/ABMT on breast cancer. This was essentially a new organization housed at BCBSA in Chicago, which developed contracts with providers and health plans to cover patient care costs "outside of usual coverage and medical necessity provisions" for eligible BCBS Plan enrollees. Because of the broad utilization of HDC/ABMT off-protocol, however, it took a long time to recruit patients for the high priority RCTs that were funded by the Demonstration Project, despite the participation of 17 BCBS Plans and the Federal Employees Program (FEP) administered by BCBSA. From about 1991 to 1999 recruitment continued but dropped off significantly when, at the May 1999 annual meeting of the American Society of Clinical Oncology (ASCO), it was demonstrated that in the two out of four high-priority trials reported, HDC/ABMT treatment resulted in no benefit to patients.

Lessons from the HDC/ABMT experience, such as early collaboration among investigators to implement needed trials with the support of payers, and independent medical review of individual cases as an appeal mechanism, remain relevant today. State mandates for coverage of HDC/ABMT for breast cancer, which numbered 15 during the mid-1990s, proved to be ill advised, as they circumvented the results of technology assessments (which showed evidence gaps) and contributed to the delay in the completion of the NCI randomized clinical trials. State mandates for coverage of qualifying clinical trials, however, have arguably promoted better evidence by funding patient care costs for well-designed clinical trials and facilitating their completion and reporting.

There continues to be public debate surrounding the evaluation, dissemination, and payment of costly medical technologies, many of them for life-threatening conditions such as cancer. This subject was highlighted by *The New York Times* in a series of summer 2008 front page articles under the series title *The Evidence Gap*. In their book *False Hope: Bone Marrow Transplantation for Breast Cancer,* the authors propose a public–private partnership for evaluation of medical procedures (Rettig et al., 2007). Because the HDC/ABMT treatment was a procedure that also used FDA-approved drugs at higher doses than standard of care, regulatory oversight does not fall under any existing governmental agency. A public–private partnership with a relevant institute at the NIH was proposed to fill this gap. In cooperation with insurers and patients, researchers would be asked to describe Phase II results with respect to the promise of particular technologies, evaluate the rationale for Phase III trials, and if necessary limit access to new procedures to these controlled trials. To address any patient concerns, review of individual cases would also be required. In addition to accelerating the production of timely data to the public on clinical effectiveness, additional benefits of this process include a mutual understanding between participants, the development of a shared interest in clinical effectiveness research, insurer funding to finance RCTs, and some protection from litigation for health plans. This concept of shared evaluation of the gaps in existing research and the design and financing of appropriate new studies could also be applied to private-sector initiatives using a neutral party rather than an NIH Institute as research coordinator.

Several lessons for coverage with evidence development can also be learned from experiences of Medicare. In 1965, Section 1862 of the Social Security Act clearly outlined Medicare's policy regarding untested treatments, with statutory language that "no payment may be made for items or services which are not reasonable and necessary for the diagnosis and treatment of illness or injury or to improve the functioning of a malformed body member." This is the "reasonable and necessary" clause of the Medicare statute, the operational definition for which has varied over the years because no coverage regulations for Medicare have ever been formally adopted. As outlined in the *Federal Register* on January 30, 1989, under a notice of proposed rulemaking (NPRM) that was never finalized, Medicare generally determined that the service was safe and effective, not experimental or investigational, and appropriate. More recently, guidelines for evaluating effectiveness developed through the MedCAC and published on the CMS website[4] include a determination that the evidence is adequate for improving net health outcomes and that the evidence is generalizable to the Medicare population. Decision memoranda for finalized NCDs also have created a form of "case law" for how CMS evaluates different services as "reasonable and necessary."

"Coverage with conditions" in Medicare emerged in the 1990s, beginning with Category A and B investigational devices, in which an HCFA (now CMS)/FDA interagency agreement allowed coverage for devices with minor incremental improvements (Category B) but not for novel devices (Category A). This permissive policy opened the door for Medicare coverage with conditions for LVRS under an NIH protocol (The National Emphysema Treatment Trial [NETT]) to evaluate its clinical effectiveness compared to intensive nonsurgical management. This was followed by the Medicare Clinical Trials Policy in 2000 that expanded Medicare coverage for qualifying clinical trials. Finally, coverage with evidence development was formalized in a CMS guidance document in 2006 (CMS coverage website). The two best examples of CED to date are ICDs for prevention of sudden cardiac death with data collection by a registry managed by the American College of Cardiology (ACC) and PET for oncology indications that were not previously approved for Medicare coverage with data collection under a registry managed by the American College of Radiology Imaging Network (ACRIN). The CMS guidance document on CED specifies that for selected national coverage decisions limited funding would be made available to support needed studies under protocol. In essence, therefore, CMS has determined that for these interventions, and for others that may follow, phased introduction and payment under protocol is "reasonable and necessary" and that national non-coverage, or unrestricted coverage, is not.

These approaches attempt to contend with the essential problem in the delivery of medical care, that for many clinical situations, evidence is insufficient to inform decision making at multiple levels: by patients, physicians, delivery systems, and policy makers. Many organizations perform systematic reviews of evidence and decision modeling, such as the AHRQ

---

[4] CMS coverage website, http://www.cms.hhs.gov/coverage.

Evidence-Based Practice Centers (EPCs), the BCBSA Technology Evaluation Center (TEC), the Drug Effectiveness Review Project (DERP) at Oregon Health and Science University (OHSU), Hayes, Inc., the ECRI Institute, the Cochrane Collaboration, and the Institute for Clinical and Economic Review (ICER). These assessments frequently identify evidence gaps on new and emerging technologies, concluding that there is not enough evidence or any relevant evidence available for decision making. Clearly there is a great need for new approaches to fill these evidence gaps, and many believe that approaches such as CED, particularly if expanded beyond CMS, offer a potential solution for at least some technologies. As a way to move this into the private sector and to ensure the opportunity for broad stakeholder input, the Center for Medical Technology Policy, a new nonprofit organization, is working with a broad group of interested parties to prioritize and facilitate research on promising emerging technologies and practices. The CMTP's approach to creating new evidence has been termed "decision-based evidence-making" as a means of promoting evidence-based medicine (EBM) by increasing the supply of useful data. By designing practical clinical trials (Tunis et al., 2003) comparing new health interventions to relevant or existing alternatives in conjunction with CED, an attempt is being made to find an optimal balance between innovation, access, evidence, and efficiency in practice. The approach is collaborative with a strong commitment to including all stakeholders in decisions and seeks to promote rapid learning through pragmatic, prospective, simpler, faster, and cheaper research studies.

A vision for a new generation of studies and approaches to assess clinical effectiveness is illustrated in Figure 5-13. Phased introduction and pay-

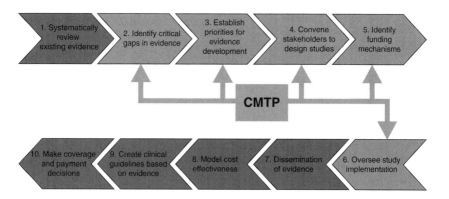

FIGURE 5-13 Where the Center for Medical Technology Policy (CMTP) fits into assessing a new generation of clinical effectiveness studies.
SOURCE: Adapted from Steve Pearson's building blocks model.

ment for interventions under protocol can contribute to each of these steps and, as indicated in Figure 5-13, the CMTP is focused on specific activities within this vision. The process could be generally described as beginning with the systematic review of existing evidence to identify critical gaps in evidence, then moving into prioritization, design, funding, study implementation, and oversight. Post-analysis, evidence would be disseminated, resulting in evidence-based clinical guidelines, coverage and payment decisions, and, in some cases, cost-effectiveness analyses by other organizations (e.g., TEC, ICER, AHRQ or its EPCs) or by other individuals.

The "priorities for evidence development (PED)" initiatives at the CMTP (and elsewhere) aim to identify evidence gaps of important technologies for conditions having a significant burden of illness or cost, using systematic reviews, technology assessments, and other types of research. One such AHRQ-funded project at the CMTP started with a Stanford EPC comparative effectiveness review of existing research comparing percutaneous coronary intervention (PCI) with CABG and identified research priorities by supplementing expert and stakeholder opinion. In developing effectiveness guidance documents (EGDs) for selected topics, the CMTP is attempting to model what the FDA and CMS have done in trying to define clear standards for different classes of technologies. Resulting guidance documents will be similar in concept to FDA guidance on evidence needed for regulatory approval but will recognize that different technologies require different types of evidence development and that decision makers often need a higher level of evidence than the FDA requires, such as for medical devices. These guidance documents will expand on information that comes out of priorities for evidence development projects and will move these projects into facilitated research. They will address several key issues, such as (1) What will it take to adequately answer these questions? and (2) What has been learned about specific technologies that might apply to all technologies in that class? Effectiveness guidance documents in development include Gene Expression Profiling in the Management of Breast Cancer and Negative Pressure Wound Therapy for Chronic Non-Healing Wounds. Finally, the CMTP has two facilitative research workgroups focused on selected questions developed through PED. Selection criteria included decision-maker interest, pragmatic design, reasonable size, and reasonable duration. Current workgroups are assessing cardiac computed tomography angiography (CTA), for which CMS recently considered for CED but did not finalize an NCD, and other forms of cardiac imaging in the management of coronary artery disease and different modalities of radiation therapy (proton beam therapy and intensity modulated radiation therapy [IMRT]) in the treatment of early-stage prostate cancer. Comprised of researchers, NIH leaders, academic physicians, professional society representatives, health plans, clinical practitioners, and patient advocates, these groups are responsible for

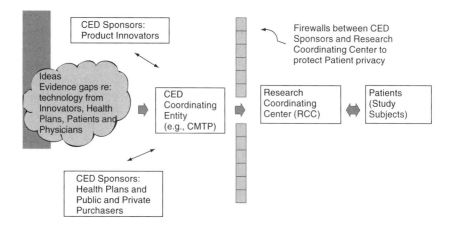

FIGURE 5-14 Schematic model of clinical study coordination under CED.

outlining and funding clinical research; they develop study designs, contract out research, oversee actual research, and disseminate results. The radiation therapy study comparing side effect profiles of proton beam versus IMRT for prostate cancer has generated the most interest and momentum to date, with the multistakeholder group developing a draft protocol, operational plan, and budget to move forward. Figure 5-14 depicts the CED model with sponsors, a coordinating entity, and privacy protections.

Another key element in promoting CED is benefit language or alternative legal mechanisms allowing health plans to participate in CED without undermining basic medical necessity provisions of their evidence of coverage documents. Historically, the Demonstration Project mechanism at BCBSA for BCBS Plan support of patient care costs for HDC/ABMT breast cancer patients outside of routine coverage addressed this issue successfully. Recently, a conceptual framework for CED with model benefit language has been developed by the CMTP as an applied policy project through a grant from the California HealthCare Foundation (Center for Medical Technology Policy, 2009) and may help to accelerate health plan interest and willingness to participate in CED. Issues addressed using a multi-stakeholder process include technology selection criteria, CED research design criteria, plan participation criteria, possible pathways to incorporate CED within a plan of benefits, and plan language. A basic issue for plans is whether to participate in CED *outside of coverage* as a special project (e.g., the BCBSA Demonstration Project) or whether to define the CED program within the benefit plan (e.g., as part of a clinical trials policy). The CED model, in conjunction with appropriate plan benefit language, completes the conceptual framework necessary for implementation of CED in commercial health plans.

In summary, although many challenges have limited progress to date on phased introduction and payment for interventions under protocol, there is optimism that the concept will continue to evolve because of Medicare experience with CED and private-sector interest. There continue to be significant barriers, however. It is difficult to reach multistakeholder consensus on study design and funding, and the most important evidence gaps may be ones that can't be filled. While ideal evidence is well understood, adequate evidence remains undefined, timing is critical (as CED is ineffective if widespread coverage exists), and CED may not be enough to encourage the conduct and completion of important clinical studies. Several strategies might help to accelerate progress, including the public–private partnership recommended for medical procedures not governed by FDA regulation, and private–sector coordination of clinical studies under CED by neutral organizations such as the nonprofit Center for Medical Technology Policy. In addition, model benefit language allowing health plans to participate in CED without undermining basic medical necessity rules is critical to facilitating their participation. Operational strategies going forward include explicit ground rules for workgroups, and separate processes for evidence gap identification, prioritization, and selection for study design and funding. CED should complement—rather than compete with—the traditional research enterprise (researchers and funding mechanisms). Finally, it is critical to look to the future and to work earlier in the product development cycle to generate evidence before widespread dissemination of the intervention in question.

RESEARCH NETWORKS

Eric B. Larson, M.D., M.P.H.
Sarah Greene, M.P.H.
Group Health Center for Health Studies

Fulfilling the Potential of the Learning Healthcare System Through Emerging Research Networks

Recent publications have acknowledged and described the limitations of our current health research enterprise (Emanuel et al., 2004; Gawande, 2002, 2007; Lenfant, 2003; Tunis et al., 2003; Zerhouni, 2005b). These limitations include structural deficiencies, insufficient generalizability, and delays in initiation and implementation from the research review system. Multi-site and network-based studies can help to make research more generalizable; but they are particularly vulnerable to slow processes. By further developing and supporting research networks that are embedded in healthcare systems, we believe we can accelerate progress toward optimal clinical care.

We need to redesign the paradigm for clinical effectiveness research to anchor it in emerging research networks that can serve as a "learning healthcare system." The notion of a learning healthcare system has gained conceptual and operational traction as a way to meet the challenges of 21st-century medical care. This care could be increasingly tailored based on rapid advances in the "omics" (genomics, proteomics, and metabolomics) and enhanced understanding of gene–environment interactions and the complex mechanisms underlying treatment responses in both infectious and chronic diseases. Taken together, the learning healthcare system and a redesigned paradigm for clinical effectiveness research hold high promise to help to meet these challenges.

A proposal to redesign the clinical effectiveness research paradigm for a learning healthcare system could draw inspiration from several existing models. These include successful initiatives such as the Cooperative Oncology Groups, large cohort studies such as the well-known Nurses' Health Study and Framingham Heart Study, as well as products of contract research organizations (CROs). They also include the large and growing work accomplished by emerging research networks in functioning delivery systems, such as the HMO Research Network and its several consortium projects already underway: the Cancer Research Network (Wagner et al., 2005), the Center for Education and Research in Therapeutics (CERT) (Platt et al., 2001), and the newly funded Cardiovascular Research Network. In this paper, we assert that emerging (and mature) networks in functioning delivery systems represent a unique opportunity, if contributing to a learning healthcare system is among the research goals. These networks have already made substantial contributions, and we believe they and their individual sites could become the mainstay of clinically relevant research that is ready to be applied to benefit both individual patients and the public's health.

Why Is the Potential of Such Networks So Great?

Being embedded in functioning delivery systems optimizes the research network's value in producing relevant and generalizable results. Population-based research is ideal for producing research results with the greatest potential for being of known generalizability and relevance. This contrasts with research from "convenience samples" (the predominant U.S. mode) or from highly specialized, typically referral-filtered populations. Examples abound. But even confining examples to the singular arena of diagnostic markers and management of Alzheimer's disease, history is littered with instances of findings that offered great hope and that both the scientific and lay communities greeted with enthusiasm, only to be ultimately found useless because they could not be confirmed and thus were not generalizable. Examples include platelet membrane fluidity (Zubenko et al., 1987), one of the first tests widely touted to be diagnostic of Alzheimer's disease—now remembered only by investigators from that time and chagrined staffers from the National Institute on Aging and other NIH Institutes who drew attention to the result as "news" of a "major breakthrough."

Looking back on over two decades of working in community-based populations, we see that much of our early work consisted not of finding new and valid markers but rather of simply demonstrating that markers from convenience samples lacked generalizability to the true population of interest. Similarly, in many instances, drug safety concerns were not evident even in very large trials from convenience samples, typically persons carefully screened and not typical of community-based everyday patients. These concerns then became evident in community-based populations, providing "poster children" for our system's failure to detect toxic effects of widely used drugs such as COX-2 inhibitors (e.g., rofecoxib) (Psaty and Furberg, 2005, 2007), thioglitazones, and epoetin alfa. Some treatments (e.g., tissue plasminogen activator for stroke) appeared effective at reducing morbidity from acute and chronic diseases in carefully conducted clinical trials, but were then reported to have dramatic adverse consequences when translated into practice (Katzan et al., 2000). Now, "pharmacovigilance" and "pharmaco-surveillance" are gaining considerable traction—and attraction—as a means of examining and ultimately preempting similar adverse drug events. A research network based in delivery systems can serve as a ready-made apparatus for this important postmarketing medication surveillance activity.

What Makes a Well-Constructed Integrated Care-Delivery System So Favorable for Producing Generalizable and Relevant Research?

First, and perhaps most critical, is the ability to conduct research—including randomized controlled trials—based in a population leading their lives as usual. Even in instances when sampling cannot be random, a population base lets researchers determine whether any characteristics differ between the population studied and the base population. This enables them to ask, even in a selected population, whether findings are generalizable and, if not, how so. One recent example involved an autopsy study set at Group Health. Subjects who end up receiving autopsy are known to be highly selected, so epidemiologists are traditionally instructed not to use autopsy data to develop inferences for more general populations. However, Sebastien Haneuse, a biostatistician working with Sonnen et al. (2007), has developed a method to determine susceptibility to selection bias in autopsy studies using a weighting scheme comparing characteristics of the living participants to those undergoing autopsy, thereby allowing adjustment if bias is present (Haneuse, 2008).

Secondly, modern integrated care delivery systems are pioneering technological and structural advancements to improve care. Web-based patient portals, secure messaging between patients and providers, and the accompanying transformation of the doctor–patient interaction may lead to dramatic changes in market dynamics, by lowering cost and ultimately improving care and health outcomes. Researchers are testing patient-directed behavior change interventions that could be integrated into the health plans' patient-facing websites. Research networks embedded in health plans have conducted RCTs and quasi-experimental studies of computerized physician order entry (CPOE) systems, including studies of various types of alerts and "academic detailing" (one-on-one education about use—and often overuse—of treatments such as medications) to reduce prescribing errors. Newer features include unfettered access to specialists, benefit redesign, and development of the "medical home" model to improve continuity of care. These innovative, testable features—if demonstrated to be successful—could become extensible platforms for U.S. healthcare reform. If not, they should be abandoned. Delivery system-based researchers are contributing to the dialogue about the infrastructure of national health information. It is crucial to develop structures, function, and standards that both meet clinical needs and facilitate a robust research enterprise. Interoperability of healthcare data (allowing data sharing among disparate systems) goes hand-in-glove with the development of this national infrastructure, and the experience of these learning healthcare systems and their researchers—who typically collaborate on multi-site, cross-platform data exchange—can inform these conversations (U.S. Department of Health and Human Services, 2008a, 2008b).

A third notable characteristic of a well-constructed, integrated care-delivery system that favors generalizable and relevant research is that it is "ecological." As a functioning system, it subjects effectiveness research to a setting that is a real, living, and breathing organization whose primary and overarching purpose is to deliver health care. Because of this purpose—which cannot be subjugated to meet the convenience that investigators often expect—their research is much more likely to be pragmatic and to reflect the extant clinical conditions in which care is (and will be) delivered. Healthcare research in these real-time learning laboratories ensures that healthcare systems and national priorities interact with each other. The reciprocal knowledge exchange between these two spheres, especially when conducted in a way that promotes both organic and systematic implementation of new knowledge, can greatly accelerate advances in health care through opportunities for translation.

Research in learning healthcare systems also affords opportunities to study not only what care should be delivered, but how it is (and should be) delivered—that is, what characteristics of providers, policies, and systems affect delivery and implementation of the research. For instance, Taplin and colleagues examined the occurrence of late-stage breast and cervical cancers in environments where women had access to screening. Their study showed the complex interplay of guidelines, contributors to effective follow-up of abnormal screens, and surprisingly more women than expected who refused care, even after learning they had suspicious lesions (Taplin et al., 2004). In another example, Simon et al. conducted a pragmatic clinical trial of antidepressants that arguably produced the best information that a clinician and patient might use to base selection of antidepressants for an individual patient or for practice guidelines. After randomly assigning more than 500 Group Health patients with depression to receive fluoxetine or tricyclic medications, the researchers found no difference in clinical or quality-of-life outcomes or overall treatment costs. They concluded that patients' and physicians' preferences are an appropriate basis for selecting initial treatment (Simon et al., 1996).

One reason trials like that of Simon et al. might be more likely to be conducted in functioning delivery systems like Group Health is the shared desire of those in the delivery system and the research unit to improve research, health care, and, of course, health outcomes. The collective goal of a learning healthcare system is to establish a reliable apparatus of evidence-based critical decision making. Over the decades, Group Health has moved from a strong commitment to the "ideal of research" to a pragmatic realization that it *needs good research on which to base clinical decisions*. Neither the clinical nor research enterprise can afford any more of the high-profile disasters that have occurred when drugs with demonstrated success in RCTs (e.g., rofecoxib and rosiglitazone) have been revealed to be too dangerous for general use because of inadequacies in the original efficacy and effectiveness research. Both researchers and clinicians realize the across-the-board risk to the clinical system and research enterprise of not anticipating and addressing these quality problems. They jointly realize that research in functioning delivery systems is an important avenue for authentic testing of effectiveness, safety, outcomes, and interactions.

Another often-overlooked characteristic of functioning care-delivery systems is the ability to exploit what we call the "bidirectionality" of research. Traditionally, the research and policy communities have stressed the need for research to go from "bench to bedside"—or from lab to clinical practice. A distinct advantage of research sites and networks embedded in functioning delivery systems is that ideas can emanate from those at the bedside: Clinicians identify critical deficiencies of care that can be researched and improved; they are poised to test novel treatment ideas, while cham-

312 REDESIGNING THE CLINICAL EFFECTIVENESS RESEARCH PARADIGM

pioning these ideas and forming ready partnerships with research teams. Similarly, researchers can refine and adapt strategies from the published literature, providing important confirmatory studies or rigorous evaluation of a natural experiment, often in larger and more representative populations. Patients—or, more typically, patient advocacy groups—may point out deficiencies or special needs that suggest research projects. Most importantly, research in a community-based delivery system can yield insights into real-world issues of highest priority to the target population.

The recently funded Clinical and Translational Science Award (CTSA) partnership between the University of Washington, Group Health, and the Northwest American Indian/Alaskan Native Network affords an unparalleled opportunity to surface the tribes' preeminent research priorities and to apply tools and strategies that the Group Health and university researchers devise to address them. We at Group Health were assuming that this network would want us to study accidents, gun safety, and maternal health in their communities. These are all areas in which we have substantial prior experience, including in American Indian and Alaskan Native communities. However, we were astounded to hear, when we spoke with them in person, that the first priority of all of the tribes was methamphetamine abuse, which they told us is destroying the life of their communities. They said, "You can study what you want, as long as you start with meth."

Ultimately, these research examples are not only bidirectional but also adaptive and iterative, as befits a more real-world and less-controlled setting. This does not detract from scientific rigor; rather, it means the protocol is more likely to be calibrated for real-world conditions. Results can be translated more effectively, since the research was conducted in the setting where the findings are applied.

What Is Our Vision to Guide the Next Generation of Studies and Exploit the Natural Advantages of Research Networks in Functioning Integrated Care-Delivery Systems?

Three general principles underlie our vision:

1. Bi-directionality—with research flowing seamlessly across bench, bedside, and community—will become an accepted aspect of most, if not all, funded health research.
2. The learning healthcare system can be seen as a catalyst, partner, and test bed for research.
3. The infrastructure needed to rapidly ramp up new research studies will evolve to meet the demands of this more complex environment.

We emphasize that the RCT will still be the cornerstone of bi-directional research. Since Archie Cochrane's seminal writing (Cochrane, 1971), we have benefited greatly from widespread acceptance that the RCT provides the most reliable evidence for judgment of effect. Effectiveness RCTs should be pragmatic, efficient, and ideally population based for better generalizability. Researchers should do more than simply communicate their results through academic manuscripts. If set in a delivery system, they have a direct route, and indeed a responsibility, to communicate results to providers and usually to participants. Consider how quickly research is translated into practice when a pharmaceutical company promotes a new drug RCT. The goal is to match this speed when we translate into practice any research that involves improving care. Yet we have not consistently done this well. An example is shared decision making for prostate surgery. This was shown in 1995 to improve outcomes and reduce costs, an ideal result (Wagner et al., 1995). However, it was not adopted or used in the delivery system where the research was conducted: Group Health.

However, traditional RCTs, which assign single patients randomly to a prespecified treatment or intervention, are expensive and time consuming. They also may be impractical for addressing many important questions. Thus, other types of studies can be valuable and informative if conducted in a well-constructed delivery system. Examples include cluster randomized trials and disease registries. Cohort studies linked to legacy medical records and electronic medical records (EMRs) in stable populations (e.g., Group Health [Smith et al., 2002] and Mayo Clinic) are quite useful for time series analyses, correlations, and quasi-experimental research using observational data generated from clinical practice—especially so-called natural experiments that occur as practice changes are instituted or external environment changes affect medical care and outcomes. We took advantage of a natural experiment when a pilot project deploying the Advanced Medical Home in a single clinic was initiated and we rapidly developed our Advanced Medical Home study. A revival of idealized primary care, the Advanced Medical Home involves a physician and healthcare team committing to serving as the home base for as much of their patients' medical care as they can provide—and as the coordinators of other care as needed (American College of Physicians, 2006). The rationale behind this model is that this coordination promises to help control costs while improving health outcomes and patient and provider satisfaction. Very preliminary results from our study suggest that the Advanced Medical Home improves the satisfaction of patients and providers without increasing costs. A study called Content of Care is another important example, in which we are using automated data to identify and address high-cost drivers of care across populations—and unwarranted variations in practice between physicians and medical centers.

What Are Some Emerging and Uniquely Important Areas Where the Theoretical Advantages of Research Networks Set in Delivery Systems Might Be Especially Valuable?

Challenging areas involve detecting drug side effects (Brown et al., 2007), vaccine safety (Hinrichsen et al., 2007), and emergence of antibiotic-resistant infectious agents. These challenges also represent an opportunity: Can research networks in functioning systems improve translation by both producing valid research findings while minimizing false starts and also by detecting side effects or changes in treatment effects more quickly after deployment? Proven examples include the Vaccine Safety Datalink (VSD) project (Centers for Disease Control and Prevention, 2008; Thompson et al., 2007), which is in the process of being emulated for infectious disease biosurveillance, e.g., using HMO Research Network sites to detect changes in antibiotic resistance among sexually transmitted diseases. Directly observing the dissemination of key clinical findings in practice also provides an effective window on translation. The up-to-the-minute, comprehensive data systems of these research networks lend themselves to examining changes in treatment, such as the use of aromatase inhibitors for adjuvant breast cancer therapy following reports of this successful therapeutic approach among referral populations in cancer trials (Aiello et al., 2008).

Genomics represents a unique opportunity for research in integrated care-delivery systems to exploit the features that make such research relevant and generalizable. Personalized medicine is an increasingly popular term in the health sector; but realizing its true promise will require working through many operational issues around the data, along with significant transformation in how care is delivered. Privacy issues and ownership considerations abound as large quantities of genomic data are being collected, analyzed, and stored. State-based regulations are likely to play a major role as data stewardship becomes a larger part of this conversation. Housing these data in delivery system-based research networks offers such clear-cut advantages as:

- Known and diverse population base
- Avoidance of referral filters
- Established and typically trusting relationship between patients and their providers in the care-delivery system
- Empiric study of consent
- Well-developed EMR to obtain phenotype information

EMRs promise a much more efficient way to determine phenotypes for research and also will be uniquely helpful when and if we can "tailor" treatment and especially prevention in a personalized way (i.e., based on known genetic risk or therapeutic responsiveness). But clinical science is hard-pressed to keep up with the pace of marketing forces and natural curiosity driving consumers to seek this information and act on it (Harmon, 2008). Notably, the National Human Genome Research Institute has significant work remaining to develop genomewide array studies based in existing cohorts. Behavioral and sociocultural examinations are accompanying the basic and preclinical research, but much work remains to fully understand the ramifications of collecting and leveraging genomic data, much less tailoring treatment based on these unique characteristics.

Is a Culture Change Under Way?

The "omics" revolution portends a cultural shift. NIH Director Zerhouni describes medicine that is not only preventive but also preemptive. He enunciates a new vision for translational research in recent publications (Zerhouni, 2005a). One outcome is the NIH Roadmap for Medical Research, a paradigm for re-engineering clinical research, which begat the NIH-funded CTSAs. This program aims to "develop a national system of interconnected clinical research networks capable of more quickly and efficiently mounting large-scale studies." One consequence of this effort is a nascent culture change and, in places, works in progress—in institutions choosing to "re-engineer" their clinical and translational research programs. Some are realizing the potential of bringing together research networks in integrated healthcare systems with university-based scientists. Reviewers of CTSA grant proposals often highlight these interfaces as particularly strong features of applications.

Given the magnitude of the CTSA program and the lofty goals related to national systems of interconnected clinical research networks, the outcomes of this Institute of Medicine (IOM) workshop should aspire to inform the NIH's CTSA program. Indeed, the IOM's proposed redesign of the clinical effectiveness research paradigm ideally would address challenges the NIH will face as it aims to re-engineer the massive biomedical research enterprise we currently enjoy in the United States. This reaffirms our second principle: that the learning healthcare system can be viewed as a catalyst, partner, and test bed for clinical research.

We believe our third principle is central to any discussion of a new vision or paradigm for research, whether in a learning healthcare system or any other setting. To meet the complex needs of researchers, care providers, and the patients we serve, the operational infrastructure needed to rapidly ramp up will need to evolve to meet the demands of new research studies in this more complex environment. The infrastructure "renovations" should consider the full gamut of opportunities to render research more efficient, including:

- Research review by Institutional Review Boards and similar ethics committees: Harmonizing regulations across federal agencies is a pivotal first step; developing stronger federal guidance about avoiding duplicative reviews of multi-institutional studies is another necessary action.
- Creating repositories of measures, surveys, and other indices, with standardized information about how these measures are used, to avoid reinventing measures de novo.
- Templates for common research processes such as gaining HIPAA authorization and developing data use agreements and similar data-sharing operations.
- A knowledge bank of effective participant recruitment strategies, analogous to the Cancer Control PLANET (Plan, Link, Act, Network with Evidence-based Tools) that the National Cancer Institute developed (National Cancer Institute Cancer Control PLANET, 2008).
- Harmonized manuscript submission procedures adopted by all publishers of medical journals.
- Continued attention to the architecture of health information—how it is collected, stored, and exchanged.

Clinical developments are outpacing our ability to implement these needed innovations. Thoughtful reconsideration of the research process, maintaining the appropriate level of attention to patient privacy, confidentiality, security, and the doctor–patient compact, will help us to close the gap between research advances and their deployment. If the nascent culture change leads to sustainable operational infrastructure, the next generation of research studies can successfully exploit the myriad advantages of emergent research networks in healthcare systems, as long as equal attention is given to the philosophical and practical tenets we have outlined here. Emerging research networks can form a reliable basis for such learning healthcare systems, which have the potential not only to accelerate the translation of research but also to ensure that it confers true benefits to patients and the public health.

REFERENCES

Aiello, E. J., D. S. Buist, E. H. Wagner, L. Tuzzio, S. M. Greene, L. E. Lamerato, T. S. Field, L. J. Herrinton, R. Haque, G. Hart, K. J. Bischoff, and A. M. Geiger. 2008. Diffusion of aromatase inhibitors for breast cancer therapy between 1996 and 2003 in the cancer research network. *Breast Cancer Research Treatment* 107(3):397-403.
Altshuler, D., J. N. Hirschhorn, et al. 2000. The common PPAR γ Pro12Ala polymorphism is associated with decreased risk of type 2 diabetes. *Nature Genetics* 26(1):76-80.

American College of Physicians. 2006. *The Advanced Medical Home: A Patient-centered, Physician-guided Model of Health Care—Policy Monograph.*

American Psychiatric Association. 2000a. *Diagnostic and Statistical Manual of Mental Disorders, 4th ed.* Washington, DC: American Psychiatric Press.

———. 2000b. Practice guideline for the treatment of patients with major depressive disorder (revision). *American Journal of Psychiatry* 157(4 Supl):1-45.

Brown, J. S., M. Kulldorff, K. A. Chan, R. L. Davis, D. Graham, P. T. Pettus, S. E. Andrade, M. A. Raebel, L. Herrinton, D. Roblin, D. Boudreau, D. Smith, J. H. Gurwitz, M. J. Gunter, and R. Platt. 2007. Early detection of adverse drug events within population-based health networks: Application of sequential testing methods. *Pharmacoepidemiology and Drug Safety* 16(12):1275-1284.

Brownstein, J. S., M. Sordo, I. S. Kohane, and K. D. Mandl. 2007. The tell-tale heart: Population-based surveillance reveals an association of rofecoxib and celecoxib with myocardial infarction. *PLoS ONE* 2(9):e840.

Byar, D. P. 1980. Why data bases should not replace randomized clinical trials. *Biometrics* 36(2):337-342.

Center for Medical Technology Policy. 2009. *Coverage for Evidence Development: A Conceptual Framework.* Oakland: California HealthCare Foundation. http://cmtpnet.org/cmtp-research/applied-policy-and-methods/coverage-with evidence-development/20090108%20-%20CMTP%20-%20CED%20Issue&20Brief.pdf/view (accessed June 21, 2010).

Centers for Disease Control and Prevention. 2008. *CDC Vaccine Safety Datalink Project.* http://www.cdc.gov/od/science/iso/vsd/ (accessed July 18, 2008).

Centers for Medicare & Medicaid Services. 2000. Medicare Coverage-Clinical Trials Program. http://www.cms.hhs.gov/ClinicalTrialPolicies/Downloads/programmemorandum.pdf (accessed June 2008).

Cochrane, A. 1971. *Effectiveness and Efficiency: Random Reflections on Health Services.* London: Royal Society of Medicine Press.

Crismon, M. L., M. Trivedi, T. A. Pigott, A. J. Rush, R. M. Hirschfeld, D. A. Kahn, C. DeBattista, J. C. Nelson, A. A. Nierenberg, H. A. Sackeim, and M. E. Thase. 1999. The Texas Medication Algorithm Project: Report of the Texas Consensus Conference panel on medication treatment of major depressive disorder. *Journal of Clinical Psychiatry* 60(3):142-156.

Emanuel, E. J., A. Wood, A. Fleischman, A. Bowen, K. A. Getz, C. Grady, C. Levine, D. E. Hammerschmidt, R. Faden, L. Eckenwiler, C. T. Muse, and J. Sugarman. 2004. Oversight of human participants research: Identifying problems to evaluate reform proposals. *Annals of Internal Medicine* 141(4):282-291.

Emrich, H. M. 1990. Studies with oxcarbazepine (trileptal) in acute mania. *International Clinical Psychopharmacology* (5):83-88.

Fava, M., A. J. Rush, M. H. Trivedi, A. A. Nierenberg, M. E. Thase, H. A. Sackeim, F. M. Quitkin, S. Wisniewski, P. W. Lavori, J. F. Rosenbaum, and D. J. Kupfer. 2003. Background and rationale for the sequenced treatment alternatives to relieve depression (STAR*D) study. *The Psychiatric Clinics of North America* 26(2):x, 457-494.

Fava, M., A. J. Rush, J. E. Alpert, G. K. Balasubramani, S. R. Wisniewski, C. N. Carmin, M. M. Biggs, S. Zisook, A. Leuchter, R. Howland, D. Warden, and M. H. Trivedi. 2008. Difference in treatment outcome in outpatients with anxious versus nonanxious depression: A STAR*D report. *American Journal of Psychiatry* 165(3):342-351.

Fontanarosa, P. B., and C. D. DeAngelis. 2002. Basic science and translational research in JAMA. *Journal of the American Medical Association* 287(13):1728.

Gawande, A. 2002. *Complications: A Surgeon's Notes on an Imperfect Science.* New York: Metropolitan Books.

————. 2007. *Better: A Surgeon's Notes on Performance.* New York: Metropolitan Books.

Haneuse, S. 2008. *Adjustment for selection bias in nueropathological studies of dementia; accounting for selection bias in a community-based neuropathological study of dementia.* Paper presented at Alzheimer's Association International Conference on Alzheimer's Disease.

Harmon, A. 2008. The DNA age: Gene map becomes a luxury item. *New York Times.* March 4, 2008.

Hinrichsen, V. L., B. Kruskal, M. A. O'Brien, T. A. Lieu, and R. Platt. 2007. Using electronic medical records to enhance detection and reporting of vaccine adverse events. *Journal of the American Medical Informatics Association* 14(6):731-735.

IOM (Institute of Medicine). 2000. *Extending Medicare Reimbursement in Clinical Trials.* Washington, DC: National Academy Press.

Jacobson, P. D., R. A. Rettig, and W. M. Aubry. 2007. Litigating the science of breast cancer treatment. *Journal of Health Politics, Policy, and Law* 32(5):785-818.

Katzan, I. L., A. J. Furlan, L. E. Lloyd, J. I. Frank, D. L. Harper, J. A. Hinchey, J. P. Hammel, A. Qu, and C. A. Sila. 2000. Use of tissue-type plasminogen activator for acute ischemic stroke: The Cleveland area experience. *Journal of the American Medical Association* 283(9):1151-1158.

Kohane, I. S., and R. B. Altman. 2005. Health-information altruists—a potentially critical resource. *New England Journal of Medicine* 353(19):2074-2077.

Kraemer, H. C., G. T. Wilson, C. G. Fairburn, and W. S. Agras. 2002. Mediators and moderators of treatment effects in randomized clinical trials. *Archives of General Psychiatry* 59(10):877-883.

Laje, G., S. Paddock, H. Manji, A. J. Rush, A. F. Wilson, D. Charney, and F. J. McMahon. 2007. Genetic markers of suicidal ideation emerging during citalopram treatment of major depression. *American Journal of Psychiatry* 164(10):1530-1538.

Lavori, P. W., A. J. Rush, S. R. Wisniewski, J. Alpert, M. Fava, D. J. Kupfer, A. Nierenberg, F. M. Quitkin, H. A. Sackeim, M. E. Thase, and M. Trivedi. 2001. Strengthening clinical effectiveness trials: Equipoise-stratified randomization. *Biological Psychiatry* 50(10):792-801.

Lenfant, C. 2003. Shattuck lecture—clinical research to clinical practice—lost in translation? *New England Journal of Medicine* 349(9):868-874.

Lumley, T. 2002. Network meta-analysis for indirect treatment comparisons. *Statistics in Medicine* 21(16):2313-2324.

March, J. S., S. G. Silva, S. Compton, M. Shapiro, R. Califf, and R. Krishnan. 2005. The case for practical clinical trials in psychiatry. *American Journal of Psychiatry* 162(5):836-846.

McKenna, R. J., A. Gelb, and M. Brenner. 2001. Lung volume reduction surgery for chronic obstructive pulmonary disease: Where do we stand? *World Journal of Surgery* 25:231-237.

Murphy, S. A., L. M. Collins, and A. J. Rush. 2007. Customizing treatment to the patient: Adaptive treatment strategies. *Drug and Alcohol Dependence* 88(Supl 2):S1-S3.

National Cancer Institute Cancer Control PLANET. 2008. *Plan, Link, Act, Network with Evidence-based Tools.* http://cancercontrolplanet.cancer.gov/ (accessed March 4, 2008).

Neaton, J. D., S. L. Normand, A. Gelijns, R. C. Starling, D. L. Mann, and M. A. Konstam. 2007. Designs for mechanical circulatory support device studies. *Journal of Cardiac Failure* 13(1):63-74.

Pearson, S. D., F. G. Miller, and E. J. Emanuel. 2006. Medicare's requirement for research participation as a condition of coverage: Is it ethical? *Journal of the American Medical Association* 296(8):988-991.

Pineau, J., M. G. Bellemare, A. J. Rush, A. Ghizaru, and S. A. Murphy. 2007. Constructing evidence-based treatment strategies using methods from computer science. *Drug Alcohol Depend* 88(Supl 2):S52-S60.

Platt, R., R. Davis, J. Finkelstein, A. S. Go, J. H. Gurwitz, D. Roblin, S. Soumerai, D. Ross-Degnan, S. Andrade, M. J. Goodman, B. Martinson, M. A. Raebel, D. Smith, M. Ulcickas-Yood, and K. A. Chan. 2001. Multicenter epidemiologic and health services research on therapeutics in the HMO Research Network Center for Education and Research on Therapeutics. *Pharmacoepidemiology and Drug Safety* 10(5):373-377.

Psaty, B. M., and C. D. Furberg. 2005. Cox-2 inhibitors—lessons in drug safety. *New England Journal of Medicine* 352(11):1133-1135.

———. 2007. The record on rosiglitazone and the risk of myocardial infarction. *New England Journal of Medicine* 357(1):67-69.

Ray, W. A. 2003. Evaluating medication effects outside of clinical trials: New-user designs. *American Journal of Epidemiology* 158(9):915-920.

Ray, W. A., P. B. Thapa, and P. Gideon. 2002. Misclassification of current benzodiazepine exposure by use of a single baseline measurement and its effects upon studies of injuries. *Pharmacoepidemiology and Drug Safety* 11(8):663-669.

Rettig, R., P. Jacobson, C. Farquhar, and W. M. Aubry. 2007. *False Hope: Bone Marrow Transplantation for Breast Cancer.* New York: Oxford University Press.

Riva, A., K. D. Mandl, D. H. Oh, D. J. Nigrin, A. Butte, P. Szolovits, and I. S. Kohane. 2001. The personal internetworked notary and guardian. *International Journal of Medical Informatics* 62(1):27-40.

Rush, A. 1999. Linking efficacy and effectiveness research in the evaluation of psychotherapies. In *Cost Effectiveness of Psychotherapy: A Guide for Practitioners, Researchers and Policymakers,* edited by N. Miller and K. Magruder. New York: Oxford University Press. Pp. 26-32.

———. 2005. Algorithm-guided treatment in depression: TMAP and STAR*D. In *Therapieresistente depressionen—aktueller wissensstand und leitlinien für die behandlung in klinik und praxis,* edited by M. Bauer, A. Berghofer, and M. Adli. Berlin-Heidelberg-New York: Springer. Pp. 459-476.

Rush, A., and D. Kupfer. 1995. Strategies and tactics in the treatment of depression. In *Treatments of Psychiatric Disorders.* Vol. 1, edited by G. Gabbard and S. Atkinson. Washington, DC: American Psychiatric Press. Pp. 1349-1368.

Rush, A. J., and R. F. Prien. 1995. From scientific knowledge to the clinical practice of psychopharmacology: Can the gap be bridged? *Psychopharmacology Bulletin* 31(1):7-20.

Rush, A. J., C. M. Gullion, M. R. Basco, R. B. Jarrett, and M. H. Trivedi. 1996. The inventory of depressive symptomatology (IDS): Psychometric properties. *Psychological Medicine* 26(3):477-486.

Rush, A. J., M. H. Trivedi, H. M. Ibrahim, T. J. Carmody, B. Arnow, D. N. Klein, J. C. Markowitz, P. T. Ninan, S. Kornstein, R. Manber, M. E. Thase, J. H. Kocsis, and M. B. Keller. 2003. The 16-item quick inventory of depressive symptomatology (QIDS), clinician rating (QIDS-C), and self-report (QIDS-SR): A psychometric evaluation in patients with chronic major depression. *Biological Psychiatry* 54(5):573-583.

Rush, A. J., M. Fava, S. R. Wisniewski, P. W. Lavori, M. H. Trivedi, H. A. Sackeim, M. E. Thase, A. A. Nierenberg, F. M. Quitkin, T. M. Kashner, D. J. Kupfer, J. F. Rosenbaum, J. Alpert, J. W. Stewart, P. J. McGrath, M. M. Biggs, K. Shores-Wilson, B. D. Lebowitz, L. Ritz, and G. Niederehe. 2004. Sequenced treatment alternatives to relieve depression (STAR*D): Rationale and design. *Controlled Clinical Trials* 25(1):119-142.

Rush, A. J., M. H. Trivedi, S. R. Wisniewski, A. A. Nierenberg, J. W. Stewart, D. Warden, G. Niederehe, M. E. Thase, P. W. Lavori, B. D. Lebowitz, P. J. McGrath, J. F. Rosenbaum, H. A. Sackeim, D. J. Kupfer, J. Luther, and M. Fava. 2006. Acute and longer-term outcomes in depressed outpatients requiring one or several treatment steps: A STAR*D report. *American Journal of Psychiatry* 163(11):1905-1917.

Rush, A. J., S. R. Wisniewski, D. Warden, J. F. Luther, L. L. Davis, M. Fava, A. A. Nierenberg, and M. H. Trivedi. 2008. Selecting among second-step antidepressant medication mono-therapies: Predictive value of clinical, demographic, or first-step treatment features. *Archives of General Psychiatry* 65(8):870-880.

Schenker, N., and T. E. Raghunathan. 2007. Combining information from multiple surveys to enhance estimation of measures of health. *Statistics in Medicine* 26(8):1802-1811.

Simon, G. E., M. VonKorff, J. H. Heiligenstein, D. A. Revicki, L. Grothaus, W. Katon, and E. H. Wagner. 1996. Initial antidepressant choice in primary care. Effectiveness and cost of fluoxetine vs tricyclic antidepressants. *Journal of the American Medical Association* 275(24):1897-1902.

Simons, W. W., K. D. Mandl, and I. S. Kohane. 2005. The ping personally controlled electronic medical record system: Technical architecture. *Journal of the American Medical Informatics Association* 12(1):47-54.

Smith, N. L., P. J. Savage, S. R. Heckbert, J. I. Barzilay, V. A. Bittner, L. H. Kuller, and B. M. Psaty. 2002. Glucose, blood pressure, and lipid control in older people with and without diabetes mellitus: The Cardiovascular Health Study. *Journal of the America Geriatric Society* 50(3):416-423.

Sonnen, J. A., E. B. Larson, P. K. Crane, S. Haneuse, G. Li, G. D. Schellenberg, S. Craft, J. B. Leverenz, and T. J. Montine. 2007. Pathological correlates of dementia in a longitudinal, population-based sample of aging. *Annals of Neurology* 62(4):406-413.

Spiegelhalter, D. J., K. R. Abrams, J. P. Myles. 2004. *Bayesian Approaches to Clinical Trials and Health-care Evaluation.* West Sussex, England: John Wiley & Sons, Ltd.

Stern, S. L., A. J. Rush, and J. Mendels. 1980. Toward a rational pharmacotherapy of depression. *American Journal of Psychiatry* 137(5):545-552.

Sung, N. S., W. F. Crowley, Jr., M. Genel, P. Salber, L. Sandy, L. M. Sherwood, S. B. Johnson, V. Catanese, H. Tilson, K. Getz, E. L. Larson, D. Scheinberg, E. A. Reece, H. Slavkin, A. Dobs, J. Grebb, R. A. Martinez, A. Korn, and D. Rimoin. 2003. Central challenges facing the national clinical research enterprise. *Journal of the American Medical Association* 289(10):1278-1287.

Taplin, S. H., L. Ichikawa, M. U. Yood, M. M. Manos, A. M. Geiger, S. Weinmann, J. Gilbert, J. Mouchawar, W. A. Leyden, R. Altaras, R. K. Beverly, D. Casso, E. O. Westbrook, K. Bischoff, J. G. Zapka, and W. E. Barlow. 2004. Reason for late-stage breast cancer: Absence of screening or detection, or breakdown in follow-up? *Journal of the National Cancer Institute* 96(20):1518-1527.

Thompson, W. W., C. Price, B. Goodson, D. K. Shay, P. Benson, V. L. Hinrichsen, E. Lewis, E. Eriksen, P. Ray, S. M. Marcy, J. Dunn, L. A. Jackson, T. A. Lieu, S. Black, G. Stewart, E. S. Weintraub, R. L. Davis, and F. DeStefano. 2007. Early thimerosal exposure and neuropsychological outcomes at 7 to 10 years. *New England Journal of Medicine* 357(13):1281-1292.

Trivedi, M. H., A. J. Rush, M. L. Crismon, T. M. Kashner, M. G. Toprac, T. J. Carmody, T. Key, M. M. Biggs, K. Shores-Wilson, B. Witte, T. Suppes, A. L. Miller, K. Z. Altshuler, and S. P. Shon. 2004a. Clinical results for patients with major depressive disorder in the Texas Medication Algorithm Project. *Archives of General Psychiatry* 61(7):669-680.

Trivedi, M. H., A. J. Rush, H. M. Ibrahim, T. J. Carmody, M. M. Biggs, T. Suppes, M. L. Crismon, K. Shores-Wilson, M. G. Toprac, E. B. Dennehy, B. Witte, and T. M. Kashner. 2004b. The inventory of depressive symptomatology, clinician rating (IDS-C) and self-report (IDS-SR), and the quick inventory of depressive symptomatology, clinician rating (QIDS-C) and self-report (QIDS-SR) in public sector patients with mood disorders: A psychometric evaluation. *Psychological Medicine* 34(1):73-82.

Trivedi, M. H., M. Fava, S. R. Wisniewski, M. E. Thase, F. Quitkin, D. Warden, L. Ritz, A. A. Nierenberg, B. D. Lebowitz, M. M. Biggs, J. F. Luther, K. Shores-Wilson, and A. J. Rush. 2006a. Medication augmentation after the failure of SSRIS for depression. *New England Journal of Medicine* 354(12):1243-1252.

Trivedi, M. H., A. J. Rush, S. R. Wisniewski, A. A. Nierenberg, D. Warden, L. Ritz, G. Norquist, R. H. Howland, B. Lebowitz, P. J. McGrath, K. Shores-Wilson, M. M. Biggs, G. K. Balasubramani, and M. Fava. 2006b. Evaluation of outcomes with citalopram for depression using measurement-based care in STAR*D: Implications for clinical practice. *American Journal of Psychiatry* 163(1):28-40.

Tunis, S. R., D. B. Stryer, and C. M. Clancy. 2003. Practical clinical trials: Increasing the value of clinical research for decision making in clinical and health policy. *Journal of the American Medical Association* 290(12):1624-1632.

U.S. Department of Health and Human Services. 2008a. *American Health Information Community.* http://www.hhs.gov/healthit/community/background/ (accessed March 4, 2008).

———. 2008b. *Office of the National Coordinator for Health Information Technology: Mission.* http://www.hhs.gov/healthit/onc/mission/ (accessed March 4, 2008).

U.S. Department of Health and Human Services, Public Health Service, and Agency for Health Care Policy and Research. 1993. Clinical Practice Guideline, Number 5: Depression in Primary Care: Volume 2. Treatment of Major Depression. Rockville, MD: U.S. Department of Health and Human Services, Public Health Service, and Agency for Healthcare Research and Quality.

Wagner, E. H., P. Barrett, M. J. Barry, W. Barlow, and F. J. Fowler, Jr. 1995. The effect of a shared decisionmaking program on rates of surgery for benign prostatic hyperplasia. Pilot results. *Medical Care* 33(8):765-770.

Wagner, E. H., S. M. Greene, G. Hart, T. S. Field, S. Fletcher, A. M. Geiger, L. J. Herrinton, M. C. Hornbrook, C. C. Johnson, J. Mouchawar, S. J. Rolnick, V. J. Stevens, S. H. Taplin, D. Tolsma, and T. M. Vogt. 2005. Building a research consortium of large health systems: The cancer research network. *Journal of the National Cancer Institute Monographs* (35):3-11.

Wideroff, L., A. N. Freedman, L. Olson, C. N. Klabunde, W. Davis, K. P. Srinath, R. T. Croyle, and R. Ballard-Barbash. 2003. Physician use of genetic testing for cancer susceptibility: Results of a national survey. *Cancer Epidemiology, Biomarkers & Prevention* 12(4):295-303.

Wilensky, G. 2006. Developing a center for comparative effectiveness information. *Health Affairs* 25(6):w572-w585.

Wisniewski, S. R., M. Fava, M. H. Trivedi, M. E. Thase, D. Warden, G. Niederehe, E. S. Friedman, M. M. Biggs, H. A. Sackeim, K. Shores-Wilson, P. J. McGrath, P. W. Lavori, S. Miyahara, and A. J. Rush. 2007. Acceptability of second-step treatments to depressed outpatients: A STAR*D report. *American Journal of Psychiatry* 164(5):753-760.

Woolf, S. H. 2008. The meaning of translational research and why it matters. *Journal of the American Medical Association* 299(2):211-213.

Zerhouni, E. A. 2005a. Translational and clinical science—time for a new vision. *New England Journal of Medicine* 353(15):1621-1623.

————. 2005b. U.S. biomedical research: Basic, translational, and clinical sciences. *Journal of the American Medical Association* 294(11):1352-1358.

Zubenko, G. S., M. Wusylko, B. M. Cohen, F. Boller, and I. Teply. 1987. Family study of platelet membrane fluidity in Alzheimer's disease. *Science* 238(4826):539-542.

6

Aligning Policy with Research Opportunities

INTRODUCTION

The scope of the reforms in clinical effectiveness research—that were the focus of the Redesigning the Clinical Effectiveness Research Paradigm workshop and that are discussed in this report—are truly broad and will deeply affect long-held practices and tenets. However, bringing such change about will require much more than new and improved methodologies. Instead, many stakeholders will need to significantly engage in reform. Cross-sector collaboration is needed to create a focus and to set priorities, to clarify the questions that must be addressed, and to marshal the resources that the reform effort requires. Moreover, the sheer scope of change needed requires stakeholders who are diverse, but working together toward common goals. A coordinated, public- and private-sector effort historically has been imperative to secure funding for such efforts and to coordinate spending strategically. Such collaborations also are vital to moving forward on the establishment of standards, such as common language for electronic health records (EHRs). Furthermore, government interventions are widely considered necessary to remove perceived policy impediments to progress. One example, stated earlier in this summary, is to address the chill on clinical research imposed by real and perceived barriers and burdens from the ways privacy rules and Institutional Review Boards (IRBs) are interpreted and structured.[1] In addition, broad partnerships are needed to effect wide access to and sharing of

---

[1] Since this workshop the Institute of Medicine (IOM) has released a report that assesses the impact of the Health Insurance Portability and Accountability Act (HIPAA) Privacy Rule on the conduct of health research and provides recommendations for ensuring the efficient conduct of research while maintaining or strengthening the privacy protections of personally

data, considered another linchpin of progress. This chapter outlines some policy levers that can drive innovative research and progress in practice-based approaches as well as the potential roles that various healthcare stakeholders can play to accelerate progress.

Focused on course-of-care data, Greg Pawlson of the National Committee for Quality Assurance describes a major opportunity to use these clinical data for "rapid learning." By capturing the experience of each patient and clinician in a structured and quantifiable manner, EHR systems have great potential to help transform our capacity to develop information that can be used as important evidence in making clinical decisions. Policy interventions will play a crucial role in improving the development of and access to databases that are suitable for clinical effectiveness research. With product approval increasingly tied to postmarket trial or database commitments to demonstrate the value of treatments, health product developers also are contending with a variety of issues related to the development and use of data for clinical effectiveness analyses. Merck's Peter K. Honig discusses several key challenges that manufacturers face in responding to these demands. Those challenges include finding a suitable balance between demands for data transparency and maintaining competitive advantage, and improving the methods used to develop clinical effectiveness information.

Recognizing that the scope and scale of existing and future evidence gaps exceed any one entity's capacity to address all of the needs related to improving evidence availability and application to improve practice, Mark B. McClellan of the Brookings Institution advocates that other approaches also are needed. These approaches should take better advantage of regulatory data that offers a rich opportunity to improve our knowledge base. McClellan cites the Food and Drug Administration Amendment Act of 2007 (FDAAA) and the Medicare Coverage with Evidence Development policy as models for how regulatory data can be integrated successfully into the ongoing capacity to develop better evidence on what works and, in turn, inform medical practice. Another speaker, J. Sanford Schwartz of the University of Pennsylvania, acknowledges that large amounts of data generated and supported by public investment provide innovative opportunities to inform clinical and comparative effectiveness assessment, but that substantial barriers must be passed for optimal use of these data. Schwartz offers a series of suggestions to mitigate the following paradox: We have large amounts of data and significant opportunities, but we are prevented from fully accessing the data and taking advantage of potential opportunities. In view of the reality that evidence-based medicine (EBM) requires integration of clinical expertise and research and depends on an infrastructure

---

identifiable health information (*Beyond the HIPAA Privacy Rule: Enhancing Privacy, Improving Health Through Research*).

that includes human capital and organizational platforms, the head of the recently created Office of Portfolio Analysis and Strategic Initiatives at the National Institutes of Health (NIH), Alan M. Krensky, describes ongoing commitments with the NIH to build a sustainable research infrastructure centered on EBM principles. Finally, Kathy Hudson of Johns Hopkins University describes work to assess public perspectives on research and efforts to engage the public and the research community in dialogue and consultation designed to weave consumer perspectives into research design, encourage consumer participation in study recruitment and retention, and generally build a relationship of enhanced trust and understanding between healthcare consumers and the research community.

COURSE-OF-CARE DATA

Greg Pawlson, M.D.
National Committee for Quality Assurance

There have been a number of conferences and publications, including an entire web *Health Affairs* volume, that have articulated the major developing opportunity to use clinical data collected for patient care (course of care data) for "rapid learning" (Etheredge, 2007; Pawlson, 2007). Rapid learning using clinical data implies that we should be able to capture the experience of each patient with each clinician in a structured and quantifiable manner similar to what we now do in formal research studies, to extend, but not entirely replace classic clinical research using randomized controlled trials (RCTs). For the purposes of this paper, we will include clinical effectiveness, health services, and other related research using large clinical databases as within the scope and definition of rapid learning. However, much of rapid learning is still far from a reality, not only because of spotty use of information technology but also because of policy and related barriers that have created a "chasm" between clinical and health services research (efforts to systematically and scientifically add to our knowledge of patient care) and the actual care of patients in practice. These barriers range from the way we fund, or in many cases do not fund, clinical and health services research, to the structure of data in most electronic records, to the form and content of health professions education. While solutions are not easy or even all that evident, we would propose the following be explored: (1) enhanced funding for health services research linked much more closely and coordinated with funding for basic and clinical research; (2) a private–public partnership, **with strong input from the research community along with others,** to set standards for what and how data is entered and retrieved from electronic medical records (EMRs), (3) an active effort to insure that data from health plans and the growing number of data consortia (Health

Information Exchanges [HIEs] and Regional Health Information Organization [RHIOs]) and similar efforts, provide more open and affordable access to legitimate researchers and educators from academic and other institutions; (4) that Health Insurance Portability and Accountability Act (HIPAA) regulations be reviewed, modified, and delimited to remove the major barriers imposed on research and rapid learning that pose NO direct risk for patients; and (5) that health professions, and especially medical, education recognize and incorporate knowledge and skills related to the use of clinical data for new knowledge.

To begin this overview, imagine a healthcare encounter in the future in which a clinician is seeing a patient with multiple cardiovascular risk factors, including obesity. The clinician records all critical parameters that are needed to follow a patient in a set of carefully structured data fields in an EMR. That data is then merged and compared to data on similar patients both within that physicians' own practice, as well as across other patients in other practices. The EMR has a decision support tool that analyzes all the data including genomic information, helps the clinician delineate and understand the precise level of the patient's cardiovascular risk (i.e., which are the critical factors to consider whether blood pressure is more of an issue than cholesterol, etc.), and provides a recommendation for treatment pathways and interventions. In this scenario, the EMR might recommend a relatively newly approved agent for hypertension as well as indicate any additional data needed to track potential treatment effects and side effects. Over the course of treatment, this patient's data is combined with those of all other patients currently taking the "new" medication in an electronic health records environment. This data (some patient identified and some de-identified depending on the need and permissions) is fed back to the individual clinician, regulatory agencies, and researchers with an interest in this medication, to provide data on how this medication, in comparison to other possible medications, is performing in actually use, both for the specific patient and for similar patients. The EHR system also could provide decision support within all attached EMRs to help clinicians to determine if the specific medication is still optimal. All of these linkages and feedback loops can be subsumed under the term "rapid learning" using health information technology (HIT).

The reality of the current situation, in most clinical settings, is far from the efficient, evidence-based practice presented in the scenario, and many barriers impede progress toward this ideal. Although a critical step, implementation of EMRs alone, or even interoperable EMRs linked in an EHR, will be sufficient to achieve this standard of care. Indeed, studies have suggested that to achieve the highest quality standard of practice today, EMRs are necessary but not sufficient (Ozcam and Kazley, 2008; Solberg et al., 2005).

Research and development funding and research focus also are major barriers to the use of electronic data for rapid learning. There is widespread acknowledgement that the current levels of funding for health services research (as contrasted with basic biological research) is far from adequate. Beyond insufficient funding, the priorities and compartmentalization of the budgets of major public (the Agency for Healthcare Research and Quality [AHRQ], NIH, Centers for Disease Control and Prevention, Department of Veteran Affairs) and private (foundations and corporations) make it difficult for researchers in a new area such as rapid learning to piece together stable funding to even begin to create the data exchange and protocols that may be required prior to initiation and testing of rapid learning. Funding for infrastructure development in the HIT area is even more problematic. While there are some efforts that are at least tangentially related to rapid learning, such as the Practice Research Network funded by the AHRQ, Aligning Forces for Quality funded by the Robert Wood Johnson Foundation, or various RHIOs and HIEs, most efforts are very underfunded and none that we are aware of directly address issues of rapid learning.

Also related to research, there continues to be a large chasm between clinical practice and even health services research. Academics often focus on datasets that are close at hand, such as those in hospitals, faculty practices, or residents' clinics. It is often challenging to identify, understand, and use data from a source outside of the academic environment, and in some instances, it is either difficult to obtain permission to use the data or substantial charges are attached to using data from private settings. However, one of the reasons that academics do tend to use available databases is the difficulty and often cost of using databases from health plans or other sources that might actually have broad and useful data.

Another barrier that presents a challenge is that electronic data standards, including those for EMRs, are still far from complete, especially the critical parameters to guide what data should be included in EMRs and how that data can be entered in fields that lend themselves to retrieval and analysis. Efforts to even do basic clinical performance measurement using EMR data (as contrasted with claims data) are often stymied by missing data (such as left ventricular ejection fraction) or fields that are non-standardized across EMRs. While several groups, including The National Quality Forum, the Office of the National Coordinator (for HIT), and a collaborative headed by the American Medical Association with the National Committee for Quality Assurance and the EMR Vendors Association (EMRVA) and others, are working on various aspects of the problem, there are few linkages of any of this work to the research community, and the work is far from complete. The issue that is perhaps the most neglected is the lack of attention to completeness of clinical data recorded on any given patient. While tangential events such as malpractice claims, audits around submitted claims for insurance or reporting for quality purposes may have some impact on efforts to have more complete data, there is little if any standardization, even within EMRs sold by a given vendor, around either defining what data elements are critical for patient care (and therefore should be nearly universally recorded) let alone in what fields or format the data are entered. Few, if any, efforts or programs are in place to enhance the training of clinicians in data entry (beyond how to enhance billing) and there are few direct rewards for enhanced data or consequences for poor data entry.

A less apparent but potentially crippling barrier is the increasing conflation of the regulation of direct human subjects in research with secondary data analysis for general knowledge. Interpretation of HIPAA, and especially the use of personal health information (PHI) is core; there are others at play as well. Since rapid learning requires secondary analysis and use of data gathered for clinical care or quality improvement purposes, how research and PHI issues are handled directly affects rapid learning. All agree that individual patients who are research subjects need to have careful oversight and protection from undue risk from all forms of research. However, it would seem that the risks to patients from data that have already been collected to monitor and assist in their own care are both quantitatively and qualitatively different from primary data collection for research purposes. Finally, there have been several incidents in which projects that have been centered on quality improvement (which is in many ways very analogous to rapid learning) have been either stopped or subject to multiple delays because they were seen or treated like primary clinical research. It is not clear how current approaches to research or PHI would treat the flow and exchange of information in our initial scenario, but there is likely to be little investment in pursuing rapid learning unless these issues are addressed.

Fortunately there are some policy interventions that could be important in overcome these barriers. With respect to the inadequacy and compartmentalization of funding, improvements are needed in the way that research and clinical learning involving HIT are funded and coordinated by both the public sector (the U.S. Department of Health and Human Services including NIH, AHRQ, and Centers for Disease Control and Prevention), Department of Defense, the Department of Veteran Affairs, and the Department of Homeland Security and the private sector, so that our overall expenditures of dollars in research and HIT better reflect national priorities. A more dramatic scenario would be to combine AHRQ and NIH budgets or to place the planning of all public-sector research and HIT development-related budgets under strong central executive branch oversight with requirements coordination for overall healthcare research budgeting. A shorter term, and more immediately critical issues is that to capitalize on the potential of greatly enhanced health care data sources, the proportion of funding for secondary database use and other health services research should be markedly increased. Calls for more funding are always viewed as easy to say but difficult to bring off given entrenched interests even within the research communities, let alone elsewhere. As it has in the past in some areas, a very clear and focused signal from the Institute of Medicine could have a substantial impact in breaking the political and policy logjam in this area.

Policy changes are also important in fostering the development of a more widely effective HIT clinical data program that might support rapid learning. Such policies should incentivize the utilization of data collected at the point of care in rapid learning and in related research efforts. Additional funding could facilitate the development of research and educational development teams that could work with health insurers, EMR vendors, and others in the creation and production of data useful for research. As previously noted, examples of this sort of linkage (e.g., HMO Research Network, AHRQ's Practice Based Research Networks [PBRNs]) are few and far between and painfully underfunded. AHRQ and NIH review panels should include more researchers and data experts with practice and clinical systems HIT backgrounds. More open and affordable access should be provided by insurers and others to large clinical databases that could be the basis of expanding opportunities for the knowledge that is critical to rapid learning. Pediatric cancer care may provide a useful example, as virtually all of the treatment provided in pediatric oncology is recorded and applied to registries or active clinical trials, which then informs the optional future care for children ongoing treatment.

To address the lack of standardization of data elements in EMRs, and to appropriately harness this resource for comparative or clinical effectiveness research or for rapid learning, researchers must be actively involved in the many discussions and organizations that are working to set standards for EMRs. In work to define common data elements, cross-link different systems, and develop approaches to the retrieval and coherent use of datasets, the input of the research community is greatly needed to ensure that critical fields, parameters, and measurements are built into the system. While there might be some hope that, as with data protocols involving ATM cards, the private sector might develop the appropriate conventions, there is a substantial presence of the public sector in health care (whether in financing such as Medicare or Medicaid or delivery of care as in the Department of Defense and the Department of Veteran Affairs). Thus only a core effort directed across multiple executive branch agencies (the U.S. Department of Health and Human Services, Department of Defense, the Department of Veteran Affairs, the Department of Homeland Security, and others) with strong and continuing liaisons and input from the private sector would seem likely to succeed. Requirements for interoperability between EMRs and other data sources; the use of standard protocols for inserting and modifying elements and extracting data related to guidelines, performance measurement, and research-knowledge expansion; and the involvement of researchers from AHRQ, NIH, and elsewhere in decisions being made about data elements in EMRs and connectivity between data sources are all areas in which a cross-departmental effort might be critical. While congressional jurisdictions might be an impediment to such an effort within the executive branch, the effects of HIT on the nearly $3 trillion healthcare sector could actually dwarf those within the banking community in the adoption of ATMs.

To address the conflation of research and quality improvement, policies are needed that protect patients but do not unduly constrain the use of secondary data that can add to our generalizable knowledge. Focused, expedited reviews of quality improvement and or research protocols that deal with secondary data could be done by groups other than the traditional IRB. To improve the clinician's ability to use data, all medical and nursing students graduating after 2015 should be required to have the equivalent of an MPH degree with a focus on population health and the use of individual and aggregated data in the care of patients. State and federal medical education funding (including Graduate Medical Education) could be tied to medical student and residency program participation in quality and resource use improvement training. Finally, a push is needed by the public and the research community to encourage boards and medical organizations to address deficiencies in the performance of practicing physicians (recertification).

Finally, to contend with the current lack of data connectivity, beyond requiring EMRs to have core capability to aggregate data across patients and to provide standardized outputs of data, the further development of HIEs, RHIOs, or other efforts at regional aggregation or exchange of clinical data is key. While supporting patient care at point of care delivery is the most important facet of this work, benchmarking, assessment, public reporting and rapid learning (both research and direct care related) should be incorporated into these efforts.

In conclusion, this appears to be a critical moment in the development of EMRs and EHRs, which have the potential to provide complete, real-world data to inform clinical practices, help to develop needed clinical effectiveness information, improve the systematic quality of care, and produce a rapid, evidence-based method of continuous practice improvement. Unless the substantial barriers to progress are addressed quickly and collectively, the United States may well fall far behind in yet another critical aspect of health care.

PHARMACEUTICAL INDUSTRY DATA

Peter K. Honig, M.D., M.P.H.
Merck Research Laboratories
Merck & Co., Inc.

The pharmaceutical industry is challenged with meeting the demands of an increasingly complex and evolving healthcare system. Regulatory, stakeholder, payer, and patient demands for increased data requirements, transparency, access, and value represent formidable issues in the areas of benefit–risk assessment, ongoing safety assessment, and comparative effectiveness. Several important initiatives are under way to address these challenges; however, significant opportunities remain that are amenable to research and policy remediation, including clinical trial and pharmaco-vigilance methodologies, data standards and access, as well as the perpetual challenge of education focused on translating evidence into behaviors.

The pharmaceutical industry is operating in a changing healthcare ecosystem. Although explicit regulatory registration evidentiary standards have not significantly changed (i.e., evidence of safety and efficacy demonstrated through adequate and well-controlled clinical investigations), regulatory and social acceptance of residual uncertainty around benefit risk has changed significantly over the past several years. Increasingly, the FDA and other regulators around the world are exercising the precautionary principle and, at times, creating barriers to new drugs reaching the market. While not affecting drugs with profound benefits in addressing unmet medical needs, some drugs occupy a grayer area of risk–benefit and are becoming harder to bring to market. Moreover the interest in risk management has led to increased postmarket clinical trial and database commitments included as a prerequisite of approval.

Payers and providers also are increasing their demands for demonstration of value. The downturn in development of "me too" drugs is, in part, an appropriate outcome of the fact that most payers will not pay for these drugs unless there is an explicit demonstration of incremental value. The commercial failure of Exubera, an inhaled insulin product, and the reimbursement challenges experienced by follow-on, TNF sequestrants for rheumatoid arthritis resulted from their perceived lack of demonstrated incremental benefit over existing therapies.

Along with these healthcare ecosystem changes, large pharmaceutical companies face continually rising costs of drug development, decreasing output of new therapeutics, and an increased number of companies competing in the fields of drug discovery and development. Basic and translational research is no longer the sole province of large integrated pharmaceutical companies but now occurs increasingly outside of the walls of industry in academic centers and smaller companies. There has been significant progress in drug development with substantial advances with regards to improved animal models of efficacy/toxicity, using system biology approaches to target identification, efficacy and safety biomarkers, dose–response methodologies, pharmacokinetic and pharmcodynamic modeling (exposure response), clinical trial simulations, disease progression models, demographic representativeness in clinical trials, and genetic and environmental predictors of pharmacodynamic response (e.g., whole genome screening). In spite of these advances, drug development remains a high-risk, high-cost proposition.

The industry is facing challenges with regard to data transparency and data access expectations. Congress recently passed the Food and Drug Administration Amendments Act of 2007, which included language about data transparency, registration, and access. Many states also are involved in this issue, developing their own laws around disclosure and transparency. Major medical journal editors also are expressing their perspectives and implanting policies around registration requirements and independent validation of results. Internationally, the World Health Organization (WHO) is also weighing in on registration transparency. The balance between transparency and proprietary considerations in a highly competitive environment remains a significant concern to industry.

Of particular interest is public- and private-sector access to utilization and claims outcome data. While a concern to the field generally, it is of particular importance to industry because of the increased need to access data to support necessary and required epidemiologic, pharmacovigilance, and outcomes research work with increasingly commoditized and proprietary data sources. Also, the data exist as decentralized and disaggregated nonstandardized clusters. This becomes a challenge, for example, in safety surveillance of rate adverse reactions, which require analysis or large number of data records across databases.

Finally, the industry faces formidable issues in the area of re-establishing trust. Trust between and among healthcare sectors including but not limited to industry is quite low. In particular, much has been done to undermine the authority and the credibility of the provider in the eyes of the patient.

To address some of these challenges, several notable initiatives are underway. Clearly the FDA's Critical Path initiative has laid the groundwork for improved science-driven regulatory evolution. Likewise, there is the Innovative Medicine Initiative (IMI) in Europe. Both exist and advocate public–private partnerships in the precompetitive space as a means of addressing significant drug discovery and development challenges (e.g., preclinical safety biomarkers). Active comparators are being increasingly incorporated into clinical registration studies and post-approval clinical trials, in part, to demonstrate incremental value. It is important to note that it is and will always remain a challenge to address every clinical question by means of randomized clinical trials. This has been recognized by the Institute of Medicine (IOM) and other groups and is the subject of a growing professional discipline around demonstration of absolute and relative clinical effectiveness. There also are some efforts underway to have more structured approaches to benefit–risk assessment. While recognizing that benefit–risk assessment will likely never be reduced to algorithmic quantitative science, it is amenable to structured methods that can inform clinical and regulatory judgment. It must be acknowledged that benefit–risk assessment is contextual and, at times, relative to currently available therapies. Clinical science still lacks the ability to quantify comparative benefits even when we believe they exist. For example there are many selective seratonin reuptake inhibitor and seratonin reuptake inhibitor on the market for the treatment of major depression, but it has never demonstrated that one works better than another or that there is variation in patient response to each drug. Lack of truly meaningful and sensitive clinical end-points, such as depression scales, can effectively blur differences. More work is need in trial methodologies and validation of sensitive and relevant end-points to address these problems. The same challenge exists for assessment of absolute and relative effectiveness. These are difficult to do before a drug comes onto the market, and better methods are needed once they come onto the market. More insight is needed on the appropriate role for natural-use studies, cluster randomization, and other types of novel trial designs.

Large, simple efficacy and safety trials are often viewed as a panacea. But little work has been done to set standards for these types of trials. Fundamental questions such as What is large? and What is simple? remain unanswered. Perceived regulatory monitoring expectations confound efforts to simplify data collection and make these less simple than they could be. They are large, but they are not so simple, and they are extremely expensive. There also are important distinctions for the design and content analysis of large simple trials for safety. Issues such as of choice of relevant patient population, relevant comparator and the adequate sizing of such studies are important considerations. There is not uniform consensus on some other basic principles around large simple trials such as whether to take an intention-to-treat (ITT) approach or a per protocol approach. For safety trials, exposure is the important variable and an ITT approach probably isn't the generally appropriate approach. This is in contradistinction to the established primary approach for evaluation of efficacy in large trials. Finally, who should conduct and pay for these trials? The NIH has historically taken up these large trials, but should others such as Centers for Medicare & Medicaid Services (CMS) or industry also contribute? These sort of fundamental issues have not been addressed.

It is encouraging that rigor and standards in pharmaco-epidemiology and meta-analysis practice have been recognized as something that continues to be addressed. Prespecification of hypotheses, scientific methods to control bias, data analysis and statistical analysis plans are now widely accepted as standard practice. Independent replication of results has long been an evidentiary standard for clinical trials and increasingly being accepted by the nonfrequentist community. Registries and sentinel and population- based pharmacovigilance systems are being developed, and equal attention is needed on improving the methodologies.

The application of Bayesian statistical approaches in the field of pharmacovigilance through the evaluation of spontaneous reports and population-based data is an active field of research. There is an initiative involving the collaboration of industry and the FDA to evaluating the potential for electronic medical records for postmarket surveillance efforts.

Finally, the ultimate challenge that faces all of us is to improve the translation of knowledge into behavior. Evidence gaps may persist, but it is still frustrating that best practices and new evidence is not optimally incorporated into patient care. New research, practice guidelines as well as medical product labeling all contain information that is important to consider in choosing patient care options. The translation of population-derived information into individual patient care is a challenge that is being addressed through EMR standards, computerized physician order entry (CPOE), and the teaching of evidence-based decision making, but there is much work to be done.

The medical education system may not adequately address needs in basic pharmacology and clinical pharmacology let alone clinical effectiveness. Concerns about new trainees' ability to interpret sophisticated analyses of the medical and pharmacologic literature have been raised, but not addressed on a national level, and currently do not include training in the incorporation of evidence into clinical practice. Changes in medical education may help advocates of evidence-based practice to achieve more improvements in care.

REGULATORY REQUIREMENTS AND DATA GENERATION

Mark B. McClellan, M.P.A., M.D., Ph.D.
Engelberg Center for Health Care Reform
The Brookings Institution

The recent public debates in Congress and in other settings on developing the capacity for comparative effectiveness research have generally focused on providing new funding and adding a new entity to the healthcare system. However, even if such an entity is established, perhaps making billions of dollars of new funding available, it is important to recognize that the scope and scale of existing and future evidence gaps exceed any single entity's capacity to address all of the needs related to improving evidence availability and application to improve practice. Other approaches are needed, and, in this respect, taking better advantage of regulatory data offers a rich opportunity to improve our knowledge base.

A major theme of the larger efforts of the IOM Roundtable on Value & Science-Driven Health Care is that the core of a learning healthcare system is not something added—through funding or new structures—but rather, is something that is built into the system that improves the efficiency, quantity, and quality of electronic data captured, enables the delivery of more sophisticated information in the actual delivery of health care, and establishes the routine capacity to learn from medical practices. Distributed data networks have been discussed as a way to facilitate these types of learnings. Because this information will not be derived from traditional randomized clinical trials, support will be needed for infrastructure, data aggregation, and analysis, and for improving the relevant statistical methods. Given the slow movement in Congress on comparative effectiveness, for the short term, a priority should be to enhance the healthcare system's capacity to generate data as a routine part of care and to use these data to learn what works in practice. This paper will highlight a couple of areas where regulatory data and prior Congressional action might help to make this happen and where it may be more feasible and may not cost billions more dollars to put this data capacity into place.

Two examples are immediately relevant to this discussion. First, the recently passed Food and Drug Administration Amendment Act of 2007 (FDAAA) envisioned a new postmarket surveillance infrastructure. Second, Medicare data that historically have primarily focused on administrative information for payment issues has the potential to be collected and used in a more sophisticated and clinically relevant way. FDAAA does more than reauthorize user fees and expand agency regulatory authority. This bill does nothing short of envision an additional built-in infrastructure in our healthcare system for developing postmarket evidence. By 2012, an active postmarket surveillance system will be available to provide information about the experience of more than 100 million Americans. This represents a fundamental change to the way we monitor and follow up on suspected safety problems with medical products; it also has the potential to serve as a first step toward introducing a more routine infrastructure into the healthcare system that can be used to address questions about the use of products in different types of patients and populations, and potentially to address effectiveness issues as well.

This kind of system is increasingly feasible as we move towards more electronic data. The pressing need to improve safety surveillance capacity has been underscored by recent shortfalls of the existing passive surveillance system. For example, the current system's dependence upon spontaneous reporting failed to detect important safety signals such as the higher rate of adverse events in the longitudinal cardiovascular outcomes related to Vioxx. Simulations carried out by the HMO Research Network have demonstrated that with an active surveillance system in place, this higher rate could have been detected in a matter of months rather than multiple years. If the vision articulated in the FDAAA is taken up and implemented effectively, the result could lead to more efficient detection and quicker action on drug labeling and use, and the ability to characterize adverse events much more quickly and precisely. These advances would, in turn, lead to more graded and timely responses from the FDA in regulatory action—not just in pulling a drug off the market, but perhaps using other kinds of labeling refinements because of increased confidence about how drugs are actually being used in the population. Finally, it opens up the opportunity for supporting improvements in evidence-based medical practices and providing some alternatives to the current approaches to addressing safety issues.

Several interesting pilot projects are under way to begin building this kind of infrastructure. Progress will require the development of standards and consistent methods for defining adverse events and pooling relevant summary data from large-scale analyses, as well as efforts to overcome issues that impede data sharing. Much can be learned about drug risks and benefits from observational studies of large population datasets; for questions that require randomization or other statistical approaches, these databases also have great potential to help design targeted trials or post-market clinical studies. Perhaps eventually with more efficient generation of information on risks and benefits, costly postmarket clinical trials can be efficiently used to augment the routine postmarket surveillance system. In sum, the passage of the FDAAA provides an immediate and rich opportunity to improve drug safety and postmarket surveillance, as well as to move the nation closer to a learning healthcare system.

The work of Medicare over the past few years provides another example of important efforts to build more evidence development into the existing healthcare system. Several national coverage decisions have utilized coverage with evidence development (CED) policy to encourage the generation of needed evidence of intervention effectiveness. As a result, some private plans—Aetna and others—have also, in some cases, provided coverage in the context of developing better evidence on how conditionally covered treatments work in clinical practice. This policy has enabled Medicare over the past few years to provide coverage a bit more broadly, specifically in areas for which the development of additional clinically relevant information was needed. Pertinent examples follow of this policy's use and impact.

One type of CED involves the establishment of clinical registries that collect and house clinically sophisticated data that augment the usual kinds of information that Medicare administrative data systems provide. Since 2005, Medicare coverage of cardioverter defibrillators is conditional on the provision of clinical information deemed necessary for future coverage decisions. In this instance, the clinical characteristics of the patients receiving the Implantable Cardioverter Defibrillator (ICD) were important in determining if the treatment should be covered, and coverage requires that such information be systematically placed in a registry in conjunction with other Medicare information such as noncomplication rates and other aspects of longitudinal care. The resulting large-scale registry is currently being analyzed to answer some important questions surrounding ICD use, including which kinds of patients are actually receiving the ICDs and how they differ from those included in clinical trials and what kind of complication rates are occurring across different settings of care; and to establish a natural history of a whole range of types of patients. Similar registries have been established as a result of CMS CED decisions for a few other cases as well, including Fludeoxyglucose Positron Emission Tomography (PET) scanning.

A second type of coverage with evidence development involves providing needed support for clinical trials. CMS has long paid for routine costs of care in clinical trials and has recently reiterated its policy to do that, but in certain cases CMS also will pay for the cost of treatment in trials conducted by the NIH and others. Examples include coverage of the use of certain biologics off-label or off-drug compendium indications for certain kinds of cancer, and, more recently, for carotid stents in some patients with moderate blockages. These decisions are being made in lieu of straight coverage denials that historically resulted when treatments did not have sufficient evidence for broad-based approval. In the context of a clinical study, CMS has more confidence that the benefits outweigh the risks and that, therefore, the treatments are reasonable and necessary for patients.

As a very helpful and inexpensive next step, Congress needs to clarify CMS's authority to use these kinds of methods to develop better evidence on what the Medicare program is paying for. It would significantly boost efforts that are already underway and help to reinforce some similar steps that are taking place in the private sector. Bariatric surgery for example has been covered in many cases by private health plans in ways that promote better evidence development.

The efforts of the FDA and Medicare demonstrate how much can currently be done to build the capacity to develop better evidence into our routine healthcare system. Obviously, better statistical methods and approaches to pooling data will be needed to fully capitalize on these efforts, but dedicated effort is needed now to develop an ongoing data capacity, so future work will not be relegated to one-off studies of particular issues in which each investigator has to pull together databases or find some subsets of data needed to answer each question. These efforts pave the way for a much more systematic approach.

Integrated or distributed data networks will be particularly helpful in addressing specific kinds of questions. Although we seem to be developing at least some relevant evidence in some areas, we don't seem to be developing very good evidence on how to get medical practitioners to follow the best available evidence. It is not enough to develop the evidence on which treatments are appropriate or may not be appropriate in particular kinds of patients. The true impact of evidence-based medicine will be through the development of evidence on what we can do to influence and support the delivery of health care that reflects best use of resources: to get the best evidence to get the best outcomes for patients at the lowest overall cost.

The work of Elliott Fisher and Jack Wennberg and his colleagues at Dartmouth have provided an in-depth analysis of the geographic variations in costs of treating Medicare beneficiaries and utilization of services. The major source of these variations is not intensive treatments like bypass operations or using one drug instead of another in a broad population of patients, but rather the many subtle and built-in differences in medical practice for patients with chronic diseases. For example, how often should patients with diabetes be referred from a primary care doctor to a specialist? How often do you see patients in follow-up? Which lab tests do you order and when? What imaging procedures are needed? What other minor procedures are needed, and how often should they be performed?

Although not high-profile intensive medical technologies, those kinds of treatments account for a surprisingly large share of the area-to-area variations and costs. These also are areas for which it has been particularly difficult to develop evidence. No medical textbooks answer the questions of which lab test should be ordered and when and how often should one see patients with diabetes. There ought to be a way to develop better evidence on approaches that can influence how patients are treated—and all of these kinds of treatments, whether lab tests or revisits, are appropriate for some kinds of patients. It would be very interesting and useful to know the answers to these types of questions. Information is needed not just on whether a patient gets a treatment or not, but what kind of interventions work in terms of payment reforms, formulary reforms, care management programs, or that other interventions that affect medical practices and populations can influence how a population of patients is being treated. These kinds of incremental differences in medical practice are very difficult to analyze through traditional randomized clinical trials; but, putting in place better infrastructure for collecting data and developing evidence longitudinally over time, on actual treatments that populations of patients are receiving, offers the opportunity to transform how care is delivered and to improve health outcomes.

There are many other examples of how regulatory data can be built into the ongoing capacity to develop better evidence on what works. But these particular examples and opportunities are worth emphasizing because of their tremendous potential for learning more about what is going on in actual medical practice.

ENSURING OPTIMAL USE OF DATA
GENERATED BY PUBLIC INVESTMENT

J. Sanford Schwartz, M.D.
School of Medicine & The Wharton School
University of Pennsylvania

Large amounts of data generated and supported by public investment provide exciting and innovative opportunities to inform clinical and comparative effectiveness assessment. Despite the potential to increase the clinical value of existing information, substantial barriers exist to optimal use of these data. Enhanced coordination in the development of publicly generated data both within and across agencies can reduce overlap and redundancy while expanding the range of issues addressed and information available. Integration of existing publicly supported research and clinical datasets should be facilitated, standardized, and routinized. Access to data generated by public investment, including those by publicly funded investigators, should be expanded through development of effective technical and support mechanisms. The increasingly restrictive interpretation and implementation of HIPAA and related privacy concerns, growth of Medicare HMOs, and the increasing commercialization of private-sector clinical databases are posing new problems for secondary data analysis, have the potential to undermine comparative effectiveness research, and threaten generalizability of research findings. Practical, less-burdensome policies for secondary data that protect patient confidentiality, expansion of Medicare claims files to incorporate new types and sources of data, and facilitated, lower cost access to private-sector secondary clinical data for publicly funded studies need to be developed and implemented.

Concerning evidence-based comparative effectiveness, if our ultimate objective is to answer clinically relevant questions, most researchers are likely in agreement that while RCTs are necessary, they are not in and of themselves sufficient to answer all of our questions. Comparative effectiveness is context dependent. The key questions can be distilled into very simple language: What is being evaluated? How is it being used? For what purpose? Why? For whom? When? Where? Our focus should not be so much on whether a study is "good" or "bad," but rather on two central, interrelated questions: What is the question we are asking, and how can we answer it in the best way? Similarly, there are no "good" or "bad" data. Again, our focus ought to be on central questions: How do we use those data, and what do we use them for? More importantly, how do we interpret them? The most significant problems in clinical effectiveness research are not that we employ poor methodology, but rather that we fail to ask the right questions.

Working backwards from a problem, one needs to structure the decision and get the information we need to identify the gaps in data needs. One of the ways to use quasi- and nonexperimental data is to inform where we should focus our clinical trials. In part, we use empiric methods and in part we use subjective expert opinion—a combination of those is probably optimal. The challenge for us is to use a whole constellation of available methods. The development of a National Problem List, which has been discussed in other contexts within the IOM, would be another avenue to push us forward.

Cost effectiveness in undertaking comparative effectiveness research is essential. We need to know how much better something is and how much more we are going to have to pay for it. Nonetheless, we do not have enough money to do all of the clinical trials that we need to do and would like to do, no matter how efficient we become in conducting RCTs.

One of the paradoxes of research today is that while we have large amounts of data and significant opportunities, there are real barriers to research effectiveness. As a key funder of research, however, the federal government can play a pivotal positive role in addressing some of these barriers and helping the research community to take full advantage of the opportunities. The government is very good, for example, in enhancing coordination and development of data within and across government and could take steps to both reduce overlap and redundancy and expand the range of issues addressed and the scope of the information available to address them. There is opportunity here for the government to formally review the type and scope of data it collects, determine where gaps exist and what opportunities exist to link databases, and then take steps to fill those gaps. Similarly, the government could expand the RCT registry to include all comparative effectiveness research—any study that says anything about safety and effectiveness should be listed. Such a registry should include the protocol, so that other researchers wouldn't have to take time to decipher whether they were looking, for example, at a post-hoc analysis, preexisting data, or preexisting hypotheses. That kind of information leads to very different implications in terms of how we interpret the information we see in front of us. Finally, the government—through AHRQ, CMS, NIH, and FDA, for example—also could play a role in defining and prioritizing research problems. We continue to struggle with the design of models—they don't so much provide answers as help us ask better questions, or they bound the estimates and give us confidence intervals rather than giving us precise answers. One of the roles that government could effectively play would be in the development of models to inform RCT priorities, needs, and design.

Originally some of us hoped that HIPAA would help make the system more rational, but in fact it is really becoming a major barrier to doing research. Part of the problem with HIPAA has to do with excessively restrictive interpretation and implementation. This exists on both the public-sector side and the private-sector side, but ultimately only the federal government can clarify and issue some guidance on how to use this appropriately. In studies using CMS data, for example, researchers are finding that it can take up to 9 months or more to clear an IRB and get through the Research Data Assistance Center. Often, there are issues with data at home institutions, too, based on fear of lawsuits. Restrictive implementation is too cumbersome and simply takes too long, in part because the system essentially asks us to start over again every time. In addition, it is expensive—some estimates are that secondary claims analyses consume some 5 percent of research budgets, due to HIPAA-related forms, processes, and regulations. In short, HIPAA has become an impediment to useful research. Moreover, HIPAA creates a very real level of risk insofar as some use it as a screen to allow them to not follow practices that they don't want to do, but that should absolutely be done. Only the federal government will be able to resolve these issues.

In terms of recommendations for privacy protection, there are viable options for practical, less-burdensome policies for secondary data that protect patient confidentiality. We can have institutionally based agreements. We can expedite IRB review for secondary data. Although it is important to remember that there is a difference between primary and secondary data and that the ethical and safety issues involved are very different. There is an order of magnitude difference between potential harm to a patient if one is looking and exploring data that has no identifying information to that patient, versus exposing someone to an active treatment; yet, most IRBs do not seem to make that distinction. It would be extremely useful to have HIPAA guidance for private data clarified and to extend federal data-use agreements regarding secondary data to institutions. There is now pressure from CMS to return data when a study is done, and we need to recognize that investigators should be able to keep data to answer questions about the study that are raised after the results are published. In addition, when researchers request data, we theoretically request only the minimal data that we need to do our study, but of course we don't always know what the minimum is—there is, therefore, always the potential of a lost opportunity to explore data in more depth.

Among other access threats to secondary data is the issue of reduced access to patient-level data. With the growth of Medicare HMOs and increasing concentration and commercialization of private-sector clinical databases, an overarching question is this: Who owns the data? Many researchers are concerned about the increasing concentration and the narrowness of the funnel to be able to get at some of these data. A junior faculty member, for example, with a simple question about the Medicare drug cap vis-à-vis copayments needs $250,000 to buy the commercial data necessary to address her problem, research that in terms of time and effort will cost just $100,000—the economics do not add up, and consequently she is unable to do her study. In fact, most investigators cannot get access to this data. The private sector sometimes uses HIPAA as an excuse not to share data. Access threats like those have the very real potential to undermine comparative effectiveness research itself and moreover to threaten research generalizability. We need to see networks opened to a broad range of investigators, and we need direct access to databases. Again a role for government would be to work with privately held databases to create processes and systems that lead to more open and affordable access and long-term, viable solutions to these problems.

In terms of recommendations to enhance data availability and access, several come to mind. We need to facilitate lower cost access to private-sector secondary clinical data for publicly funded studies. We need to increase public–private partnerships (e.g., the Interagency Registry for Mechanically Assisted Circulatory Support—INTERMACS). We need to develop standardized data elements and definitions across payers and providers. We need to actively explore future opportunities for data aggregation and sharing. We need to incentivize sharing and access.

Finally, an effectiveness study registry is needed and could be substantially supported by the development of better data files at the NIH. It is the requirement of every NIH grant that data from that grant are supposed to be made available to colleagues for as long as 2 years after a trial ends, yet this practice is not widely followed. The NIH should develop reasonable guidelines for data sharing and then enforce that requirement, perhaps even with modest financial incentives as a carrot, and perhaps on a per-use basis. In general, we as investigators have to be more willing to share our data. How one protects intellectual property is one thing, but we need to understand that just because we collect data does not necessarily mean that we own it forever.

Medicare data can and should be enhanced. For example Medicare claims files data sources could be expanded to include lab values, imaging results, and Part D. Disease cohorts could be created by expanding the creation of integrated public-use data, using the Surveillance, Epidemiology and End Results (SEER) Program, CMS, and Department of Veteran Affairs as models. And electronic data transmission should be supported.

In terms of data linkage and integration, support for effectiveness-related data collection and analysis for publicly accessible, federally funded data is needed, especially for prospectively collected data. Government should do a much better job of routinely integrating databases. One approach would be to give a government panel the responsibility of identifying that data that can be integrated across surveys and with Medicare data and seeing that that is done unless there is a compelling reason not to. Routine linkage of clinical and research data also could be facilitated—in NIH-sponsored RCTs, for example, and in public-use versions of registries and surveys (NIH, AHRQ, CMS, VA, Centers for Disease Control and Prevention, National Center for Health Statistics, and possibly FDA). Medicare ought to be the model and the routine.

Finally, investment in methods is needed at the federal level—particularly for the development and evaluation of innovative methods to assess comparative effectiveness. The validity of quasi- and nonexperimental methods—including simple and complex models, adjustment procedures, and Bayesian approaches—in conjunction with RCTs also need to be assessed. For clinical trials, there should be a policy for funding some of these methods concurrently to see what these methods would have shown compared to what the trial is going to show. Broad experimentation with quasi-experimental and practical RCTs is also needed.

Einstein said that in the midst of every challenge lies opportunity. So it is today, with respect to the optimal use of health data. We must find ways to contend with the current stalemate between the great potential of large amounts of existing data and the many barriers that prevent the access needed to explore their utility for comparative effectiveness research.

BUILDING THE RESEARCH INFRASTRUCTURE

Alan M. Krensky, M.D.[2]
Office of Portfolio Analysis and Strategic Initiatives, NIH

Abstract

Evidence-based medicine requires integration of clinical expertise and research and is dependent upon an infrastructure that includes human capital and organizational platforms. The National Institutes of Health (NIH) is committed to supporting a stable, sustainable scientific workforce. Continu-

---

[2] I thank Drs. Barbara Alving, Director, National Center for Research Resources, NIH; Jeffrey Bluestone, University of California San Francisco, Director, Immune Tolerance Network, and Norka Ruiz-Bravo, Deputy Director for Extramural Research, NIH, for their helpful comments and data.

ity in the pipeline and the increasing age at which new investigators obtain independent funding are the major threats to a stable workforce. To address these concerns, the NIH is developing new programs that target first time R01 equivalent awardees with programs such as the Pathway to Independence and NIH Director's New Innovator Awards, with approximately 1,600 new R01 investigators funded in 2007. NIH-based organizational platforms are intra- and inter-institutional. The Clinical and Translational Science Awards (CTSAs) fund academic health centers to create homes for clinical and translational science, from informatics to trial design, regulatory support, education and community involvement. The NIH is in the midst of building a national consortium of CTSAs that will serve as a platform for transforming how clinical and translational research is conducted. The Immune Tolerance Network (ITN), funded by the National Institute of Allergy and Infectious Diseases (NIAID), the National Institute of Diabetes & Digestive & Kidney Diseases (NIDDK), and the Juvenile Diabetes Research Foundation (JDRF), is an international collaboration focused on critical path research from translation to clinical development. The ITN conducts scientific review, clinical trials planning and implementation, tolerance assays, data analysis, and identification of biomarkers, as well as provides scientific support in informatics, trial management, and communications. Centralization, standardization, and the development of industry partnerships allow extensive data mining and specimen collection. Most recently, the nonprofit Immune Tolerance Institute (ITI) was created at the intersection of academia and industry to speed scientific discoveries into marketable therapeutics. Policies aimed at building a sustainable research infrastructure are critical to support evidence-based medicine.

Progress in modern science is increasingly dependent upon robust infrastructure, including human capital, facilities, and organizational structure. Policies aimed at recognizing gaps and redundancies and improving infrastructure are fundamental to advance knowledge and translation to human disease. Evidence-based medicine requires close attention to infrastructure needs. I highlight three areas: (1) the pipeline of investigators, (2) "homes" for clinical and translational medicine, and (3) a model for translational and developmental networking.

The Pipeline

The NIH is committed to supporting a stable and sustainable workforce. Recent analyses raise concerns about the increasing age at which new investigators are able to become independent and the general "aging" of the scientific workforce (Figure 6-1 and Table 6-1). These findings raise the question as to whether we have a sufficient number of new investigators to carry out health-related research in the future. Close attention to this issue

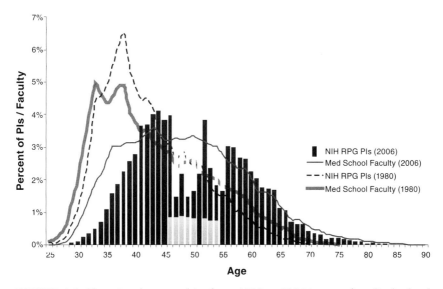

FIGURE 6-1 Changing demographics from 1980 to 2006 in age of medical school faculty and principal investigators (PIs) of NIH research project grants (RPGs). SOURCE: Derived from IMPAC II Current History and Files and AAMC Faculty Roster System.

TABLE 6-1 Summary of Changes in NIH Principal Investigators (PI) and Medical School Faculty Pools from 1980–2006

Year	1980	1998	2006
No. and Avg. Age of NIH PI	14,887 (39.1)	17,761 (42.7)	25,419 (50.8)
Number and Average Age of NIH New PI	1,843 (37.2)	1,355 (39.0)	1,346 (42.4)
No. of Med. School Faculty Positions	53,552	73,413	121,468
Avg. Age of Med. School Faculty	43.1	45.2	48.7
Avg. Age of First-time Assist. Prof.	33.9	35.4	37.7

and implementation of appropriate interventions are required. The goal is to move new investigators to R01-type support and independence earlier in their careers. Strategies to accomplish this goal include accelerated notification of review outcome to permit a more rapid response and turn-around time for revised applications and the specific targeting of 1,500 new R01 investigators for 2007 and the 5-year rolling average in subsequent years.

Award mechanisms aimed at developing new investigators include: (1) the Pathway to Independence (K99/R00), (2) NIH Director's New Innovator Award, and (3) Career Development Awards.

The Pathway to Independence Award recognizes the challenges of transitioning from a postdoctoral trainee to an independent scientist. Reports from the National Research Council of the National Academies (*Bridges to Independence: Fostering the Independence of New Investigators in Biomedical Research*[3] and *Advancing the Nation's Health Needs: NIH Research Training Program*[4]) highlighted the need for enhanced efforts to foster the transition of postdoctoral scientists from mentored environments to independence (National Research Council, 2005a, 2005b). The K99/R00 award provides up to 5 years of support in two phases. The initial award (K99) provides 1 to 2 years of mentored, postdoctoral support. The second phase (R00) provides up to 3 years of independent research support and is activated when the awardee accepts a full-time tenure track (or equivalent) faculty position. Applicants must be in postdoctoral positions and may be at nonprofit, for-profit, or governmental agencies, including intramural NIH laboratories. Both U.S. citizens and non-U.S. citizens are eligible.

The NIH Director's New Innovator Award is designed to support new investigators who propose bold and highly innovative new research approaches with the potential to produce major impacts on broad, important problems in the biological, behavioral, clinical, social, physical, chemical, computational, engineering, and mathematical sciences. The NIH Director's Pioneer Award[5] was created in 2004 to provide additional means to identify scientists with ideas that have the potential for high impact, but that may be too novel, span too diverse a range of disciplines, or be at a stage too early to fare well in the traditional peer review process. The NIH Director's New Innovator Award[6] was created in 2007 to support a small number of new investigators of exceptional creativity.[7]

Up to 24 awards of up to $1.5 million for a 5-year period (an average annual budget of up to $300,000 direct costs) plus applicable facilities and administrative costs are planned for Fiscal Year 2008.

In addition to these new initiatives, NIH Institutes and Centers support a variety of mentored career development programs designed to foster the transition of new investigators to research independence. These programs span research career development opportunities for investigators who have made a commitment to focus on patient-oriented research through the

---

[3] See http://books.nap.edu/catalog/11249.html.
[4] See www.nap.edu/booksearch.php?term=%22nrc+analysis%22&isbn=0309094275.
[5] See http://nihroadmap.nih.gov/pioneer/.
[6] See http://grants.nih.gov/grants/new_investigators/innovator_award/.
[7] See http://grants.nih.gov/grants/new_investigators/innovator_award/.

Mentored Patient-Oriented Research Career Development Award (K23)[8] to research career development opportunities for individuals with highly-developed quantitative skills seeking to integrate their expertise in research relevant to the mission of NIH (K25).[9] All NIH Career Development Award programs are described in detail at the K kiosk Internet site.[10]

Clinical and Translational Research: Creating a New Discipline

The NIH developed the Roadmap for Biomedical Research to speed scientific discovery and its efficient translation to patient care by providing an incubator space for funding innovative programs to address scientific challenges (Zerhouni, 2003, 2007). Roadmap initiatives are expected to (1) have a high potential to transform how biomedical research is conducted, (2) synergistically promote and advance individual missions of the NIH Institutes and Centers to benefit health, (3) apply to issues beyond the scope of any one or small number of Institutes and Centers, (4) be unlikely to be undertaken by other entities, and (5) demonstrate a public health benefit in the public domain. The CTSA, which arose from the Roadmap processes, are designed to eliminate barriers between clinical and basic research, to address the increasing complexities involved in conducting clinical research, and to help institutions nationwide create an academic home for clinical and translational science.

Each applicant academic health center creates an individualized home for clinical and translational science, challenging some traditional approaches to link clinical trial design, implementation, and regulation with biostatistics, informatics, ethics, training, and community. These new entities serve as platforms for healthcare organizations, industry, and government to synergize their efforts to shepherd biomedical discoveries to clinical applications. They offer new philanthropic opportunities for development of cures for human disease. The NIH is in the midst of building a national consortium of 60 units with an annual budget of $500 million. Priority topics for the consortium include (1) creating open and interoperable information systems, (2) ensuring patient safety and openness to new approaches via Institutional Review Boards, (3) developing a new discipline of researchers with degrees in clinical and translational science, and (4) establishing a network of community engagement research resources and evaluate its impact. This experiment is forging new partnerships, encouraging new methods and approaches, and providing a platform for a coordi-

---

[8] See http://grants.nih.gov/grants/guide/pa-files/PA-05-143.html.
[9] See http://grants.nih.gov/grants/guide/pa-files/PA-06-087.html.
[10] See http://grants.nih.gov/training/careerdevelopmentawards.htm.

nated nationwide network aimed at efficiently bringing new treatments to patients.

The Immune Tolerance Network: A Model for Critical Path Research

The ITN, established in 1999 with funding from NIAID, NIDDK, and JDRF, is an international collaboration focused on critical path research from translation to clinical development (Bluestone et al., 2000; Rotrosen et al., 2002). The ITN solicits, develops, implements, and assesses clinical strategies and biologic assays in order to induce, maintain, and monitor immune tolerance in human disease.[11] In May 2007, the ITN received a $220 million, 7-year renewal of its contract from the NIAID, which will be used to continue the ITN research mission world-wide.[12] It is a model for a team approach for critical path research and development, a key infrastructure for drug development. If "translational research" involves moving basic discoveries from concept to clinical evaluation, the critical path involves drug development via "proof of principle" studies, including clinical trials, assay development, and evaluation tools.

The ITN aggregates more than 75 clinicians, investigators, and government officials to provide the infrastructure to review and develop grant proposals, fund clinical trials and assay development, and provide infrastructure required to test the applicability of basic discovery to human disease. This includes scientific support via information systems, management and operations, and communications as well as business development and financial administration.[13] The network provides centralization and standardization of all activities, including data and specimen acquisition, handling, storage, and evaluation. Quality assessments and validation techniques meet industry standards. Industry partners in clinical research, technology, and drug development and supply have aligned to support more than 25 clinical trials. Standardization and reproducibility allow extensive data and specimen analysis both within and across clinical trials.

Challenges addressed by the network include mining of data, team development, development of new biomarkers and therapeutics, and enhancement of the commercial and intellectual potential of mechanism-based clinical research. Academics are working with industry and government to blur the boundaries that often constrain free movement from discovery to drug development. This new approach specifically addresses the growing concerns that despite increasing global expenditures in drug

---

[11] See www3.niaid.nih.gov/research/topics/immune/clinical.htm.
[12] See http://pub.ucsf.edu/newsservices/releases/200705032/.
[13] See www.immunetolerance.org.

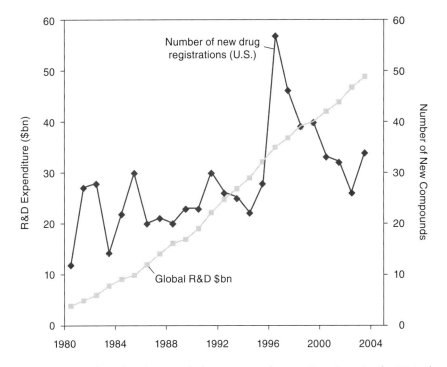

FIGURE 6-2 There has been a decline in new drug registrations in the United States despite a continued, dramatic increase in research and development (R&D) expenditures since 1995.
SOURCE: McKinnon, R., K. Worzel, G. Rotz, and H. Williams. 2004. *Crisis? What crisis? A fresh diagnosis of big pharma's R&D productivity crunch.* New York: Marakon Associates.

research and development, the number of new drugs registered continues to decline since 1996 (Figure 6-2).

The Immune Tolerance Institute: Completing the Task

Despite the progress in developing the ITN structure and function over the past 7 years, it became clear that the route from academia to industry was not completely bridged. To address this gap, the Immune Tolerance Institute (ITI) was forged to support academic–industrial collaboration to leverage discoveries into marketable therapeutics. It includes programs and services supporting the continuum from research and development, mechanistic assays, and standardization of data and specimen handling and analysis to intellectual property and product development (Figures 6-3, 6-4, and 6-5).

Transforming Critical Path Science

Current Structure/Challenges	ITI Strengths	Opportunities
Consortium-driven/Decentralized	• Centralized resources and expertise	• Economies of scale • Streamlined processes (SOPs) • Higher quality, more reproducible data • Enhanced business service
Single investigator studies/ Lack robustness	• High throughput, highly standardized technologies	• More effective data integration maximizes interpetive power • Scalability, reproducibility • Quality assurance and control
Manual processing of patient samples/ Inefficiencies	• Centralized processing • Sample tracking system • Data visualization	• Reproducibility/standardization • Quality control • Cost effectiveness • Customer service • Better data management
Limited business development resources/ Hampers product development	• Dedicated, focused business development and intellectual property infrastructure	• More effective intellectual property development • Productive collaborations, i.e., public–private, industry–academic partnerships • Efficient product development • Enhanced translation to patient benefit

FIGURE 6-3 ITI strengths and opportunities to transform critical path science.

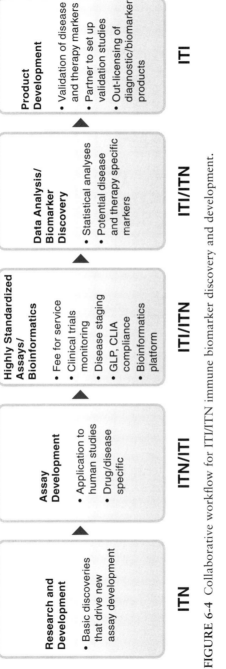

FIGURE 6-4 Collaborative workflow for ITI/ITN immune biomarker discovery and development.

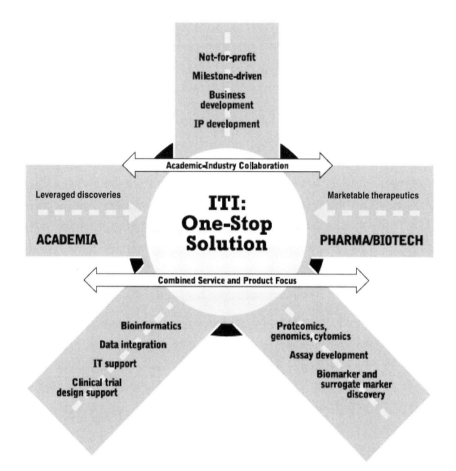

Positioned at the intersection of academia and industry, ITI's programs and services support Critical Path goals by speeding scientific discoveries from bench to bedside with greater precision and cost efficiency.

FIGURE 6-5 ITI: At the intersection of academia and industry.

Together the ITN and ITI couple clinical trials and discovery research with milestone-oriented industry standards for quality control, standard operating procedures, and validated production methodologies. An integrated multidisciplinary organization has evolved to foster the team-building and collaborations required across many disciplines and areas of expertise. A solid platform of clinical service, mechanistic and informatics support, and an array of professional expertise extend the capabilities of the organization beyond either classical academic or pharmaceutical entities. This experiment has built new functionality aimed at improving drug development.

Practical Next Steps

1. Monitor workforce status and proactively provide for a robust and appropriate pipeline of human capital.
2. Develop the CTSA consortium as a platform for clinical and translational medicine.
3. Expand the ITN/ITI model to drug development in general, transcending the divisions between academics, government, and industry.

ENGAGING CONSUMERS

Kathy Hudson, Ph.D.
Johns Hopkins University
Rick E. Borchelt
Shawna Williams
Genetics and Public Policy Center[14]

The Human Genome Project created a wealth of genetic data, breathtaking in its promise but potentially overwhelming in its scope. Data generated by the Human Genome Project and successor projects already are transforming the practice of medicine, enabling better medical diagnoses and informing treatment options, including drug choices and dosage. Less than a decade ago, the hunt for genes responsible for illness was a painstakingly slow process limited primarily to identifying single genes that caused disease, such as Huntington disease and cystic fibrosis. The cost of DNA sequencing was so astronomical it required vast infusions of federal money. Today genomewide association studies point to whole complexes of genes that interact with each other and with the environment to affect human health, and the cost of sequencing an individual human genome in its entirety is widely anticipated to drop below $1,000 in the near future.

[14] The Genetics and Public Policy Center (GPPC) thanks its funders, The Pew Charitable Trusts and the National Human Genome Research Institute, for making possible its public engagement work. Gail Geller, David Kaufman, Lisa LeRoy, Juli Murphy, and Joan Scott each played invaluable roles in its focus groups. Most importantly, the GPPC would like to thank those who have participated in its public engagement activities.

Absent from most discussions around how to harness these technical advances to accelerate discoveries and their translation into treatments has been the evolving relationship between researcher and study participant. Genomewide association studies themselves are large in scope and complex in nature: Conducting meaningful clinical effectiveness research requires collecting, sharing, and analyzing large quantities of health information from many individuals, potentially for long periods of time. To be truly successful, this research needs the support and active involvement of participants. As defined by current practice, however, the relationship between scientists and the public and between researcher and research participant is ill-suited to successfully leverage such active participation.

The roots of this uneasy relationship lie in the historical reliance that the biomedical community—and the science and technology community more generally—traditionally has placed in a "deficit model" of interaction with the public (Ziman, 1991). The basic assumption behind this model is that there is a linear progression from public education to public understanding to public support, and that this model—if followed—would cultivate a public enthusiastically supportive of research with "no questions asked."

The science community has since the era of World War II been operating under this information-deficit model, built on a one-way flow of information from the expert to the public with very little information flowing back the other way. This model has driven communication of science and technology for so long despite its very obvious shortcoming: Neither public support for research nor scientific literacy has increased notably in all of that time.

In fact, asymmetric communications practices have cultivated a public wary and mistrustful of the scientific enterprise (Millstone and van Zwanenberg, 2000), in part because they exacerbate the disconnect between scientists' perceptions of the public, and the public's perceptions of scientists. A quote from a series of scientist interviews we conducted some years ago encapsulates the engrained thinking of too many scientists: "I don't think that the general uninformed public should have a say, because I think there's a danger. There tends to be a huge amount of information you need in order to understand. It sounds really paternalistic, but I think this process should not be influenced too much by just the plain general uninformed public" (Mathews et al., 2005).

The dim view that scientists have of the public's ability to contribute to science and science policy is reciprocated by public attitudes toward scientists; as Bauer et al. note: "Mistrust on the part of scientific actors is returned in kind by the public. Negative public attitudes, revealed in large-scale surveys, confirm the assumptions of scientists: a deficient public is not to be trusted" (Bauer et al., 2007). More than 40 percent of respondents in a 2004 national survey of some 4,600 U.S. residents, for example, did not trust scientists "to put society's interest about their personal goals" (Kalfoglou et al., 2004). Specifically in the context of proposed genetic research, more than 40 percent of respondents in a national survey agreed with the statement that "Researchers these days don't pay enough attention to the morals of society," and nearly half believed that "Researchers are biased" and do studies to support what they already believe.[15]

This observation frequently is born out in focus groups on genetics conducted by the GPPC; one quote, representing what we hope is an extreme point of view, comes from a focus group conducted a couple of years ago in connection with reproductive genetic technologies: "We are all responsible people here but some of them scientists, because of the science and because of their warped minds, will do something stupid."

Clearly, one-way or highly asymmetric communication with the public is just not working. Writing in *Science* in 2003, American Association for the Advancement of Science Chief Executive Officer Alan Leshner summarized the problem eloquently: "Simply trying to educate the public about specific science-based issues is not working. . . . We need to move beyond what too often has been seen as a paternalistic stance. We need to engage the public in a more open and honest bidirectional dialogue about science and technology" (Leshner, 2003).

As a consequence, research-performing institutions increasingly are turning to public engagement and public consultation approaches to enlist public support (Bauer et al., 2007), a concept Jasanoff terms "the participatory turn" in science and technology (Jasanoff, 2003). One reason that probably motivates scientists to look to new approaches in communication and engagement is the continued belief that if the public really understood, it would support increased budgets, and grants would have a higher likelihood of being funded. This may well be true. Certainly awareness is a prerequisite to advocacy, although evidence is sorely lacking about how these two variables interact—the only thing that is clear is that the relationship isn't a direct one (Lynch, 2001). But better public understanding of science can add value to science in many other ways (Mathews et al., 2005), leading to better-informed health decision making and to better recruitment for research studies, not to mention recruitment for the science and technology workforce. A better-informed public could provide meaningful input to help shape better policy and even to help design more meaningful public information efforts. Finally, a better-informed public could become more engaged in research and related policy and claim its rightful role as partner in this effort.

The goal of these two-way, symmetric communications models is

---

[15] Unpublished data, Genetics and Public Policy Center.

mutual satisfaction of *both* parties, the research enterprise and its public—in this case, the researcher and the study subject—with the relationships that exist between them. This mutual-satisfaction approach emphasizes true bi-directional interaction and requires a commitment to transparency on the part of the organization; negotiation, compromise, and mutual accommodation; and institutionalized mechanisms of hearing from and responding to the public. It places a premium on long-term relationship building with all of the strategic publics: research participants, certainly, but also media, regulators, community leaders, policy makers, and others (Borchelt, 2008). These emerging models offer promise for scientists and the public to engage more fully and productively.

Unlike the unidirectional and hierarchal communication that characterize past efforts, public engagement can result in demonstrable shifts in knowledge and attitudes among participants. This shift may not always be in the direction scientists might expect or prefer, however. The expected outcome is different, as well: Rather than aspiring solely for or insisting upon the public's deeper understanding of science, a primary goal of public engagement is scientists' deeper understanding of the public preferences and values.

While it has become fashionable for many scientific organizations to say they're doing "public engagement," few encourage or engage in true dialogue with the public or publics. Unfortunately, they treat public engagement or public consultation as a box-checking exercise necessary before they get on with their "real" work (Leshner, 2006). Organizations rarely devote significant resources to meaningful symmetric communication (Grunig et al., 2002).

In terms of the translation of human genetics from research to clinical practice, public engagement can be undertaken at a number of points along the discovery pipeline (Figure 6-6). The beginning of this pipeline is happily bloated as the discovery of genes and variants is currently expanding at a mind-boggling velocity. Using new knowledge of the human genome and these advanced technologies, scientists have developed genetic tests for more than 1,200 genetic conditions, and these genetic tests are available in clinics (or, sometimes, even directly to consumers over the Internet). In genomics today, you can pay to have a million of your genetic variants analyzed, then can sit at your computer and read your results. Companies such as deCODE, 23andMe, and Navigenics recently grabbed headlines when they announced their whole-genome scanning services.

Although we see as yet very little in terms of an impact of genetics on public health at the end of this pipeline, we remain extremely enthusiastic about new thinking that is emerging in this area. For example, a Centers for Disease Control and Prevention (CDC)-funded effort titled Evaluation of Genomic Applications and Practice and Prevention (EGAPP) is looking

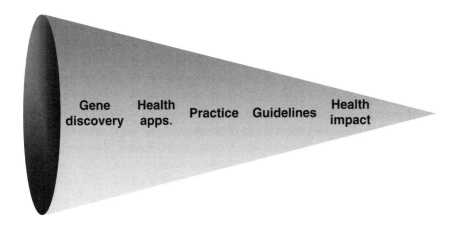

Gene discovery **Health apps.** **Practice** **Guidelines** **Health impact**

FIGURE 6-6 Translational pipeline compared to public participation.

very carefully at genetic tests. Its goal is to use a systematic, evidence-based process to assess genetic tests and other applications of genomic technology in transition from research to clinical and public health practice. This past December, for example, EGAPP published its first major set of recommendations regarding the appropriate use of genetic testing to guide treatment of depression and identified gaps in knowledge (Evaluation of Genomic Applications in Practice and Prevention [EGAPP] Working Group, 2007). Importantly, the CDC simultaneously made available funding to specifically fill identified knowledge gaps (Centers for Disease Control and Prevention, 2008).

The public interface with research is seldom encountered in the "upstream" end of the research process, where knowledge gaps are identified and research designed to address them. Rather, public engagement if it exists at all is clustered almost exclusively around health outcomes, principally comprising such items as information, advertising, and health campaigns. The next level upstream from simply informing is to consult, to obtain meaningful feedback from the public, and then to collaborate, to a point where the public is involved in issue identification, framing, prioritization, and agenda setting for research.

The GPPC has been involved in a pilot public consultation project well upstream in the pipeline. This project seeks to inform the design and implementation of a large, prospective cohort study proposed by the NIH and other federal healthcare agencies to look at the effects of genes, environment, diet, and lifestyle, and to dissect how they interact with one another and contribute to health and disease. This study would enroll 500,000 individuals representative of the U.S. population, collect DNA and other specimens from them, conduct age-appropriate physical/developmental exams of each participant, interview them for lifestyle and behavioral information and to discern environmental exposures, then follow the cohort for at least a decade. The collected data would be coded and entered into a very large database, which would be mine-able by researchers for the study of complex diseases. Research results would be fed back into the database (Collins, 2004).

Advisory committees have suggested to the NIH that it would be a good idea to talk to the public first about the project (National Human Genome Research Institute, 2004; Secretary's Advisory Committee on Genetics, 2007). Accordingly, the GPPC entered into a cooperative agreement with the National Human Genome Research Institute at the NIH to learn what the public knows and thinks about large-scale genetic databases and to pilot test engagement strategies; as part of this effort we are conducting interviews, surveys, focus groups, and town hall meetings. Ultimately these efforts will develop and evaluate informational materials for the public, assess public attitudes, engage citizens and community leaders, and test methods for initiating community-based dialogue.

A preliminary glimpse at results from just-completed focus groups for this project is telling. The public is far more science-savvy than we may have given them credit for—about the role of genes in disease, and about the interactions between genes, environment, and lifestyle. Focus group participants were able to appreciate the overall value of the study and the need for a large and representative study. They recognized that scientific research is an iterative process that sometimes gives false leads that draw researchers down the wrong path and that subsequent studies can provide contradictory results. A representative quote comes from a focus group participant in Philadelphia:

> [There is] this "news flash" . . . but then they come out a couple of weeks later and they will say well "this is good to eat." And then a couple of weeks later they will say "this goes as heart disease." And then they say, "no, now new research has discovered this doesn't." You know, they do that all the time. Within a certain amount of time they come up with conflicting reports.

Our work with the focus groups provided some insights into general public attitudes toward participation in scientific research. Altruism is alive and well, albeit not in everyone. Views on participation were tied to general trust of science and government and concerns about loss of confidentiality and misuse of information. Whether the majority of people would participate hinges on the level of burden participation would impose, consideration of incentives or compensation offered for participation, and—the strongest predictor of people's willingness to participate—what they would receive in terms of return of research results. A universal refrain in the focus groups was "show me the data." Clearly, we are past the point of no return of results. If one participates in a population-based research study today, however, under the prevailing researcher–participant compact, odds are very good that personal research results will not be disclosed to study participants. This is clearly a challenge, but it also presents an opportunity for reassessing the nature of the communication flow in a research setting.

The ethos of many participants can be summarized in this quote from one of our focus groups: "If you're in this whole study, I want to know everything that you all find out about me." Of course, not everyone would want or demand access to their research results. For some, those results would be "too much information." This view is summarized in this quote: "I don't want to know everything little thing that is wrong with me because I already have so much wrong with me to begin with. If I know more, I am just, people are going to be like wow, how do you live your life."[16]

We heard over and over again that people want choices in their participation. They want to set their preferences—and that exact phrase was used over and over again—analogous to how we set preferences on our computers. They want to be able to make decisions about how their samples and information would be used, about what kind of information they would get back, and how it would be returned.

The importance of being an informed and active participant was underscored by focus group discussions about the nature of the consent they would provide for their participation. While researchers typically view consent as the process by which participants understand and agree to what they are getting in to, focus group members felt that it is (or should be) a reciprocal documentation of the roles and obligations of both the participant and the research team. This speaks to the underlying distrust among the public of science and its practitioners and a desire to reflect on and protect their own interests. Perhaps most importantly, we heard desire on the part of the public to be active participants, if not partners, with researchers.

Obviously, these early findings are qualitative data. The next steps in the project are to test the findings quantitatively in a survey of 5,000 Americans.

In addition to the NIH, the GPPC is working with the Department of Veterans Affairs (VA) on engagement around a project to build a research database of genetic samples linked to a medical records system. They asked us to talk first about the project with veterans. This quote from a veteran shows again the value of symmetric communication: "The fact that they have people sitting around talking about this in advance of even starting to

---

[16] Unpublished data, Genetics and Public Policy Center.

build it tells me that they're paying attention. . . . This right here is oversight, you know, at the get-go. So I think that that's a really good thing; and I think ultimately it's going to be one more way that veterans give something from themselves to make this country better."

The NIH and VA are to be applauded for their commitment to consultation and engagement of potential research participants in the design and implementation of large-cohort genetic studies. But it should be remembered that simply obtaining information from the public is not sufficient either to claim that the public has been "engaged" or to engender public trust in or support of proposed research. Profound ethical issues attend the meaningful practice of public engagement: One cannot promise engagement but only make a show of listening. The commitment to symmetric communication falls short if the organization hears, but does not respond to, the concerns or issues of its publics. Mutual satisfaction requires that researchers be open to reasonable changes requested of them, just as effective—and ethical—public engagement programs in science should signal a willingness to incorporate public input in science policy, regulatory programs, or research design.

REFERENCES

Bauer, M., N. Allum, and S. Miller. 2007. What can we learn from 25 years of PUS survey research? Liberating and expanding the agenda. *Public Understanding of Science* 16(79).

Bluestone, J. A., J. B. Matthews, and A. M. Krensky. 2000. The immune tolerance network: The "Holy Grail" comes to the clinic. *Journal of the Americal Society Nephrology* 11(11):2141-2146.

Borchelt, R. 2008. Public relations in science: Managing the trust portfolio. In *Handbook of Public Communication of Science and Technology*, edited by M. Bucchi and B. Trench. New York: Routledge.

Centers for Disease Control and Prevention. 2008. *Genomic Applications in Practice and Prevention (GAPP): Translation Research (U18)*. http://www.cdc.gov/od/pgo/funding/GD08-001.htm (accessed February 20, 2008).

Collins, F. S. 2004. The case for a US prospective cohort study of genes and environment. *Nature* 429(6990):475-477.

Etheredge, L. M. 2007. A rapid-learning health system. *Health Affairs (Millwood)* 26(2): w107-w118.

Evaluation of Genomic Applications in Practice and Prevention (EGAPP) Working Group. 2007. Recommendations from the EGAPP working group: Testing for cytochrome p450 polymorphisms in adults with nonpsychotic depression treated with selective serotonin re-uptake inhibitors. *Genetics in Medicine* 9:819-825.

Grunig, L., J. Grunig, and D. Dozier. 2002. *Excellent Public Relations and Effective Organizations: A Study of Communication Management in Three Countries*. Mahwah, NJ: Lawrence Erlbaum Associates.

Jasanoff, S. 2003. Technologies of humility: Citizens participation in governing science. *Minerva* 41(3):223-244.

Kalfoglou, A., J. Scott, and K. Hudson. 2004. *Reproductive Genetic Testing: What America Thinks*. Washington, DC: Genetics and Public Policy Center.

Leshner, A. I. 2003. Public engagement with science. *Science* 299(5609):977.
Leshner, A. 2006. Science and public engagement. *Chronicle of Higher Education* B20.
Lynch, M. 2001. Managing the trust portfolio. Paper read at PCST2001 Conference.
Mathews, D. J., A. Kalfoglou, and K. Hudson. 2005. Geneticists' views on science policy formation and public outreach. *American Journal of Medical Genetics A* 137(2):161-169.
McKinnon, R., K. Worzel, G. Rotz, and H. Williams. 2004. *Crisis? What crisis? A Fresh Diagnosis of Big Pharma's R&D Productivity Crunch*. New York: Marakon Associates.
Millstone, E., and P. van Zwanenberg. 2000. A crisis of trust: For science, scientists or for institutions? *Nature Medicine* 6(12):1307-1308.
National Human Genome Research Institute. 2004. *Design Considerations for a Potential United States Population-based Cohort to Determine the Relationships Among Genes, Environment, and Health: Recommendations of an Expert Panel*. Bethesda, MD: U.S. Department of Health and Human Services.
National Research Council. 2005a. *Advancing the Nation's Health Needs: NIH Research Training Programs*. Washington, DC: The National Academies Press.
———. 2005b. *Bridges to Independence: Fostering the Independence of New Investigators in Biomedical Research*. Washington, DC: The National Academies Press.
Ozcam, Y., and A. Kazley. 2008. Do hospitals with electronic medical records (EMRS) provide higher quality care? An examination of three clinical conditions. *Medical Care Research and Review* 65:496-517.
Pawlson, L. G. 2007. Health information technology: Does it facilitate or hinder rapid learning? *Health Affairs (Millwood)* 26(2):w178-w180.
Rotrosen, D., J. B. Matthews, and J. A. Bluestone. 2002. The Immune Tolerance Network: A new paradigm for developing tolerance-inducing therapies. *Journal of Allergy and Clinical Immunology* 110(1):17-23.
Secretary's Advisory Committee on Genetics, Health and Society. 2007. *Policy Issues Associated with Undertaking a New Large U.S. Population Cohort Study of Genes, Environment, and Disease*. Bethesda, MD: U.S. Department of Health and Human Services.
Solberg, L. I., S. H. Scholle, S. E. Asche, S. C. Shih, L. G. Pawlson, M. J. Thoele, and A. L. Murphy. 2005. Practice systems for chronic care: Frequency and dependence on an electronic medical record. *Americal Journal of Managed Care* 11(12):789-796.
Zerhouni, E. 2003. Medicine. The NIH roadmap. *Science* 302(5642):63-72.
Zerhouni, E. A. 2007. Translational research: Moving discovery to practice. *Clinical Pharmacology and Therapeutics* 81(1):126-128.
Ziman, J. 1991. Public understanding of science. *Science, Technology, & Human Values* 16:99-105.

7

Organizing the Research
Community for Change

INTRODUCTION

In the context of a compelling, and rapidly growing, need for better approaches to develop and apply evidence about the comparative effectiveness of healthcare choices, the workshop Redesigning the Clinical Effectiveness Research Paradigm: Innovation and Practice-Based Approaches explored opportunities presented by emerging research networks and data resources, innovative study designs, and new methods of analysis and modeling that might help to address the evidence gaps. Participants in the meeting examined broadly the role of innovative research designs and tools that can expedite the development of evidence on clinical effectiveness by streamlining approaches and bringing research and practice closer together.

Comments throughout the workshop also highlighted system fragmentation and misaligned incentives that limit capacity to conduct timely research that addresses practical clinical questions. Cross-discipline and cross-sector work was emphasized as essential to shaping and supporting the development of an efficient and robust clinical effectiveness research enterprise. Ensuring research that focuses on producing evidence for physicians, patients, and policy makers; draws upon expertise from many different disciplines and fields (e.g., clinical trialists, epidemiologists, and health services and outcomes researchers); and functions to capture, extend, and apply learnings throughout an intervention's lifecycle (e.g., development, approval, postmarket refinement) will require reevaluation and adjustment to many facets of the existing research enterprise (e.g., emphasis on postmarket evaluations in broad populations as well as approval studies, cross-disciplinary education and training, alignment of policy goals with funding, publication and career advancement opportunities, improved linkages with healthcare delivery systems).

The final workshop sessions were dedicated to discussion of how the research community might be organized, mobilized, and supported to effect broad changes needed. Common themes and follow-up opportunities for the Roundtable, noted throughout the discussion are also summarized here.[1]

INCREASING KNOWLEDGE FROM PRACTICE-BASED RESEARCH

The multifaceted, practice-oriented approach to clinical effectiveness research discussed at the workshop complements and blends with traditional trial-oriented clinical research and may be represented as a continuum in which evidence is continuously produced by a blend of experimental studies with patient assignment (clinical trials); modeling, statistical, and observational studies without patient assignment; and monitored clinical experience (see Figure 7-1).

The ratio of the various approaches will vary with the nature of the intervention, as does the weight given to the available studies. This enhanced flexibility and range of research resources is facilitated by the development of innovative study design and analytic tools, and by the growing potential of electronic health records to allow much broader structure access to the results of the clinical experience. The ability to draw on real-time clinical insights will naturally improve over time.

The research community will play a vital role in developing a clinical effectiveness research enterprise that provides timely, reliable information that can be used in clinical decision making. Discussions throughout the workshop not only highlighted current shortfalls in the quality, quantity, and efficiency of this current research, but also explored many opportunities to develop incentives for the changes needed and to support those changes once they have been implemented. As reviewed in previous chapters, many elements are being developed and used to ensure research can be used more effectively to make evidence-based decisions in a clinical setting. These elements include innovative tools, techniques, and strategies that improve the efficiency and reliability of study methodologies; vastly larger and clinically richer datasets; and advances in information technology that will connect researchers and information, thus enabling studies not possible before. In some respects the largest challenge is engaging the research community

---

[1] This chapter is drawn from the panel discussion and concluding summary comments at the workshop made by Michael McGinnis and the submitted comments of participants during and following the meeting. They do not constitute consensus findings or recommendations of the Institute of Medicine or the National Academies.

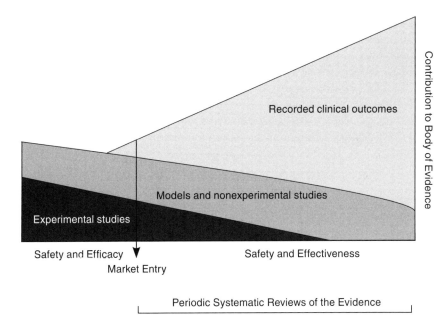

FIGURE 7-1 Evidence development in the learning healthcare system.

in efforts to resolve key technical and policy challenges, including removing barriers to coordination and implementation of research and research results. For example, improved understanding is needed of when and how the various methods are best applied to different research questions and which measures will improve study validation and reporting. Standardization of data and other efforts to improve data utility through coordination and linkage, as well as attention to issues related to data transparency and privacy or proprietary concerns are also priority areas. Because these issues often span disciplines and healthcare sectors, participants in the last session of the workshop were asked to suggest opportunities to foster the collaboration needed across the public and private sectors to drive change.

OPPORTUNITIES FOR ACTION

Mark B. McClellan, Brookings Institution;
Alan M. Krensky, National Institutes of Health;
Garry Neil, Johnson & Johnson;
John Niederhuber, National Cancer Institute;
Lewis Sandy, United Health Care

The five panelists opened the final workshop session by discussing some key needs and opportunities for the future of clinical effectiveness research.

They explored guiding principles for the research community; opportunities to use a lifecycle approach to help clinical research evolve into evidence development; and infrastructure needs and key challenges. To sharpen the focus on immediate opportunities, participants were asked to suggest activities that could be started in the next 12–18 months, in the absence of new legislation, funding, or creation of a central coordinating capacity. Following are summaries of comments from the panel and the subsequent open discussion.

Guiding Principles

Several panelists commented on the dramatic potential of the emerging era of research to accelerate the transfer of knowledge between basic research and clinical practice. Recent advances in genetics and genomics mark the "beginning of the beginning," with the past decade of research providing a rich catalog of information that potentially can be translated into interventions with clinical use. Taking advantage of such opportunity will require the current system of clinical research—in use for the past 50 years—to evolve into one that makes better use of the power of technology to gather and use data to improve patient care and outcomes. As the pace of research and product development accelerates, the creation of systems to help track the effects of these agents in real time will be especially important. Guiding such dramatic reform will require a clarification of the mission, focus, and approaches to clinical effectiveness research and a greater emphasis on supporting innovation.

Clarify the Mission and Focus of Clinical Effectiveness Research

The fundamental mission of research is to help patients, yet there has been a detectable shift away from this basic tenet, as research organizations focus more on economics and less on impacting health outcomes. The identification of priority areas for research presents the opportunity to force greater focus on key issues, and a clear prioritization approach to identify issues with the greatest impact on the nation's health and healthcare system would help decision makers to allocate limited resources more effectively (e.g., where limited evidence exists and there is high variability in practice; high costs and growth potential; or large populations are affected).

Along with the development of strategic initiatives to identify and address evidence gaps, consideration is needed on how to establish appropriate evaluation components. Developing metrics not only will help to track progress but also will illustrate the impact of focused research efforts. Demonstrating that research is practical, relevant, and effective enough to have a tangible impact on practice is crucial to organizing the research community for change. It was stressed that marking such early successes will help to generate additional resources and sustained support for expanded clinical effectiveness research.

Develop a Research Paradigm That Strengthens Research Capacity

The goal of clinical effectiveness research is to provide information on the effects of interventions on treatment outcomes in routine care. From hybrid studies and the mining of large databases to practices such as cluster randomization, pragmatic trials, and practice-based investigations and new study designs (e.g., equipoise stratified randomized designs and adaptive treatment studies) or posthoc data analyses (e.g., moderator analyses), clearly many paths provide answers to clinically important questions. The research paradigm needs to provide a framework that emphasizes best practices in methodologies while strengthening overall research capacity. Research methods should be defined clearly (e.g., strengths, weaknesses, appropriateness), with unmistakable expectations for conduct and reporting of results. The research community must invest more of its talent in the evaluation of methodologies and in the establishment of clear guidelines on the standards of evidence that must be met by research—whether for approval, coverage, or publication.

Greater attention to matching study design to appropriate research questions also will allow a broader use of methods and drive improvements in the approaches and data resources needed to support a new generation of research. For example, as the number of databases and clinical registries has increased, researchers have developed new means to deal with threats to validity—both external validity, as in the development of effectiveness research, and internal validity—including approaches that exploit the concepts of proxy variables using high-dimensional propensity scores and exploiting provider variation in prescribing preference using instrumental variable analysis. New study designs such as adaptive trials and genome-wide association studies are being developed to exploit diverse information sources. A framework that embraces these new tools and techniques and that focuses on understanding the best approach to answering key questions will enable the research community to not only probe questions of clinical effectiveness but also to explore opportunities to extend and improve the overall approach to research.

Likewise, a paradigm that focuses on state-of-the-art design and conduct of methods will drive needed improvements in emerging data resources. Research will continue to benefit more from having large data streams, registries, and billing databases, but only if we contend with important statistical and data aggregation issues. In particular, new methods are needed to pool data from diverse sources. Detailed documentation of sources and quality control also will be needed to ensure data integrity and use. The structure of these data resources must be considered to minimize false discovery rates.

Supporting Innovation

Several participants stressed the importance of efforts to supply the talent, resources, and opportunities needed for innovation. Faced with the growing diversity and quantity of data available, it was noted that developing approaches to integrating data—that do not depend on tools or specific standards—would truly transform our ability to harness these data. This and other emerging technical challenges underscore the importance of generating a cadre of investigators and innovators who can take on these and other obstacles to matching the capacity for discovery with the astounding rate at which data are generated.

The research community also needs opportunities and incentives to test tools such as hybrid, preference-based, or quasi-experimental designs, statistical tools, and modeling approaches to better understand their appropriate use. Some of these new analytic tools are already adding to our knowledge base, but with sufficient innovation incentives researchers can define a new generation of studies that make even greater gains in efficiency and accuracy. To ensure that these new techniques are fully developed, tested, and appropriately adopted, funding might be redirected to accommodate greater experimentation with methodologies. Traditional approaches to research funding and policy will need to shift to support innovation.

Lifecycle Approach to Evidence Development

The efficacy assessments that lead to a product's approval traditionally have been considered the end stage of evidence development. However, a lifecycle approach to evidence development begins with efficacy testing in the preapproval stage and continues throughout the postmarket environment. This shows the findings, often significant, that often occur when a product is given to real-world patient populations. Throughout a product's lifecycle, new questions emerge on efficacy and effectiveness. Randomized controlled trials (RCTs) provide information about efficacy, and hybrid approaches that combine the best attributes of RCTs with complementary methodology have been employed to develop more information on effectiveness. The recently completed National Institute of Mental Health-sponsored comparative effectiveness trials of antipsychotic medications in patients with schizophrenia (the CATIE trials), for example, blended features of efficacy studies and large, simple trials to provide extensive information. Staging or sequencing methods is an opportunity to better integrate trials and studies for clinical effectiveness evidence development across a product's lifecycle. Several participants raised the prospects of coverage with evidence development approaches and support of specialty society registries to support these types of postmarket evidence generation.

Infrastructure

The postmarket environment will become increasingly important in clinical research. It was suggested that realizing the potential for personalized medicine is predicated on the development of a system that will support research that is increasingly bidirectional, drawing from and contributing to clinical care. Similarly, other participants noted, in many cases sufficient evidence exists to guide practice, yet that evidence is not applied enough. Identification and exploration of evidence-based "best practices" will improve understanding of barriers to effective application of evidence. Additional knowledge also might inform the research community about the system components needed to capture information at the point of care for continuous refinement of practice guidelines and decision support tools. Drawing research closer to practice will require new approaches to practice and funding as well as to infrastructure improvement.

To turn genetic findings into knowledge that can be applied at the patient level, for example, researchers will need to use information technology to collect, catalog, organize, and analyze data on genotype, biodata, and phenotype. A long-term vision for the infrastructure required is of robust and standardized electronic health records (EHRs) deployed nationwide that are designed for research as well as of patient and provider support. A tool that captures information systematically and aggregates, normalizes, and synthesizes data in ways that enable efficient analyses is still a distant prospect. However, specialty society registries offer opportunities for immediate progress. These clinical data resources have been used to conduct postmarket studies as well as large-scale trials. Considerable progress is being made in the development of tools, strategies, and policies that will enable multiple users from different sites, perhaps even competitors, to access some of the large databases. A key improvement to these resources would be greater linkage and horizontal integration to ensure the focus is on patient care rather than on a single disease.

The need for greater linkage and greater coordination between efforts was also a strong theme in discussions of infrastructure needs. Several examples of networked resources, such as the HMO Research Network (HMORN) and the Clinical and Translational Science Awards (CTSAs) institutions, were suggested as important infrastructures on which to build. Coordination capacity and platforms for collaboration on issues of mutual interest for collaboration also were viewed as needed infrastructure. For example, the National Institutes of Health (NIH), Agency for Healthcare Research and Quality, payers, and manufacturers might be convened to identify priority areas for methods advancement and enhancement. Opportunities to strengthen collaborative efforts of academia, industry, and government, perhaps through public–private partnerships, were also suggested, with several panelists viewing the public sector as critical in providing an enabling platform between academics and the private sector.

There was also an emphasis on supporting and reinforcing existing and planned infrastructure to strengthen research capacity. Collaboration will be needed in efforts to aggregate data from diverse sources, construct measures consistently, and better use existing data resources. Other efforts to move to more integrated data capabilities, including the addition of clinical data to administrative databases will expand research capacity. Another key opportunity for collaboration was around coverage with evidence development. From the private-sector perspective, such efforts are complicated by the approval needed from all impacted states. Although coverage conditional on the development of needed evidence would ideally be supported by all payers, regulatory issues need to be resolved, including those related to collusion. Related areas for collaborative work included developing a common language for contracting and intellectual property issues and addressing privacy and security issues to facilitate more efficient research while protecting the patient. Although broad-scale change on these dimensions may require legislation, in the near term, collaboration between relevant parties could serve to identify and resolve the many inconsistencies and inefficiencies that now present unnecessary obstacles to important research efforts. Clarification of the interpretation of Institutional Review Boards was viewed as a particularly pressing example of an area in need of collaborative work.

Infrastructure currently in development, such as that for postmarket surveillance, was also discussed as a key opportunity. These postmarket, or Phase IV, studies are typically carried out in a fragmented fashion, with multiple organizations conducting separate investigations. If developed and supported carefully and adequately, this infrastructure will enable a more thorough approach to evidence development.

COMMON THEMES[2]

The presentations and discussions were rich and stimulating and elicited important insights on our evolving clinical research capacity. The following

---

[2] The material presented expresses the general views and discussion themes of the participants of the workshop, as summarized by staff, and should not be construed as reflective of conclusions or recommendations of the Roundtable or the Institute of Medicine.

BOX 7-1
Redesigning the Clinical Effectiveness Research Paradigm

- Address current limitations in applicability of research results
- Counter inefficiencies in timeliness, costs, and volume
- Define a more strategic use to the clinical experimental model
- Provide stimulus to new research designs, tools, and analytics
- Encourage innovation in clinical effectiveness research conduct
- Promote the notion of effectiveness research as a routine part of practice
- Improve access and use of clinical data as a knowledge resource
- Foster the transformational research potential of information technology
- Engage patients as full partners in the learning culture
- Build toward continuous learning in all aspects of care

---

highlights a number of common themes heard throughout the course of the workshop (Box 7-1), as well as possible multistakeholder activities for consideration by the IOM Roundtable on Value & Science-Driven Health Care and its members.

- *Address current limitations in applicability of research results.* Because clinical conditions and their interventions have complex and varying circumstances, there are different implications for the evidence needed, study designs, and the ways lessons are applied: the internal and external validity challenge. In particular given our aging population, often people have multiple conditions—co-morbidities—yet study designs generally focus on people with just one condition, limiting their applicability. In addition, although our assessment of candidate interventions is primarily through pre-market studies, the opportunity for discovery extends throughout the lifecycle of an intervention—development, approval, coverage, and the full period of implementation.
- *Counter inefficiencies in timeliness, costs, and volume.* Much of current clinical effectiveness research has inherent limits and inefficiencies related to time, cost, and volume. Small studies may have insufficient reliability or follow-up. Large experimental studies may be expensive and lengthy but have limited applicability to practice circumstances. Studies sponsored by product manufacturers have to overcome perceived conflicts and may not be fully used. Each incremental unit of research time and money may bring greater con-

fidence but also carries greater opportunity costs. There is a strong need for more systematic approaches to better defying how, when, for whom, and in what setting an intervention is best used.

- *Define a more strategic use to the clinical experimental model.* Just as there are limits and challenges to observational data, there are limits to the use of experimental data. Challenges related to the scope of possible inferences, to discrepancies in the ability to detect near-term versus long-term events, to the timeliness of our insights and our ability to keep pace with changes in technology and procedures, all must be managed. Part of the strategy challenge is choosing the right tool at the right time. For the future of clinical effectiveness research, the important issues relate not to whether randomized experimental studies are better than observational studies, or vice versa, but to what's right for the circumstances (clinical and economic) and how the capacity can be systematically improved.

- *Provide stimulus to new research designs, tools, and analytics.* An exciting part of the advancement process has been the development of new tools and resources that may quicken the pace of our learning and add real value by helping to better target, tailor, and refinc approaches. Use of innovative research designs, statistical techniques, probability, and other models may accelerate the timeliness and level of research insights. Some interesting approaches using modeling for virtual intervention studies may hold prospects for revolutionary change in certain clinical outcomes research.

- *Encourage innovation in clinical effectiveness research conduct.* The kinds of "safe harbor" opportunities that exist in various fields for developing and testing innovative methodologies for addressing complex problems are rarely found in clinical research. Initiative is needed for the research community to challenge and assess its approaches—a sort of meta-experimental strategy— including those related to analyzing large datasets, in order to learn about the purposes best served by different approaches. Innovation is also needed to counter the inefficiencies related to the volume of studies conducted. How might existing research be more systematically summarized or different research methods be organized, phased, or coordinated to add incremental value to existing evidence?

- *Promote the notion of effectiveness research as a routine part of practice.* Taking full advantage of each clinical experience is the theoretical goal of a learning healthcare system. But for the theory to move closer to the practice, tools and incentives are needed for caregiver engagement. A starting point is with the anchoring of the focus of clinical effectiveness research planning and priority setting on the point of service—the patient–provider interface—as the source of attention, guidance, and involvement on the key questions to engage. The work with patient registries by many specialty groups is an indication of the promise in this respect, but additional emphasis is necessary in anticipation of the access and use of the technology that opens new possibilities.

- *Improve access and use of clinical data as a knowledge resource.* With the development of bigger and more numerous clinical data sets, the potential exists for larger scale data mining for new insights on the effectiveness of interventions. Taking advantage of the prospects will require improvements in data sharing arrangements and platform compatibilities, the addressing of issues related to real and perceived barriers from interpretation of privacy and patient protection rules, enhanced access for secondary analysis to federally sponsored clinical data (e.g., Medicare part D, pharmaceutical, clinical trials), the necessary expertise, and stronger capacity to use clinical data for postmarket surveillance.

- *Foster the transformational research potential of information technology.* Broad application and linkage of electronic health records holds the potential to foster movement toward real-time clinical effectiveness research that can generate vastly enhanced insights into the performance of interventions, caregivers, institutions, and systems—and how they vary by patient needs and circumstances. Capturing that potential requires working to better understand and foster the progress possible, through full application of electronic health records, developing and applying standards that facilitate interoperability, agreeing on and adhering to research data collection standards by researchers, developing new search strategies for data mining, and investing patients and caregivers as key supporters in learning.

- *Engage patients as full partners in the learning culture.* With the impact of the information age growing daily, access to up-to-date information by both caregiver and patient changes the state of play in several ways. The patient sometimes has greater time and motivation to access relevant information than the caregiver, and a sharing partnership is to the advantage of both. Taking full advantage of clinical records, even with blinded information, requires a strong level of understanding and support for the work and its importance to improving the quality of health care. This support may be the most important element in the development of the learning enterprise. In addition, the more patients understand and communicate with their caregivers about the evolving nature of evidence, the less disruptive will be the frequency and amplitude of public response to research results that find themselves prematurely, or without appropriate interpretative guidance, in the headlines and the short-term consciousness of Americans.

- *Build toward continuous learning in all aspects of care.* This foundational principle of a learning healthcare system will depend on system and culture change in each element of the care process with the potential to promote interest, activity, and involvement in the knowledge and evidence development process, from health professions education to care delivery and payment.

ISSUES FOR POSSIBLE ROUNDTABLE FOLLOW-UP

Among the range of issues engaged in the workshop's discussion were a number that could serve as candidates for the sort of multistakeholder consideration and engagement represented by the Roundtable on Value & Science-Driven Health Care, its members, and their colleagues.

Clinical Effectiveness Research

- *Methodologies.* How do various research approaches best align to different study circumstances—e.g., nature of the condition, the type of intervention, the existing body of evidence? Should Roundtable participants develop a taxonomy to help identify the priority research advances needed to strengthen and streamline current methodologies and to consider approaches for their advancement and adoption?
- *Priorities.* What are the most compelling priorities for comparative effectiveness studies, and how might providers and patients be engaged in helping to identify them and set the stage for research strategies and funding partnerships?
- *Coordination.* Given the oft-stated need for stronger coordination in the identification, priority setting, design, and implementation of clinical effectiveness research, what might Roundtable members do to facilitate evolution of the capacity?
- *Clustering.* The National Cancer Institute is exploring the clustering of clinical studies to make the process of study consideration and launching quicker and more efficient? Should this be explored as a model for others?
- *Registry collaboration.* Since registries offer the most immediate prospects for broader "real-time" learning, can Roundtable participants work with interested organizations on periodic convening

of those involved in maintaining clinical registries, exploring additional opportunities for combined efforts and shared learning?

- *Phased intervention with evaluation.* How can progress be accelerated in the adoption by public and private payers of approaches to allow phased implementation and reimbursement for promising interventions for which effectiveness and relative advantage has not been firmly established? What sort of neutral venue would work best for a multistakeholder effort through existing research networks (e.g., CTSAs, HMORN)?
- *Patient preferences and perspectives.* What approaches might help to refine practical instruments to determine patient preferences— such as the NIH's PROMIS (Patient-Reported Outcomes Measurement Information System)—and apply them as central elements of outcome measurement?
- *Public–private collaboration.* What administrative vehicles might enhance opportunities for academic medicine, industry, and government to engage cooperatively in clinical effectiveness research? Would development of common contract language be helpful in facilitating public–private partnerships?
- *Clinician engagement.* Should a venue be established for periodic convening of primary care and specialty physician groups to explore clinical effectiveness research priorities, progress in practice-based research, opportunities to engage in registry-related research, and improved approaches to clinical guideline development and application?
- *Academic health center engagement.* With academic institutions setting the pattern for the predominant approach to clinical research, drawing prevailing patterns closer to broader practice bases will require increasing the engagement with community-based facilities and private practices for practice-based research. How might Roundtable stakeholders partner with the Association of American Medical Colleges and Association of Academic Health Centers to foster the necessary changes?
- *Incentives for practice-based research.* Might an employer–payer working group from the Roundtable be useful in exploring economic incentives to accelerate progress in using clinical data for new insights by rewarding providers and related groups working to improve knowledge generation and application throughout the care process?
- *Condition-specific high-priority effectiveness research targets.* Might the Roundtable develop a working group to characterize the gap between current results and what should be expected, based on current treatment knowledge, strategies for closing the

gap, and collaborative approaches (e.g., registries) for the following conditions:
— Adult oncology
— Orthopedic procedures
— Management of co-occurring chronic diseases?

Clinical Data

- *Secondary use of clinical data.* Successful use of clinical data as a reliable resource for clinical effectiveness evidence development requires the development of standards and approaches that assure the quality of the work. How might Roundtable members encourage or foster work of this sort?
- *Privacy and security.* What can be done within the existing structures and institutions to clarify definitions and reduce the tendencies for unnecessarily restrictive interpretations on clinical data access, in particular related to secondary use of data?
- *Collaborative data mining.* Are there ways that Roundtable member initiatives might facilitate the progress of EHR data mining networks working on strategies, statistical expertise, and training needs to improve and accelerate postmarket surveillance and clinical research?
- *Research-related EHR standards.* How might EHR standard-setting groups be best engaged to ensure that standards developed are research friendly, developed with the research utility in mind, and have the flexibility to adapt as research tools expand?
- *Transparency and access.* What vehicles, approaches, and stewardship structures might best improve the receptivity of the clinical data marketplace to enhanced data sharing, including making federally sponsored clinical data more widely available for secondary analysis (data from federally supported research, as well as Medicare-related data)?

Communication

- *Research results.* Since part of the challenge in public misunderstanding of research results is a product of "hyping" by the research community, how might the Roundtable productively explore the options for "self-regulatory guidelines" on announcing and working with media on research results?
- *Patient involvement in the evidence process.* If progress in patient outcomes depends on deeper citizen understanding and engagement as full participants in the learning healthcare system—both

as partners with caregivers in their own care, and as supporters of the use of protected clinical data to enhance learning—what steps can accelerate?

As interested parties consider these issues, we need to remember that the focus of the research discussed at the workshop is, ultimately, for and about the patient. The goals of the work are fundamentally oriented to bringing the right care to the right person at the right time at the right price. The fundamental questions we seek to answer for any healthcare intervention are straightforward: Can it work? Will it work—for *this* patient in *this* setting? Is it worth it? Do the benefits outweigh any harms? Do the benefits justify the costs? Do the possible changes offer important advantages over existing alternatives?

Finally, despite the custom of referring to "our healthcare system," the research community in practice functions as a diverse set of elements that often seems to connect productively only by happenstance. Because shortfalls in coordination and communication impinge on the funding, effectiveness, and efficiency of the clinical research process—not to mention its progress as a key element of a learning healthcare system—the notion of working productively together is vital for both patients and the healthcare community. Better coordination, collaboration, public–private partnerships, and priority setting are compelling priorities, and the attention and awareness generated in the course of this meeting are important to the Roundtable's focus on redesigning the clinical effectiveness research paradigm.

Appendixes

Appendix A

Workshop Agenda

Redesigning the Clinical Effectiveness Research Paradigm:
Innovation and Practice-Based Approaches
A Learning Healthcare System Workshop
IOM Roundtable on Evidence-Based Medicine

December 12-13, 2007
Lecture Room
The National Academy of Sciences Building
2100 C Street, NW
Washington, DC 20037

Issues motivating the discussion:
1. Need for substantially improved understanding of the comparative clinical effectiveness of healthcare interventions.
2. Strengths of the randomized controlled trial muted by constraints in time, cost, and limited applicability.
3. Opportunities presented by the size and expansion of potentially interoperable administrative and clinical datasets.
4. Opportunities presented by innovative study designs and statistical tools.
5. Need for innovative approaches leading to a more practical and reliable clinical research paradigm.
6. Need to build a system in which clinical effectiveness research is a more natural by-product of the care process.

Goal: To explore these issues, identify potential approaches, and discuss possible strategies for their engagement.

DAY ONE

8:30   WELCOME AND OPENING REMARKS
        *Denis A. Cortese, Mayo Clinic and Chair, IOM Roundtable
        on Evidence-Based Medicine*

9:00   KEYNOTE: CLINICAL EFFECTIVENESS RESEARCH—PAST,
        PRESENT, AND FUTURE
        Overview of the evolution of clinical effectiveness research,
        current state of play, key challenges (e.g., keeping pace,
        inference gap, cost, policy), and future opportunities to
        generate reliable insights.
        Harvey V. Fineberg, Institute of Medicine

9:30   SESSION 1: CASES IN POINT—LEARNING FROM EXPERIENCE
        This session will present several case examples of high
        profile issues—some linked to delayed applications
        of effective treatments or to premature adoption of
        unwarranted treatments—that hold important lessons for
        future work in the design and interpretation of clinical
        effectiveness studies.
        *Chair: Joel Kupersmith, Veterans Health Administration
        and IOM Roundtable on Evidence-Based Medicine*

        • Hormone replacement therapy
          JoAnn E. Manson, Harvard Medical School
        • Drug-eluting coronary stents
          Ashley B. Boam, Food and Drug Administration
        • Bariatric surgery
          David R. Flum, University of Washington

[10:15 to 10:30 Break]

        • Antipsychotic therapeutics
          Philip S. Wang, National Institute of Mental Health
        • Cancer screening
          Peter B. Bach, Memorial Sloan-Kettering Cancer Center

        Respondent: Brian G. Firth, Cordis
        General discussion

12:00   LUNCH
        (Box lunches are available in the Executive Dining Room)

12:45   Session 2: Taking advantage of new tools and
techniques
Where might we expect improvements from analytic tools,
sample size, and data quality and availability? What novel
techniques could researchers use in conjunction with new
information, models, and tools?
*Chair: Donald M. Steinwachs, Johns Hopkins University
and IOM Roundtable on Evidence-Based Medicine*

- Innovative approaches to clinical trials
  Robert M. Califf, Duke University
- Innovative analytic tools for large clinical and
  administrative databases
  Sebastian Schneeweiss, Harvard Medical School
- Adaptive and Bayesian approaches to study design
  *Donald A. Berry, University of Texas, M.D. Anderson
  Cancer Center*
- Simulation and predictive modeling
  Mark S. Roberts, University of Pittsburgh, Archimedes Inc.
- Emerging genetic information
  *Teri A. Manolio, National Human Genome Research
  Institute*

*Respondent: Michael Lauer, National Heart, Lung, and
Blood Institute*
General discussion

[2:45 to 3:00 Break]

3:00   Session 3: Organizing and improving data utility
What are the research implications of the development of
much larger, electronically accessible health records and
administrative and clinical databases? How might they most
appropriately be applied to clinical effectiveness research?
What rules of engagement are needed to harness emerging
data sources?
*Chair: Denis A. Cortese, Mayo Clinic and IOM Roundtable
on Evidence-Based Medicine*

- Electronic health records/point of care data
  Ronald A. Paulus, Geisinger Health System

- Administrative and claims data
  Alexander M. Walker, Harvard School of Public Health & Worldwide Health Info. Science Consultants
- Registries
  Alan J. Moskowitz, Columbia University
- Distributed research model
  Richard Platt, Harvard Pilgrim Health Care and Harvard Medical School

  Respondent: William H. Crown, Ingenix
  General discussion

4:45   GENERAL DISCUSSION OF THE KEY POINTS OF THE DAY
Chair: Denis A. Cortese, Mayo Clinic and IOM Roundtable on Evidence-Based Medicine

5:15   RECEPTION—GREAT HALL

DAY TWO

8:45   WELCOME AND SHORT RECAP OF DAY ONE
J. Michael McGinnis, Institute of Medicine

9:00   KEYNOTE: RESEARCH THAT MEETS EVIDENCE NEEDS
Evidence gaps and research challenges. Insights on how the approach to clinical effectiveness research can better take advantage of emerging tools and study designs to address the challenges, including those related to generalizability, heterogeneity of treatment effects, and multiple co-morbidities?
Chair: Carolyn M. Clancy, Agency for Healthcare Research and Quality and IOM Roundtable on Evidence-Based Medicine

9:30   SESSION 4: MOVING TO THE NEXT GENERATION OF STUDIES
What are the key opportunities and needed advancements to improve our approach to clinical effectiveness research? How might we take better advantage of emerging resources to plan, develop, and sequence studies that are more timely, relevant, efficient, and generalizable—and account for lifecycle variation of the conditions and interventions in play?
Chair: Robert M. Califf, Duke University

- Large data streams and the power of numbers
  Sharon-Lise T. Normand, Harvard Medical School
- Observational studies
  Wayne A. Ray, Vanderbilt University
- Experimental and hybrid studies
  A. John Rush, University of Texas Southwestern Medical Center

[10:15 to 10:30 Break]

- Accommodating genetic variation as a standard feature of clinical research
  Isaac S. Kohane, Harvard Medical School
- Phased introduction and payment for interventions under protocol
  Wade M. Aubry, Center for Medical Technology Policy
- Research networks
  Eric B. Larson, Group Health Cooperative

Respondent: Joe V. Selby, Kaiser Permanente
General discussion

12:00   LUNCH
           (Box lunches are available in the Executive Dining Room)

12:45   SESSION 5: ALIGNING POLICY WITH RESEARCH
           OPPORTUNITIES
           What policy levers can drive innovative research and
           progress in practice-based approaches? What barriers need
           to be addressed to accelerate the progress?
           *Chair: Richard Platt, Harvard Pilgrim Health Care and
           IOM Roundtable on Evidence-Based Medicine*

- Course-of-care data
  Greg Pawlson, National Committee for Quality Assurance
- Manufacturer data
  Peter K. Honig, Merck
- Regulatory requirements and data generation
  Mark B. McClellan, Brookings Institution
- Publicly sponsored health data
  J. Sanford Schwartz, University of Pennsylvania
- Building the research infrastructure
  Alan M. Krensky, National Institutes of Health

 • **Engaging consumers**
   Kathy Hudson, Johns Hopkins University

   Respondent: Jerry Avorn, Harvard Medical School
   General discussion

3:15   SESSION 6: ORGANIZING THE RESEARCH COMMUNITY FOR
       CHANGE—DISCUSSION PANEL
       What guiding principles are important in refining the
       clinical effectiveness research paradigm and in fostering
       the necessary changes? What issues need to be addressed
       in integrating trials into a lifecycle approach to evidence
       development? What expertise and training might be needed?
       What are some of the political challenges?
       Chair: J. Michael McGinnis, Institute of Medicine

       Panel discussion
       *Panel: Alan M. Krensky (NIH), Mark B. McClellan
       (Brookings Institution), Garry Neil (Johnson & Johnson),
       John Niederhuber (NCI), Lewis Sandy (United HealthCare)*

4:30   CONCLUDING SUMMARY REMARKS AND ADJOURNMENT
       J. Michael McGinnis, Institute of Medicine

Workshop Planning Committee
Robert M. Califf, MD, Duke Clinical Research Institute, Duke University
Lynn Etheredge, George Washington University
Kim Gilchrist, MD, AstraZeneca LP
Bryan Luce, PhD, MBA, United Biosource Corporation
Jonathan Perlin, MD, PhD, MSHA, FACP, HCA Inc.
Richard Platt, MD, MS, Harvard Medical School and Harvard Pilgrim

Appendix
B

Biographical Sketches of
Workshop Participants

Wade M. Aubry, M.D., has had experience in technology assessment, coverage decisions, and research with a number of different organizations in the private and public sectors. He is Associate Director of the Center for Medical Technology Policy (CMTP), which provides a neutral forum for payers, manufacturers, researchers, clinicians, and patients to work together to identify evidence gaps and fund prospective, real-world research to inform healthcare decisions. He is also Senior Medical Advisor for the California Technology Assessment Forum, an open forum process of technology assessment using evidence-based criteria. Dr. Aubry has twice been a member of the CMS MEDCAC, is a former Chair of the national BCBSA TEC Medical Advisory Panel, and has recently been appointed to a 2-year term on the AHRQ Effective Health Care Stakeholder Group. He is Associate Clinical Professor of Medicine at the UCSF Institute for Health Policy Studies, where he works on the California Health Benefits Review Program, an assessment program for proposed health plan mandates for the California legislature. Previously, he was Senior Advisor for the Health Technology Center (HealthTech), Vice President of the Lewin Group, Senior Vice President and Chief Medical Officer for Blue Shield of California, and Medicare Part B Medical Director for Northern California. He has served on numerous national advisory committees for the NIH, IOM, NCQA, and others. Dr. Aubry received his B.S. degree Phi Beta Kappa from Stanford University, his M.D. degree from the UCLA School of Medicine, and his postgraduate training in internal medicine and endocrinology at Cedars-Sinai Medical Center. Among his publications on medical technology, he is co-author of a comprehensive case study on bone marrow transplants for breast cancer, which was published in January 2007 by Oxford University Press and titled *False Hope: Bone Marrow Transplantation for Breast Cancer.*

Jerry Avorn, M.D., is Professor of Medicine at Harvard Medical School and Chief of the Division of Pharmaco-epidemiology and Pharmaco-economics in the Department of Medicine at Brigham and Women's Hospital. An internist, geriatrician, and drug epidemiologist, he studies the intended and adverse effects of drugs, physician prescribing practices, and medication policy. Dr. Avorn pioneered the "academic detailing" approach in which evidence-based information about drugs is provided to doctors through educational outreach programs run by noncommercial sponsors; such programs are now in widespread use throughout the United States, Canada, Australia, Europe, and the developing world. He completed his undergraduate training at Columbia University in 1969, received an M.D. from Harvard Medical School in 1974, and was a resident in internal medicine at the Beth Israel Hospital in Boston. He has served on several national and international panels as an expert on the determinants and consequences of medication use, and is a past President of the International Society of Pharmaco-Epidemiology. Dr. Avorn is the author of more than 200 papers in the medical literature on medication use and its outcomes, and he is one of the most highly cited researchers working in the area of medicine and the social sciences. His book, *Powerful Medicines: The Benefits, Risks, and Costs of Prescription Drugs,* was published by Knopf in 2004 and re-issued in 2005.

Peter B. Bach, M.D., is Associate Attending Physician at Memorial Sloan-Kettering Cancer Center in New York and is board certified in internal medicine, pulmonary medicine, and critical care medicine. He is a National Institutes of Health-funded researcher with expertise in quality of care and epidemiologic research methods. His research on health disparities, variations in healthcare quality, and lung cancer epidemiology has appeared in *The New England Journal of Medicine,* the *Journal of the American Medical Association,* and the *Journal of the National Cancer Institute.* Bach served as a senior adviser to the Administrator of the Centers for Medicare & Medicaid Services from February 2005 through November 2006, where his work focused on improving evidence about the effect of therapies and devices and revising payment to enhance care quality. He was the agency lead on cancer policy. During the Rwandan Civil War, he was a camp physician in Goma, Zaire, caring for refugees. Bach received his bachelor's degree in English and American Literature from Harvard College, his M.D. from the University of Minnesota, and his master's degree in public policy from the University of Chicago, where he was also a Robert Wood Johnson

Clinical Scholar. He completed his clinical training in internal medicine, pulmonary and critical care at the Johns Hopkins Hospital.

Donald A. Berry, Ph.D., is Head and Chair of the Division of Quantitative Sciences in the Department of Biostatistics at the University of Texas M.D. Anderson Cancer Center and an international expert in the field of biostatistics. He holds the Frank T. McGraw Memorial Chair for Cancer Research at The University of Texas M.D. Anderson Cancer Center. His primary interest is the prevention and treatment of breast cancer. He serves as the faculty statistician on the Breast Cancer Committee of the Cancer and Leukemia Group B (CALGB), a national oncology group. In this role he designs and supervises the conduct and analysis of clinical trials in breast cancer. A native of Massachusetts, Dr. Berry received his Ph.D. in statistics from Yale University and previously served on the faculty at the University of Minnesota and at Duke University, where he held the Edger Thompson Professorship in the College of Arts and Sciences. The author of more than 200 published articles as well as several books on biostatistics in medical research, Dr. Berry has been the principal investigator for numerous medical research programs funded by the National Institutes of Health and the National Science Foundation. A current project funded by the National Cancer Institute (NCI) describes the usage and benefits of breast cancer treatment. He was also the principal investigator of an NCI project CISNET: Cancer Intervention and Surveillance Network. This project focused on statistical modeling to assess the relative contribution of screening mammography, tamoxifen, and chemotherapy to the drop in breast cancer mortality observed in the United States since 1990. Another focus of Dr. Berry's statistical research is designing clinical trials that utilize patients more efficiently and that treat patients in the trials more effectively. Dr. Berry is a statistics editor for the *Journal of the National Cancer Institute* and associate editor for *Breast Cancer Research and Treatment* and also for *Clinical Cancer Research*, and he is a Fellow of the American Statistical Association and of the Institute of Mathematical Statistics.

Ashley B. Boam, M.S., currently serves as Acting Deputy Director for Science and Review Policy in the Office of Device Evaluation at FDA's Center for Devices and Radiological Health. Ms. Boam earned her B.S.E and M.S.B.E. in biomedical engineering from Tulane University and the University of Alabama at Birmingham, respectively. She joined the FDA in 1993 as a scientific reviewer in the Division of Ophthalmic and ENT Devices. In 2002, she joined the Division of Cardiovascular Devices as Chief of the Interventional Cardiology Devices Branch. Products reviewed by the branch include drug-eluting stents, embolic protection devices, cardiac occluders, and other devices associated with coronary percutaneous interventional procedures.

Robert M. Califf, M.D., is currently Vice Chancellor for Clinical Research, Director of the Duke Translational Medicine Institute (DTMI), and Professor of Medicine in the Division of Cardiology at the Duke University Medical Center in Durham, North Carolina. For 10 years he was Director of the Duke Clinical Research Institute, a premier academic research organization. A native of South Carolina, Dr. Califf graduated from Duke University, summa cum laude and Phi Beta Kappa, in 1973 and from Duke University Medical School in 1978, where he was selected for Alpha Omega Alpha. He performed his internship and residency at the University of California at San Francisco and his fellowship in Cardiology at Duke University. He is board certified in internal medicine (1984) and cardiology (1986) and is a Fellow of the American College of Cardiology (1988). Dr. Califf has served as an editor for the first and second editions of the landmark textbook, *Acute Coronary Care*, published by Mosby, Inc., and is the Editor-in Chief of Mosby's *American Heart Journal*. He is a section editor for the *Textbook of Cardiovascular Medicine* and has been an author or coauthor of more than 600 peer-reviewed journal articles. He is a contributing editor for theheart.org, an online information resource for academic and practicing cardiologists. Dr. Califf has led the Duke Clinical Research Institute (DCRI) efforts for many of the best-known clinical trials in cardiovascular disease. With his colleagues from the Duke Databank for Cardiovascular Disease, he has written extensively about clinical and economic outcomes in chronic heart disease. He is considered an international leader in the fields of health outcomes, quality of care, and medical economics. Dr. Califf has served on the Cardiorenal Advisory Panel of the U.S. FDA and the Pharmaceutical Roundtable of the Institute of Medicine (IOM). He also served on the IOM Committee that recommended Medicare coverage of clinical trials, which Congress recently approved. He is director of the coordinating center for the Centers for Education & Research on Therapeutics™ (CERTs), a public–private partnership among AHRQ, DCRI, academia, industry, and consumer groups. This partnership focuses on research and education that will advance the best use of medical products.

Carolyn M. Clancy, M.D., is Director of the Agency for Healthcare Research and Quality (AHRQ). Prior to 2002 she was Director of the Agency's Center for Outcomes and Effectiveness Research (COER). Dr. Clancy, a general internist and health services researcher, is a graduate of Boston College and the University of Massachusetts Medical School. Following clinical training in internal medicine, Dr. Clancy was a Henry J. Kaiser Family Foundation Fellow at the University of Pennsylvania. She was also an assistant professor in the Department of Internal Medicine at the Medical College of Virginia in Richmond before joining AHRQ in 1990. Dr. Clancy holds an academic appointment at George Washington University School of Medicine (Clinical Associate Professor, Department of Medicine), and she is the Senior Associate Editor of *Health Services Research* and serves on multiple editorial boards (currently *Annals of Family Medicine, American Journal of Medical Quality,* and *Medical Care Research and Review*). Dr. Clancy has published widely in peer-reviewed journals and has edited or contributed to seven books. She is a member of the Institute of Medicine and was elected a Master of the American College of Physicians in 2004.

Denis A. Cortese, M.D., is President and Chief Executive Officer of Mayo Clinic and Chair of the Executive Committee. He has been a member of the Board of Trustees since 1997 and previously served on that Board from 1990 to 1993. Following service in the U.S. Naval Corps, he joined the staff of the Mayo Clinic in Rochester, Minnesota, in 1976 as a specialist in pulmonary medicine. He was a member of the Board of Governors in Rochester before moving to the Mayo Clinic in Jacksonville, Florida, in 1993. From 1999 to 2002 he served as Chair of the Board of Governors at the Mayo Clinic and Chair of the Board of Directors at St. Luke's Hospital in Jacksonville, Florida. He is a Director and former President of the International Photodynamic Association and has been involved in the bronchoscopic detection, localization, and treatment of early-stage lung cancer. He is a member of the Healthcare Leadership Council and the Harvard/Kennedy School Healthcare Policy Group, and he is a former member of the Center for Corporate Innovation. He served on the Steering Committee for the RAND Ix Project, "Using Information Technology to Create a New Future in Healthcare," and the Principals Committee of the National Innovation Initiative. He also is a charter member of the Advisory Board of World Community Grid and a founding member of the American Medical Group Association Chairs/Presidents/CEOs Council. Dr. Cortese is a graduate of Temple University, completed his residency at the Mayo Graduate School of Medicine, and is a professor of medicine in Mayo Clinic College of Medicine. Dr. Cortese is a member of the Institute of Medicine, a Fellow of the Royal College of Physicians in England, and an honorary member of the Academia Nacional de Mexicana (Mexico).

William H. Crown, Ph.D., is President of i3 Innovus, the Health Economics and Outcomes Research division of Ingenix. From 1982 to 1995, Dr. Crown was a faculty member at the Florence Heller Graduate School, Brandeis University, where he taught graduate courses in statistics and conducted research on the economics of aging and long-term care policy. Prior to joining Ingenix in 2004, Dr. Crown was Vice President of Outcomes Research and Econometrics at Medstat, where he conducted numerous retrospective database analyses of the burden of illness associated with various diseases—particularly respiratory and mental health conditions.

Dr. Crown's work in the area of depression was one of the first applications of econometric techniques in outcomes research to control for the effects of selection bias when using retrospective data to evaluate drug technologies. He has 25 years of experience conducting health policy and income maintenance research for private-sector and public-sector clients. Dr. Crown is author or co-author of four books and more than 90 refereed journal articles, book chapters, and other publications.

Brian G. Firth, M.D., Ph.D., is Worldwide Vice President, Health Affairs, Cordis Corporation, a Johnson & Johnson company. Cordis develops and markets devices for circulatory disease management. Among Dr. Firth's responsibilities are worldwide strategic medical input for the corporation and liaison with major medical societies, publishing results of Cordis' clinical research articles, and inter-company cardiovascular research and health policy activities within Johnson & Johnson. He was appointed to this position in August 2007. Dr. Firth began his career at Johnson & Johnson in 1995 as Vice President, Research and Development, Johnson & Johnson Interventional Systems, now part of Cordis. He was named Vice President, Research and Development at Cordis in 1996, and the following year, was appointed Worldwide Vice President, Medical Affairs and Chief Scientific Officer. From June 1999 to July 2007, he served as Worldwide Vice President of Medical Affairs and Health Economics. In this capacity, he was one of the chief architects behind the successful launch of the CYPHER® Sirolimus-eluting stent. Dr. Firth obtained his medical degree (bachelor of medicine; bachelor of surgery) with honors from the University of Cape Town in South Africa. He then attended Oxford University as a Rhodes Scholar where he obtained a doctorate of philosophy in cardiovascular physiology. He completed his residency in internal medicine and fellowship in cardiology at the Groote Schuur Hospital in Cape Town. He also completed a fellowship in cardiology at the University of Texas Southwestern Medical Center in Dallas, Texas, and then served as a cardiologist and Professor of Medicine at that institution for more than 10 years. He received his master of business administration from Amber University in Dallas. He is also a Fellow of the Royal College of Physicians, UK, The American College of Cardiology, and the American Heart Association. A member of many professional medical societies, committees, and educational boards, Dr. Firth has published more than 80 manuscripts and co-authored several books on cardiology.

David R. Flum, M.D., M.P.H., is a gastrointestinal surgeon and outcomes researcher at the University of Washington. He holds the rank of Associate Professor in the Schools of Medicine and Public Health and serves as the Director of the Surgical Outcomes Research Center (SORCE) at the

University of Washington. He is one of the Principal Investigators of the Longitudinal Assessment of Bariatric Surgery (LABS) study and the Medical Director of the Surgical Clinical Outcomes Assessment Program (SCOAP), a statewide surgical QI activity. He is also a contributing editor for the *Journal of the American Medical Association*. Dr. Flum's areas of particular expertise include surgical management of gastrointestinal disorders and advanced laparoscopy with an interest in biliary tract disorders and complex abdominal wall hernias.

Annetine C. Gelijns, Ph.D., is Co-Director (with Alan Moskowitz) of the International Center for Health Outcomes and Innovation Research (InCHOIR) and a Professor of Surgical Sciences and Public Health in the Department of Surgery, College of Physicians and Surgeons, and the Division of Health Policy and Management of the Mailman School of Public Health, Columbia University, New York City. She is also a Division Chief in the Department of Surgery. Her current research focuses on measurement of the long-term clinical outcomes and economic impact of clinical interventions, patient safety research, and the factors driving the development and diffusion of medical technology. She has special expertise in cardiovascular disease, particularly in the design, coordination, and analysis of multicenter left ventricular assist devices (LVAD) trials. She has been the Director of the Data Coordinating Center for the NHLBI-sponsored REMATCH trial, is the PI of the DCC for a SCCOR grant on the biology of long-term LVAD implantation, and co-PI for the NHLBI-sponsored CT Surgery Network. She co-chairs the cost-effectiveness section of the INTERMACS registry of mechanical circulatory support devices.

Peter K. Honig, M.D., M.P.H., is Executive Vice President for Global Regulatory Affairs, Global Clinical Research Operations and Data Management, Product Safety, Quality Assurance and OTC Development at Merck Research Laboratories. He is former Director of the Office of Drug Safety in FDA's Center for Drug Evaluation and Research (CDER). He joined CDER as a medical officer in the Division of Oncology and Pulmonary Drug Products in 1993 and assumed many roles and responsibilities during his FDA career, including FDA representative to the CERTs Steering Committee, and CDER liaison to the Harvard and Johns Hopkins Clinical Investigators fellowship training programs. Dr. Honig was also active internationally as the FDA representative to the International Conference on Harmonization (ICH) MedDRA (Medical Dictionary for Regulatory Activities) Management Board and the E2B Expert Working Group and currently serves as PhRMA member of the ICH Steering Committee. Dr. Honig received his baccalaureate, medical, and public health degrees from Columbia University in New York. He has postgraduate training and is board certified in internal medicine and clinical pharmacology and was elected a Fellow of the American College of Physicians (FACP). Dr. Honig retains faculty appointments at the Uniformed Services University of the Health Sciences and Georgetown University Medical School. He is a past President of the American Society of Clinical Pharmacology and Therapeutics (ASCPT).

Kathy Hudson, Ph.D., is the founder and Director of the Genetics and Public Policy Center (GPPC) and an Associate Professor in the Berman Bioethics Institute, Institute of Genetic Medicine, and the Department of Pediatrics at Johns Hopkins University. Hudson founded the GPPC to fill an important niche in the science policy landscape and to focus exclusively on public policy issues raised by advances in human genetics. She leads the GPPC's efforts to address legal, ethical, and policy issues related to human reproductive genetic technologies, genetic testing quality and oversight, and public engagement in genetic research. Hudson serves on the boards of the Health Privacy Project, the Guttmacher Institute, the Annual Review of Genomics and Human Genetics and PXE International, the Personalized Healthcare Working Group for the U.S. Department of Health and Human Services, the Committee on Science, Engineering and Public Policy for the American Association for the Advancement of Science, and the Social Issues Committee for the American Society of Human Genetics. She has published articles about and is a frequent speaker on issues related to biotechnology, genetics, and public policy. Before founding the GPPC, Hudson was the Assistant Director of the National Human Genome Research Institute (NHGRI) responsible for communications, legislation, planning, and education activities. Previously, Hudson served as a Senior Policy Analyst in the U.S. Department of Health and Human Services and worked on Capitol Hill. She holds a Ph.D. in molecular biology from the University of California at Berkeley, an M.S. in microbiology from the University of Chicago, and a B.A. in biology from Carleton College.

Isaac S. Kohane, M.D., Ph.D., is the director of the Children's Hospital Informatics Program and is the Henderson Associate Professor of Pediatrics and Health Sciences and Technology at Harvard Medical School (HMS). He is also the co-Director of the HMS Center for Biomedical Library and Director of the HMS Countway Library of Meidicine. Dr. Kohane leads multiple collaborations at Harvard Medical School and its hospital affiliates in the use of genomics and computer science to study cancer and the development of the brain (with emphasis on autism). He also has developed several computer systems to allow multiple hospital systems to be used as "living laboratories" to study the genetic basis of disease while preserving patient privacy. Dr. Kohane has published more than 160 papers in the medical literature and authored a widely used book on microarrays for an integrative genomics. He has been elected to multiple honor societies including the American Society for Clinical Investigation and the American College of Medical Informatics. He leads a doctoral program in genomics and bioinformatics at MIT. He is also a practicing pediatric endocrinologist.

Alan M. Krensky, M.D., is the first Director of the Office of Portfolio Analysis and Strategic Initiatives (OPASI) and a Deputy Director of the National Institutes of Health. He was at Stanford University for 23 years where he served as the Shelagh Galligan Professor of Pediatrics, Associate Dean for Children's Health, Associate Chair for Research, Chief of the Division of Immunology and Transplantation Biology, and Executive Director of the Children's Health Initiative. A medical graduate of the University of Pennsylvania in 1977, he trained in pediatrics and nephrology at Boston Children's Hospital and immunology at the Dana-Farber Cancer Institute. He moved to Stanford as Assistant Professor of Pediatrics in 1984, was appointed Shelagh Galligan Professor in 1995, and has been at the NIH since July 2007. Dr. Krensky's research program was continuously funded by the NIH from 1984 to his assumption of the NIH post. He has made important contributions to understanding the role of human T lymphocytes in disease and applying this information to the development of new diagnostic and therapeutic approaches. He has published more than 250 scientific articles, served on numerous editorial and scientific advisory boards, and holds 10 patents. Dr. Krensky is a member of the American Society of Clinical Investigation and Association of American Physicians, and he served as President of the Society for Pediatric Research and Secretary-Treasurer of the American Society of Nephrology.

Joel Kupersmith, M.D., is the Chief Research and Development Officer of the Department of Veterans Affairs. He is a graduate of New York Medical College where he also completed his residency in internal medicine. Subsequently, he completed a cardiology fellowship at Beth Israel Medical Center/Harvard Medical School, after which he joined the faculty of the Mt. Sinai School of Medicine where he rose to the rank of Professor and Director of the Clinical Pharmacology section. After this he became Chief of Cardiology and V.V. Cooke Professor of Medicine at the University of Louisville, Professor and Chairperson, Department of Medicine at the College of Human Medicine at Michigan State University, and then Dean, School of Medicine and Graduate School of Biomedical Sciences, Vice President for Clinical Affairs at Texas Tech University as well as CEO of the Faculty Practice. In this position there were many advances in the medical center, including a marked stepwise drop in the faculty attrition rate; legislative initiatives; growth of the research enterprise; important recruitments; many educational initiatives; construction projects; improved scores of entering students; and increased number of minority students. Subsequently, Dr. Kupersmith was a Scholar-in-Residence at both the Institute of Medicine and the Association of American Medical Colleges before assuming duties as Chief Research and Development Officer at VHA. Dr. Kupersmith has 154 publications and 2 books. His earlier research interests were in the area of electrophysiology, the causes and treatment of heart rhythm abnormalities, and implantable cardioverter defibrillators. Subsequently, he published on cost effectiveness of heart disease treatments, and most recently his work has been on health policy issues. Dr. Kupersmith has been on many national and international committees involved in heart disease and journal editorial boards. He is a member of numerous professional organizations including the American Society for Clinical Investigation. Dr. Kupersmith also has been a Visiting Scholar at the Hastings Center for Ethics.

Eric B. Larson, M.D., M.P.H., M.A.C.P., is Executive Director of Group Health's Center for Health Studies. A graduate of Harvard Medical School, he trained in internal medicine at Beth Israel Hospital in Boston, completed a Robert Wood Johnson Clinical Scholars and M.P.H. program at the University of Washington, and then served as Chief Resident of University Hospital in Seattle. He served as Medical Director of the University of Washington Medical Center and Associate Dean for Clinical Affairs from 1989 to 2002. His research spans a range of general medicine topics and has focused on aging and dementia, including a long-running study of aging and cognitive change set in the Group Health Cooperative—The UW/Group Health Alzheimer's Disease Patient Registry/Adult Changes in Thought Study. He has served as President of the Society of General Internal Medicine, Chair of the OTA/DHHS Advisory Panel on Alzheimer's Disease and Related Disorders and was Chair of the Board of Regents (2004–2005) of the American College of Physicians. He is an elected member of the Institute of Medicine.

Michael Lauer, M.D., joined NHLBI in July 2007 as Director of the Division of Prevention and Population Science. A board-certified cardiologist, he received his M.D. from Albany Medical College in 1985 and underwent postgraduate training within the Harvard University system at Massachusetts General Hospital, Boston Beth Israel Hospital, and the Harvard School of Public Health. After completing specialized research training in Cardiovascular Epidemiology at the Framingham Heart Study, he joined the staff at the Cleveland Clinic in 1993. During 14 years at the clinic, he established a world-renowned clinical epidemiology research program with primary focus on diagnostic testing and comparative effectiveness. His research led to more than 150 publications in top medical journals, grant support from the American Heart Association and the NIH, and election to the American Society of Clinical Investigation. Dr. Lauer has served as Contributing Editor for *JAMA*, co-Director of the Cleveland Clinic Coronary Care Unit, Director of Cardiac Clinical Research, and as first Vice-Chair of the Cleveland Clinic IRB. He achieved distinction in medical education, leading the development of a clinical research curriculum at the newly founded Cleveland Clinic Lerner Medical College at Case Western Reserve University, where he was Professor of Medicine, Epidemiology, and Biostatistics. In his current position at NHLBI, Dr. Lauer is leading a $300 million per year research division that oversees major programs in cardiovascular epidemiology and prevention.

Teri Manolio, M.D., Ph.D., is Director of the Office of Population Genomics of the National Human Genome Research Institute (NHGRI) at the NIH. She received her M.D. from the University of Maryland in 1980 and her Ph.D. in human genetics/genetic epidemiology from Johns Hopkins University in 2001. She joined the National Heart, Lung, and Blood Institute in 1987 where she was heavily involved in large-scale cohort studies such as the Cardiovascular Health Study and the Framingham Heart Study. She moved to NHGRI in 2005 to lead efforts in applying genomic technologies to population research, including the Genetic Association Information Network (GAIN) and the Genes and Environment Initiative (GEI). She is the author of more than 190 original research papers and has research interests in the epidemiology of subclinical cardiovascular disease, ethnic differences in disease risk, and genomewide association studies of complex diseases.

JoAnn E. Manson, M.D., Dr.P.H., is Professor of Medicine and the Elizabeth Fay Brigham Professor of Women's Health at Harvard Medical School, Chief of Preventive Medicine at Brigham and Women's Hospital (BWH), and co-Director of the Connors Center for Women's Health and Gender Biology at BWH. An endocrinologist and epidemiologist, Dr. Manson is actively involved in women's health research, including several large-scale clinical trials and observational studies of cardiovascular disease, diabetes, cancer, and osteoporosis. Her research has focused on the role of reproductive and hormonal factors, lifestyle variables such as diet and physical activity, and novel plasma and genetic markers as predictors of CVD and diabetes. Dr. Manson is Principal Investigator of the Boston center for the Women's Health Initiative (WHI), the CVD component of the Harvard Nurses' Health Study, the Boston site for the Kronos Early Estrogen Prevention Study (KEEPS), the Women's Antioxidant and Folic Acid Cardiovascular Trial, and other studies. She has published more than 600 articles in medical/scientific journals. Dr. Manson is the recipient of numerous awards, including the "Woman In Science Award" from the American Medical Women's Association, the Bowditch Award for Excellence in Public

Health from the Massachusetts Medical Society, the Postmenopausal Cardio-vascular Health Research Award from the North American Menopause Society, the International Prize "Premio Benessere Stresa" for "Women's Wellbeing and Health in Midlife," and was included in the National Library of Medicine's exhibit "History of American Women Physicians."

Mark B. McClellan, M.D., Ph.D., became the Director of the Engelberg Center for Healthcare Reform at the Brookings Institution in July 2007. The Center studies ways to provide practical solutions for access, quality, and financing challenges facing the U.S. healthcare system. In addition, Dr. McClellan is the Leonard D. Schaeffer Chair in Health Policy Studies. Dr. McClellan has a highly distinguished record in public service and in aca-demic research. He is the former administrator for the Centers for Medicare & Medicaid Services (2004–2006) and the former Commissioner of the Food and Drug Administration (2002–2004). He also served as a member of the President's Council of Economic Advisers and Senior Director for Health Care Policy at the White House (2001–2002). In these positions, he developed and implemented major reforms in health policy. Dr. McClellan was also an associate professor of economics and associate professor of medicine (with tenure) at Stanford University, from which he was on leave during his government service. He directed Stanford's Program on Health Outcomes Research, and he was also associate editor of the *Journal of Health Economics* and co-Principal Investigator of the Health and Retire-ment Study (HRS), a longitudinal study of the health and economic status of older Americans. His academic research has been concerned with the effectiveness of medical treatments in improving health, the economic and policy factors influencing medical treatment decisions and health outcomes, the impact of new technologies on public health and medical expendi-tures, and the relationship between health status and economic well being. Dr. McClellan is a Member of the Institute of Medicine of the National Academies and a Research Associate of the National Bureau of Economic Research. A graduate of the University of Texas at Austin, Dr. McClellan earned his M.P.A. from Harvard's Kennedy School of Government in 1991, his M.D. from the Harvard-MIT Division of Health Sciences and Technol-ogy in 1992, and his Ph.D. in economics from MIT in 1993.

J. Michael McGinnis, M.D., M.P.P., is Senior Scholar at the Institute of Medicine of the National Academy of Sciences, leading its initiative on evidence-based medicine. From 1999 to 2005, he served as Senior Vice President and founding Director of the Health Group and as Counselor to the President at the Robert Wood Johnson Foundation. From 1977 to 1995, he held continuous appointments as Assistant Surgeon General, Deputy Assistant Secretary for Health, and founding Director, Disease

Prevention and Health Promotion, through the Carter, Reagan, Bush and Clinton Administrations. Programs and policies created and launched at his initiative include the Healthy People process on national health objectives, now in its third decade; the U.S. Preventive Services Task Force, now in its fourth iteration; the Dietary Guidelines for Americans (with USDA), now in its sixth edition; the RWJF Health & Society Scholars Program; the RWJF Young Epidemiology Scholars Program; and the RWJF Active Living family of programs. His international service includes appointments as Chair of the World Bank/European Commission Task Force on post-war reconstruction of the health sector in Bosnia (1995–1996) and State Coordinator for the World Health Organization smallpox eradication program in Uttar Pradesh, India (1974–1975). He is an elected member of the IOM, Fellow of the American College of Epidemiology, and Fellow of the American College of Preventive Medicine. Current and recent board memberships include the Nemours Foundation Board of Directors; the IOM Committee on Children's Food Marketing (Chair); the NIH State-of-the-Science Panel on Multivitamins in Chronic Disease Prevention (Chair); the Health Professionals Roundtable on Preventive Services (Chair); the FDA Food Advisory Committee/Subcommittee on Nutrition; and the Board of the United Way of the National Capital Area (Chair, Resource Development).

Alan J. Moskowitz, M.D., F.A.C.P., co-directs (with Annetine Gelijns) the International Center for Health Outcomes and Innovation Research (InCHOIR) and is a practicing internist at Columbia University. His academic appointments are in the College of Physicians and Surgeons and Mailman School of Public Health of Columbia University, where he is a Professor of Clinical Medicine, Surgery and Health Policy and Management. His research is focused in the areas of cardiovascular and cerebrovascular diseases. He is a principal investigator in the NINDS-supported ARUBA trial, an international RCT comparing watchful waiting to lesion eradication for unruptured brain arteriovenous malformations, co-Principal Investigator on an NHLBI-sponsored SCCOR grant studying mechanical circulatory support devices in advanced heart failure patients, and co-Principal Investigator on the NHLBI-sponsored cardio-thoracic surgery network. Dr. Moskowitz is a member of the Institutional Review Board of Columbia University and co-chairs the cost-effectiveness section of the INTERMACS registry of mechanical circulatory support devices.

Garry Neil, M.D., is Corporate Vice President, Corporate Office of Science and Technology (COSAT), Johnson & Johnson (J&J). In this role, Garry leads a team that catalyzes sustained growth for J&J by identifying and launching emerging technologies that underpin the creation of future businesses. Neil has broad experience in science, medicine, and pharmaceutical development. He has held a number of senior positions within J&J, most recently Group President, J&J Pharmaceutical Research and Development, where he was responsible for maximizing existing strengths and leveraging collective resources to bring innovative new molecular entities (NMEs) to market quickly and cost effectively. Through a number of new initiatives he helped transform J&J's pharmaceutical R&D to a much more capable and productive organization and helped to recruit a number of top scientists. Under his leadership a number of important new medicines for the treatment of cancer, anemia, infections, central nervous system and psychiatric disorders, pain, and genitourinary and gastrointestinal diseases gained initial or new and/or expanded indication approvals. Before joining J&J, he held senior-level positions with Astra Merck Inc., Astra Pharmaceuticals, Astra Zeneca, and Merck KGaA. Neil has written more than 50 articles and book chapters. He holds an M.D. from the University of Saskatchewan, College of Medicine and completed his postdoctoral clinical training in internal medicine and gastroenterology at the University of Toronto. He is a Fellow of the American College of Physicians, a Fellow of the American College of Gastroenterology, a member of the American Association of Immunologists, and the Society for Clinical Trials. He is a member of the Board of the Reagan-Udall Foundation and the J&J Development Corporation, and he is J&J's representative to and Vice Chairman of the Pharmaceutical Research and Manufacturers Association (PhRMA) Science and Regulatory Committee.

John E. Niederhuber, M.D., is the Director of the National Cancer Institute (NCI). Both a surgeon and researcher, Dr. Niederhuber has dedicated his four-decade career to the treatment and study of cancer—as a professor, cancer center director, National Cancer Advisory Board chair, external advisor to the NCI, grant reviewer, and laboratory investigator supported by NCI and the NIH. In addition to his management of NCI, Dr. Niederhuber remains involved in research, through his laboratory on the National Institutes of Health campus. Under his leadership, the Laboratory of Tumor and Stem Cell Biology, which is a part of the Cell and Cancer Biology Branch of NCI's Center for Cancer Research, is studying tissue stem cells as the cell-of-origin for cancer. He is working to identify, fully characterize, and isolate this population of cells, with the hypothesis that they might become a therapeutic target. Dr. Niederhuber also holds a clinical appointment on the NIH Clinical Center Medical Staff. As a surgeon, Dr. Niederhuber's clinical emphasis is on gastrointestinal cancer, hepatobiliary cancer, and breast cancer. Prior to his appointment, Dr. Niederhuber was NCI's Chief Operating Officer and Deputy Director for Translational and Clinical Sciences, a position he assumed in September 2005. In June 2002, President Bush appointed Dr. Niederhuber as Chair of the National Cancer Advisory Board. He resigned that position in order to become NCI's Deputy Director.

Sharon-Lise T. Normand, Ph.D., is a Professor of Biostatistics in the Department of Health Care Policy, Harvard Medical School and in the Department of Biostatistics at the Harvard School of Public Health. Dr. Normand's methodological research focuses on Bayesian biostatistics with special emphasis on statistical methods for health services and outcomes research including assessment of quality of care, medical guideline construction, profiling, and meta-analysis. Normand has developed a long line of research on methods for the analysis of patterns of treatment and quality of care for patients with cardiovascular disease and patients with mental disorders. Her work in the area of profiling medical care providers involves developing analytic methods for (1) comparing providers using outcomes-based measures and for (2) determining the appropriate unit of analysis, e.g., health plan-level analysis or physician-level analysis, using process-based measures.

Ronald A. Paulus, M.D., M.B.A., is Geisinger's Chief Technology and Innovation Officer, responsible for ensuring system-wide innovation. His responsibilities include Geisinger Ventures, the system's new business formation and intellectual property commercialization function; and Clinical Innovation, leading the system's initiatives focused on care transformation through patient activation, novel technologies, and care redesign. Prior to joining Geisinger Health System, Dr. Paulus was Chief Healthcare Officer for Quovadx, Inc. (NASDAQ: QVDX), which acquired CareScience, Inc., a NASDAQ company providing clinical solutions to improve healthcare quality and efficiency where he had been President and CEO. Before joining CareScience, Dr. Paulus served as Vice President, Operations of Salick Health Care, Inc., a NASDAQ company providing oncology and dialysis services, which was subsequently acquired by AstraZeneca Pharmaceuticals. Dr. Paulus received his M.D. degree from The School of Medicine, University of Pennsylvania, and his M.B.A., concentration in healthcare management, and B.S. in economics from The Wharton School, University of Pennsylvania.

Greg Pawlson, M.D., M.P.H., is the Executive Vice President of National Committee for Quality Assurance (NCQA). NCQA is a leading evaluator of healthcare services and is especially well known for its development of HEDIS® clinical performance measures. At NCQA, beyond his role as a senior member of the leadership team, Dr. Pawlson has oversight and responsibility for research and analysis, federal and state contracting, and performance measure development. While at NCQA, Dr. Pawlson has played a major role in development and maintenance of the current set of HEDIS® measures and other NCQA measures including those used in physician recognition programs and pay for performance projects. Before joining NCQA in January 2000, Dr. Pawlson was Senior Associate Vice President for Health Affairs and worked with the quality and utilization management efforts of the GW Health Plan and Faculty Practice. Prior to that Dr. Pawlson had served as Chairman of the Department of Health Care Sciences (DHCS) and Director of the Institute for Health Policy, Outcomes and Human Values at GW. During a sabbatical year at GW in 1987, Dr. Pawlson served as a Robert Wood Johnson Health Policy Fellow and health policy aide on the staff of Senator George Mitchell (D-Maine), and in 1997–1998 he was a scholar in residence at the American Association of Medical Colleges, at its Center for the Assessment and Management of Change in Academic Medicine. Within organized medicine Dr. Pawlson served as president or on the board of a number of organizations including the American Geriatrics Society, the Society for General Internal Medicine, the Bon Secours Health System, and the American College of Medical Quality. Dr. Pawlson has more than 100 publications in peer-reviewed journals and has received numerous awards and citations for his teaching and research.

Richard Platt, M.D., M.S., is a Professor and Chair of the Department of Ambulatory Care and Prevention. He is an internist trained in infectious diseases and epidemiology. He is a member of the Association of American Medical Colleges Advisory Panel on Research and the IOM Roundtable on Evidenced-Based Medicine, and he currently chairs the FDA Drug Safety and Risk Management Advisory Committee. He has chaired the Executive Committee of the HMO Research Network, was co-chair of the Board of Scientific Counselors of the CDC's Center for Infectious Diseases, chaired the NIH study section, Epidemiology and Disease Control 2, and the CDC Office of Health Care Partnerships Steering Committee. His research focuses on developing multi-institution automated record linkage systems for use in pharmacoepidemiology and for population-based surveillance, reporting, and control of both hospital- and community-acquired infections, including bioterrorism events. He is Principal Investigator of the CDC-sponsored Center of Excellence in Public Health Informatics, the AHRQ sponsored HMO Research Network Center for Education and Research in Therapeutics (CERT), co-Principal Investigator of a Modeling Infectious Disease Agent Study (MIDAS), and the CDC-sponsored Eastern Massachusetts Prevention Epicenter.

Wayne A. Ray, Ph.D., is a Professor of Preventive Medicine and the Director of the Division of Pharmacoepidemiology at Vanderbilt University School of Medicine. His undergraduate work was in Mathematics at the University of Washington (1971) and he has a master's degree in biostatistics (1974) and computer science (1981), both from Vanderbilt. He is a Fellow of the International Society for Pharmacoepidemiology. Dr. Ray also founded and directs the master of public health program at Vanderbilt. Dr. Ray has had a long-standing research interest in population-based studies of therapeutic interventions and has published more than 150 studies that use observational methods to assess safety and efficacy or seek to define and improve suboptimal use of therapeutic interventions. Dr. Ray pioneered the methodology for using large automated databases, particularly Medicaid, for these types of studies. His work includes fundamental studies of psychotropic drugs and injuries, nonsteroidal anti-inflammatory drugs (NSAIDs) and upper gastrointestinal disease, NSAIDs/coxibs and the risk of coronary heart disease, and medications and sudden cardiac death. He also has been a strong advocate of the need to reform the present drug regulatory system to better protect public health.

Mark S. Roberts, M.D., M.P.P., is an internist and Professor of Medicine, Health Policy and Management and Industrial Engineering at the University of Pittsburgh, where he is Chief of the Section of Decision Sciences and Clinical Systems Modeling. He earned a B.A. in economics from Harvard College, completed medical school at Tufts University and a masters in public policy (MPP) from the Kennedy School of Government. After residency and fellowship in internal medicine, he joined the Harvard Medical School faculty until moving to Pittsburgh in 1993. He has spent his entire academic career in decision sciences and health policy, and he is the author of more than 100 papers and book chapters. His research has been directed toward developing and enhancing decision analytic methods in order to build models that are more clinically realistic and directed towards clinical and policy decisions. The modeling of complex biologic processes and evaluating the tension between realistic models of clinical process and their analytic tractability is a major area of interest and expertise. Over the past 10 years, he has helped to advance the applications of analytic techniques from industrial engineering and management science, such as simulation and optimization to problems in health and medicine. He has served as a consultant to Archimedes, Inc. on multiple projects.

A. John Rush, M.D., is Vice Chair for the Department of Clinical Sciences, Rosewood Corporation Chair in Biomedical Science and Professor of Psychiatry at the University of Texas Southwestern Medical Center at Dallas. His research has focused on the development and testing of innovative treatments for mood disorders including medications, medication combinations, somatic treatments and psychotherapy, as well as disease management protocols (treatment algorithms) for severe and persistent mental illnesses, especially mood disorders. He has authored more than 470 papers and chapters and 10 books and has received continuous NIMH research support for 30 years. He was Principal Investigator on the NIMH-sponsored STAR*D (Sequenced Treatment Alternatives to Relieve Depression) trial. He presently directs the NIMH Depression Trials Network (DTN), which conducts efficacy-effectiveness research with depressed patients. His past awards include the Mood Disorders Research Award of the American College of Psychiatrists, the Paul Hoch Award from the American Psychopathological Association, the Edward J. Sachar Visiting Scholar Award from Columbia, the Nola Maddox Falcone Prize from NARSAD, the American Psychiatric Association Award for Research in Psychiatry, and the Gold Medal Award from the Society of Biological Psychiatry. He is past President of the Society of Biological Psychiatry and the Society for Psychotherapy Research.

Lewis G. Sandy, M.D., M.B.A., of UnitedHealth Group (United Health-Care), has been with UnitedHealth Group since 2003. He is currently Senior Vice President of clinical advancement, where he leads efforts to promote efficient and effective health care, provide tools and information to doctors and patients to promote health, and foster the growth of evidence-based medicine. From 1997 to 2003, he was Executive Vice President of the Robert Wood Johnson Foundation (RWJF), the nation's largest health-focused private foundation. At RWJF, he was responsible for the foundation's program development and management, strategic planning, and administrative operations. An internist and former Health Center Medical Director at the Harvard Community Health Plan in Boston, Massachusetts, Dr. Sandy received his B.S. and M.D. degrees from the University of Michigan and an M.B.A. degree from Stanford University.

Sebastian Schneeweiss, M.D., Sc.D., is Associate Professor of Medicine at Harvard Medical School and Associate Professor of Epidemiology at the Harvard School of Public Health. He is Director for Drug Evaluation and Outcomes Research and Vice-Chief of the Division of Pharmacoepidemiology and Pharmacoeconomics, Department of Medicine, Brigham and Women's Hospital in Boston. After his medical training he received a doctorate in pharmacoepidemiology from Harvard. He served on the faculty of the University of Munich Medical School before leading a research group in Boston. His current NIH-funded research in pharmacoepidemiology and pharmaceutical outcomes research uses large claims databases and pharmacoepidemiologic methods. He is Director of the Brigham and Women's Hospital DEcIDE Research Center funded by AHRQ that conducts studies and develops methods on the comparative effectiveness of biopharmaceuticals. Dr. Schneeweiss has published more than 150 articles in peer-reviewed journals, received several research merit awards, and is Fellow of the American College of Epidemiology and the International Society for Pharmacoepidemiology.

J. Sanford (Sandy) Schwartz, M.D., is Leon Professor of Medicine and Health Management and Economics, School of Medicine and Wharton School; Senior Fellow, Leonard Davis Institute of Health Economics (LDI); and Senior Scholar, Center for Clinical Epidemiology/Biostatistics. Former Executive Director, LDI (University of Pennsylvania's center for health services and policy research), Schwartz is a clinically oriented health services researcher focusing on assessment of medical interventions (including cost/quality trade-offs and healthcare disparities), medical decision making, and medical innovation adoption/diffusion. Dr. Schwartz has served as advisor to federal agencies (NIH, AHRQ, CDC, IOM, NAS, CMS, DOD); nonprofit groups (Robert Wood Johnson, W.K. Kellogg, John A. Hartford, AAMC, NCQA); pharmaceutical, insurance, and managed care organizations; and state health/regulatory agencies. Founding Director of American College of Physicians' Clinical Efficacy Assessment Project (the medical profession's first evidence-based guideline program) and past-President of the American Federation of Clinical Research and Society for Medical Decision Making, he served in editorial capacities for the *American Journal of Managed Care, Journal of General Internal Medicine and Medical Decision Making*. Dr. Schwartz is a member of the NHLBI Adult Treatment Panel III National Cholesterol Education Program; Blue Cross and Blue Shield Associations Medical Advisory Panel; CMS Medicare Coverage Advisory Committee (MCAC); and several policy-related American Heart Association Disease Management, Reimbursement and Policy Workgroups.

Joe V. Selby, M.D., M.P.H., has been the Director of the Division of Research (DOR), Kaiser Permanente, Northern California, since 1998. He is a family physician, clinical epidemiologist, and health services researcher. Prior to becoming DOR Director, Dr. Selby served for 7 years as DOR's Assistant Director for Health Services Research. He also serves as Lecturer in the Department of Epidemiology and Biostatistics, University of California, San Francisco School of Medicine, and as a Consulting Professor, Health Research and Policy, Stanford University School of Medicine. Dr. Selby is a member of the Agency for Healthcare Policy and Research study section for Health Care Quality and Effectiveness. He was a commissioned officer in the Public Health Service from 1976 to 1983 and received the Commissioned Officer's Award in 1981. Dr. Selby has authored or co-authored more than 100 peer-reviewed scientific publications and has written numerous book chapters. His publications cover a spectrum of topics from colon cancer screening and diabetes complications to the delivery of primary care.

Donald M. Steinwachs, Ph.D., is the Chair of the Department of Health Policy and Management at Johns Hopkins University. He also holds the Fred and Julie Soper Professorship of Health Policy and Management. Dr. Steinwachs's current research includes studies of medical effectiveness and patient outcomes for individuals with specific medical, surgical, and psychiatric conditions; studies of the impact of managed care and other organizational and financial arrangements on access to care, quality, utilization, and cost; and studies to develop better methods to measure the effectiveness of systems of care, including case mix (e.g., Ambulatory Care Groups), quality profiling, and indicators of outcome. He has a particular interest in the role of routine management information systems (MIS) as a source of data for evaluating the effectiveness and cost of health care. This includes work on the integration of outcomes management systems with existing MIS in managed care settings.

Alexander M. Walker, M.D., Dr.P.H., is Adjunct Professor of Epidemiology at Harvard School of Public Health, where he was formerly a professor and Chair of the Department of Epidemiology. His research encompasses the safety of drugs, devices, vaccines, and medical procedures. Current studies include postmarketing safety studies for recently approved drugs, natural history of disease studies to provide context for Phase III clinical trials, studies of the impact of drug labeling and warnings on prescribing behavior, and determinants of drug uptake and discontinuation. Additional areas of research and expertise include health effects of chemicals used in the workplace and statistical methods in epidemiology. Dr. Walker received an M.D. degree from Harvard Medical School in 1974 and a doctorate of public health in epidemiology from the Harvard School of Public Health in 1981. Dr. Walker is associate editor of *Pharmacoepidemiology and Drug Safety*, and he is on the Board of Directors of the International Society for Pharmacoepidemiology, for which he also served as President in 1995–1996. He was a statistical consultant for the *New England Journal of Medicine* from 1992 through 1996 and a Contributing Editor of *The Lancet* from 1999 through 2001. From 2000 through 2007, he served as Senior Vice President for Epidemiology at Ingenix. Dr. Walker has written or contributed to more than 250 peer-reviewed articles in drug safety, epidemiology, and occupational health, and is the author of a book of essays, *Observation and Inference: An Introduction to the Methods of Epidemiology*.

Philip S. Wang, M.D., Dr.P.H., is the Director of the Division of Services and Intervention Research at the National Institute of Mental Health. He also remains on leave from his faculty appointments at Harvard Medical School. He completed his undergraduate, medical school, psychiatry residency, as well as doctoral training in epidemiology, all at Harvard University. His research has focused on three areas: psychopharmacoepidemiology; psychopharmacoeconomics; and mental health services research. He was the Principal Investigator of the NIMH-sponsored Work Outcomes Research and Cost-effectiveness Study (WORCS), a large-scale trial to examine the return-on-investment of enhanced depression care for workers. Dr. Wang has served as a voting member on the FDA Psychopharmacologic Drugs Advisory Committee, FDA Neurological Devices Panel, and FDA Endocrinologic and Metabolic Drugs Advisory Committee. He also served on the NIMH Services Research and Clinical Epidemiology Study Section. He is currently Chair of the WHO World Mental Health Study Services Research Work Group. He is a member of the American Psychiatric Association's DSM-V Task Force and has consulted on several APA work groups to develop evidence-based treatment guidelines. Dr. Wang is an author of approximately 140 scientific publications.

Appendix C

Workshop Attendee List

Patricia Adams
National Pharmaceutical Council

Deborah Ascheim
Columbia University

Carol Ashton
University of Alabama,
  Birmingham

David Atkins
Agency for Healthcare Research
  and Quality

Wade Aubry
Health Technology Center

Jerry Avorn
Harvard Medical School

Peter Bach
Memorial Sloan-Kettering Cancer
  Center

Mara Baer
Blue Cross Blue Shield Association

Bob Ball
Food and Drug Administration

Michael Banyas
U.S. Department of Health and
  Human Services

Dennis Barbour
Society for Investigative
  Dermatology

Bart Barefoot
GlaxoSmithKline

Barbara A. Bartman
Agency for Healthcare Research
  and Quality

Rachel Behrman
Food and Drug Administration

Rami Ben-Joseph
sanofi-aventis

Debra Berlanstein
University of Maryland, Baltimore

Elise Berliner
Agency for Healthcare Research
   and Quality

Donald Berry
The University of Texas M.D.
   Anderson Cancer Center

Richard Billingsley
George Washington University
   Medical Center

Ashley Boam
Food and Drug Administration

Douglas Boenning
U.S. Department of Health and
   Human Services

Rosemary Botchway
Primary Care Coalition of
   Montgomery County

Mary Jo Braid-Forbes
The Moran Company

Amanda Brodt
AcademyHealth

Lynda Bryant-Comstock
GlaxoSmithKline

Jonca Bull
Genentech

David Burns
National Institute of Allergy and
   Infectious Diseases

Dale Burwen
Food and Drug Administration

Robert Califf
Duke University Medical Center

James Carey
Novartis Pharmaceuticals
   Corporation

Kristin Carman
American Institutes for Research

Linda Carter
Johnson & Johnson

Stephanie Chang
Agency for Healthcare Research
   and Quality

Yen-pin Chiang
Agency for Healthcare Research
   and Quality

Grace Chow
National Institutes of Health

Carolyn Clancy
Agency for Healthcare Research
   and Quality

Alex Clyde
Medtronic, Inc.

Andrew Cohen
AGC & Associates

Perry D. Cohen
Parkinson Pipeline Project

Denis Cortese
Mayo Clinic

Kenyatta Cosby
Johns Hopkins Medical Institute

Catherine Craven
Johns Hopkins University

Thomas Croghan
Mathematica Policy Research

William Crown
i3 Innovus

Frederick Curro
New York University

J. Nico D. de Neeling
Health Council of the Netherlands

Vicky Debold
National Vaccine Information
   Center

Donald DeNucci
National Institutes of Health and
   Department of Veterans Affairs

Nancy Derr
Food and Drug Administration

Kelly Devers
Virginia Commonwealth
   University

Deirdre DeVine
Tufts-New England Medical
   Center

Christopher Dezii
Bristol-Myers Squibb Company

Louis Diamond
Thomson Healthcare

Denise Dougherty
Agency for Healthcare Research
   and Quality

Clay Dunagan
BJC HealthCare

Philip Duvall
Avalere Health

Jill Eden
Institute of Medicine

Maggie Elestwani
Memorial Hermann-Texas
   Medical Center

Lynn Etheredge
George Washington University

Frank Evans
National Institutes of Health

Christina Farup
Novartis

Shamiram Feinglass
Centers for Medicare & Medicaid
   Services

Karen Wolk Feinstein
Jewish Healthcare Foundation

Harvey Fineberg
Institute of Medicine

Brian Firth
Cordis
Johnson & Johnson

Leslye Fitterman
Centers for Medicare & Medicaid
Services

David Flum
University of Washington

Steven Fox
Agency for Healthcare Research
and Quality

Susan Friedman
American Osteopathic Association

Richard Fry
Foundation for Managed Care
Pharmacy

Jean Paul Gagnon
sanofi-aventis

Dan Galper
American Psychological
Association

Annetine Gelijns
Columbia University

Sharon Gershon
Food and Drug Administration

Kim Gilchrist
AstraZeneca

Don Goffena
WL Gore and Associates, Inc.

Mark Gorman
National Coalition for Cancer
Survivorship

Tina Grande
Healthcare Leadership Council

Mark Grant
Blue Cross Blue Shield Association

Mary Grealy
Healthcare Leadership Council

Lea Greenstein
Institute of Medicine

Jerry Grossman
Health Care Delivery Project

Joao Guerra
Hospital Reynaldo Santos

Stuart Guterman
The Commonwealth Fund

Kara Haas
Ethicon Endo-Surgery

J. Michael Hall
American Liver Foundation

Andrea Harabin
National Heart, Lung, and Blood
Institute

Nancy Hardt
Office of Speaker Nancy Pelosi

Alex Hathaway
GlaxoSmithKline

Anthony Hayward
National Institutes of Health

Erin Holve
AcademyHealth

Peter Honig
Merck & Co., Inc.

Mary Horlick
National Institutes of Health

Jane Horvath
Merck & Co., Inc.

Lia Hotchkiss
Agency for Healthcare Research
   and Quality

Julianne Howell
Centers for Medicare & Medicaid
   Services

Kathy Hudson
Genetics and Public Policy Center

Belinda Ireland
BJC HealthCare

Gretchen Jacobson
Congressional Research Service

Laura Johnson
National Institutes of Health

Mary Joyce
National Heart, Lung, and Blood
   Institute

Peter Juhn
Johnson & Johnson

Elisabeth Kato
Hayes, Inc.

Bruce Kelly
Mayo Clinic

Grace Kelly
National Institutes of Health

Ruth Kirby
National Heart, Lung, and Blood
   Institute

Isaac Kohane
Harvard Medical School

Rachel Kramer
The Moran Company

Alan Krensky
National Institutes of Health

Nora Kronenthal
National Science Foundation

Cara Krulewitch
Food and Drug Administration

Joel Kupersmith
Department of Veterans Affairs

Hanns Kuttner
Office of Senator Orrin Hatch

Arnold Kuzmack
Food and Drug Administration

William Lang
American Association of Colleges
   of Pharmacy

Jeanne Larsen
Georgetown University Medical
   Center

Eric Larson
Group Health Cooperative

Michael Lauer
Division of Prevention and
   Population Science

Cato Laurencin
University of Virginia

Martha Lee
Food and Drug Administration

Teresa Lee
AdvaMed

Anna Legreid Dopp
Office of Senator Lieberman

Carole Lever
MedStar—Union Memorial
    Hospital

Allyson H. Lewis
American Liver Foundation

Kenneth Lin
Agency for Healthcare Research
    and Quality

Susan Lin
National Center for Health
    Statistics

Tsai-Lien Lin
Center for Biologics Evaluation
    and Research

Keith Lind
AARP

Anne Linton
The George Washington University

Alicia Livinski
National Institutes of Health

Kathleen Lohr
RTI International

Ruth Lopert
George Washington University

Bryan Luce
United BioSource Corporation

Carole Magoffin
National Minority Quality Forum

Michele Malloy
Georgetown University Medical
    Center

Teri Manolio
National Human Genome
    Research Institute

JoAnn Manson
Harvard Medical School

Norman Marks
Food and Drug Administration

Ivonne Martinez
Georgetown University

Noel Mazade
National Association of State
    Mental Health Program
    Directors Research Institute,
    Inc.

Mark McClellan
Brookings Institution

Kathleen McCormick
Science Applications International
    Corporation

Newell McElwee
Pfizer, Inc.

Scott McKenzie
Johnson & Johnson

Kathryn McLaughlin
America's Health Insurance Plans

Robert Mechanic
Brandeis University

Carolyn Miles
National Institutes of Health

Amy Miller
Personalized Medicine Coalition

Wilhelmine Miller
George Washington University

Kelly Montgomery
American Diabetes Association

Hazel Moran
Mental Health America

Alan Moskowitz
Columbia University

Esther Myers
The American Dietetic Association

Garry Neil
Johnson & Johnson

David Nexon
AdvaMed

George Neyarapally
Agency for Healthcare Research
  and Quality

John Niederhuber
National Cancer Institute

Sharon-Lise Normand
Harvard Medical School

Parivash Nourjah
Agency of Healthcare Research
  and Quality

Patrick O'Connor
Food & Drug Administration

Keith Ortiz
VantagePoint Consulting Group

Awo Osei-Anto
Avalere Health

Dina Paltoo
National Institutes of Health

Ronald Paulus
Geisinger Health System

L. Gregory Pawlson
National Committee for Quality
  Assurance

Stephen Pelletier
Pelletier Editorial

Eleanor M. Perfetto
Pfizer, Inc.

Gary Persinger
National Pharmaceutical Council

Sarah Pitluck
Genentech

Rich Platt
Harvard Medical School and
  Harvard Pilgrim Health Care

Janet Prvu-Bettger
University of Pennsylvania

Antonello Punturieri
National Heart, Lung, and Blood
   Institute

G. Gregory Raab
Raab & Associates, Inc.

Gurvaneet Randhawa
Agency for Healthcare Research
   and Quality

Purva Rawal
Office of Senator Lieberman

Wayne Ray
Vanderbilt University School of
   Medicine

John Rayburn
Healthcare Leadership Council

Carolina Reyes
Genentech, Inc.

John C. Ring
American Heart Association

Mark Roberts
Center for Research on Health
   Care

Yves Rosenberg
National Heart, Lung, and Blood
   Institute

Wayne Rosenkrans
AstraZeneca Pharmaceuticals

John Rush
University of Texas Southwestern
   Medical Center

Stephen Ryan
AstraZeneca

Susan Samson
University of California San
   Francisco

Karen Sanders
American Psychiatric Association

Lewis Sandy
United Healthcare

Phil Sarocco
Boston Scientific

Jyme Schafer
Centers for Medicare & Medicaid
   Services

Donna Schaffer
Center for Medical Technology
   Policy

Kristin Schneeman
FasterCures

Sebastian Schneeweiss
Harvard Medical School

Lawrence Schott
Centers for Medicare & Medicaid
   Services

David Schulke
American Health Quality
   Association

Sandy Schwartz
University of Pennsylvania

Art Sedrakyan
Agency for Healthcare Research
   and Quality

Jodi Segal
Johns Hopkins University School
   of Medicine

Joe Selby
Kaiser Permanente

Steve Severance
Vivalog

Gail Shearer
Consumers Union

George Silberman
Cancer Policy Group, LLC

Rebecca Singer Cohen
United BioSource Corporation

Jean Slutsky
Agency for Healthcare Research
   and Quality

Scott Smith
Agency for Healthcare Research
   and Quality

Melissa Stegun
George Washington University

Donald Steinwachs
Johns Hopkins University

Melissa Stevens
FasterCures

Ansalan Stewart
Office of the Assistant Secretary
   for Policy and Planning

Catherine Stoney
National Institutes of Health

Michael Stoto
Georgetown University

Paul Strasberg
National Center for Education
   Evaluation

David Sugano
Schering-Plough Pharmaceuticals

Kara Suter
The Moran Company

Betty Tai
Center of Clinical Trials Network

Jorge Tavel
National Institute of Allergy and
   Infectious Diseases

Robert Temple
Food and Drug Administration

Anne Trontell
Agency for Healthcare Research
   and Quality

Sean Tunis
Center for Medical Technology
   Policy

Karen Ulisney
National Institutes of Health

Craig Umscheid
University of Pennsylvania Health
    System

Douglas Varner
Georgetown University Medical
    Center

Don Vena
The EMMES Corporation

Corinne Vosmer
Science Applications International
    Corporation

Alec Walker
Harvard University

Marc Walton
Food and Drug Administration

Cunlin Wang
Food and Drug Administration

Philip Wang
National Institute of Mental
    Health

Gretchen Wartman
National Minority Quality Forum

Brian Waterman
BJC HealthCare

Kathleen Weis
Pfizer, Inc.

Sue West
University of North Carolina

Karen Williams
National Pharmaceutical Council

Todd Williamson
sanofi-aventis

Michael Wittek
Medtronic, Inc.

Kim Wittenberg
Agency for Healthcare Research
    and Quality

Hui-Hsing Wong
Office of the Assistant Secretary
    for Planning and Evaluation

Nelda Wray
University of Alabama,
    Birmingham

Laura Zick
Eli Lilly and Company

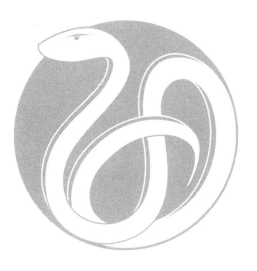

OTHER PUBLICATIONS IN THE
LEARNING HEALTHCARE SYSTEM SERIES